IMMUNOLOGY AND IMMUNE SYSTEM DISORDERS

VACCINES

OPERATION WARP SPEED, REGULATION AND SAFETY

IMMUNOLOGY AND IMMUNE SYSTEM DISORDERS

Additional books and e-books in this series can be found on Nova's website under the Series tab.

IMMUNOLOGY AND IMMUNE SYSTEM DISORDERS

VACCINES

OPERATION WARP SPEED, REGULATION AND SAFETY

OLIVER HUERTA
EDITOR

snova
New York

Additional color graphics may be available in the e-book version of this book.

Library of Congress Cataloging-in-Publication Data

ISBN: 978-1-53619-059-5

Published by Nova Science Publishers, Inc. † New York

CONTENTS

PREFACE

In recent months, the Coronavirus Disease 2019 (COVID-19) pandemic has spread globally, with the United States now reporting the highest number of cases of any country in the world. Currently, there are few treatment options available to lessen the health impact of the disease and no vaccines or other prophylactic treatments to curb the spread of the virus. Researchers and product developers are testing numerous types of vaccines—both in the laboratory and in some early-stage testing in humans. This book answers frequently asked questions about current efforts related to research and development of vaccines, their regulation, and related policy issues.

Chapter 1 - This chapter to Congress details a strategy to achieve the principal purpose and objective of Operation Warp Speed (OWS): ensuring that every American who wants to receive a COVID-19 vaccine can receive one, by delivering safe and effective vaccine doses to the American people beginning January 2021. The leadership of OWS has committed to being transparent with Congress, the media, and the American people. OWS has provided regular briefings on topics of interest to Congress and the media and will continue to provide updates and announcements as OWS reaches new milestones. Congress has been a vital partner in the all-of-America response to the COVID-19 pandemic. With support provided through emergency supplemental and flexible discretionary funding, OWS has now made strong progress toward a safe and effective COVID-19 vaccine, with multiple candidates in Phase 3 clinical trials. Simultaneously, OWS and partners are developing a plan for delivering a safe and effective product to Americans as quickly and reliably as possible. Experts from the Department of Health and Human Services (HHS) are leading vaccine development, while experts from the Department of Defense (DoD) are partnering with the Centers for Disease Control and Prevention (CDC) and other parts of HHS to coordinate supply, production, and distribution of vaccines. Successful implementation of the national COVID-19 vaccination program requires precise coordination across federal, state, local, tribal, and territorial governments and among many public and private partners. Cooperation on each of these fronts has already begun, as detailed throughout this strategy document. OWS is harnessing the strength of existing vaccine delivery infrastructure while leveraging innovative strategies, new public-private partnerships, and robust engagement of state, local, tribal, and territorial health departments to ensure efficient, effective, and equitable access to COVID-19 vaccines. Some variables that will impact the planning of this vaccination program are unknown until a vaccine is authorized or approved by the Food and Drug Administration (FDA), such as populations for whom a given vaccine is most appropriate, distribution and storage requirements, dosage requirements, and other variables. This document lays out a flexible strategy that can accommodate a range of scenarios. Through the COVID-19 vaccination program, OWS seeks to achieve maximum uptake of the vaccine across all population groups. The eventual objective of the vaccination program is to leave the U.S. government and commercial infrastructure better able to respond to pandemics and public health crises in the future.

Chapter 2 - Operation Warp Speed's goal is to produce and deliver 300 million doses of safe and effective vaccines with the initial doses available by January 2021, as part of a broader strategy to accelerate the development, manufacturing, and distribution of COVID-19 vaccines, therapeutics, and diagnostics (collectively known as countermeasures).

Chapter 3 - This is an edited, reformatted and augmented version of U.S. Department of Health and Human Services Publication.

Chapter 4 - In recent months, the Coronavirus Disease 2019 (COVID-19) pandemic has spread globally, with the United States now reporting the highest number of cases of any country in the world. Currently, there are few treatment options available to lessen the health impact of the disease and no vaccines or other prophylactic treatments to curb the spread of the virus. The biomedical community has been working to develop new therapies or vaccines, and to repurpose already approved therapeutics, that could prevent COVID-19 infections or lessen severe outcomes in patients. In addition, efforts have been underway to develop new diagnostic tools (i.e., testing) to help better identify and isolate positive cases, thereby reducing the spread of the disease. To this end, Congress has appropriated funds for research and development into new *medical countermeasures* (MCMs) in several recent supplemental appropriations acts. MCMs are medical products that may be used to treat, prevent, or diagnose conditions associated with emerging infectious diseases or chemical, biological, radiological, or nuclear (CBRN) agents. MCMs include biologics (e.g., vaccines, monoclonal antibodies), drugs (e.g., antimicrobials, antivirals), and medical devices (e.g., diagnostic tests). This chapter answers frequently asked questions about current efforts related to research and development of medical countermeasures, their regulation, and related policy issues. Although several efforts are underway, medical product research, development, and approval is a difficult and high-risk endeavor that takes years in typical circumstances. In response to COVID-19, this process has been expedited, including through several federal programs and mechanisms covered in this chapter. However, expedited medical product development can carry certain risks, such as a more limited safety profile for new products upon approval.

Chapter 5 - In the race to develop a Coronavirus Disease 2019 (COVID-19) vaccine, several pharmaceutical companies, governments, and educational institutions around the world have begun testing their potential COVID-19 vaccines in clinical trials. Clinical trials are used to assess whether a new pharmaceutical product, such as a vaccine, is safe for humans and effective in achieving its intended purpose. Companies must generally test new pharmaceutical products on humans through clinical trials to obtain U.S. Food and Drug Administration (FDA) approval to market the product. But using human subjects to test these novel products exposes them to unknown health and safety risks, raising ethical considerations for FDA and for the sponsors and Institutional Review Boards (IRBs) overseeing the investigations. These stakeholders—sponsors, IRBs, and FDA—aim to balance the need to ensure that the product is safe and effective against the desire to bring the product to market quickly, tensions that are heightened during a worldwide pandemic. Existing law requires FDA and IRBs to weigh these considerations when evaluating proposed clinical trial designs for COVID-19 vaccines. This chapter describes the legal and regulatory framework that governs clinical trials for pharmaceutical products, such as vaccines, and some avenues researchers and Congress may consider for accelerating that process during the COVID-19 pandemic. (For ease of reference, this Sidebar uses the term *drugs* includes both traditional drugs and biological products, including vaccines.)

Chapter 6 - SARS-CoV-2 causes COVID-19, and developing a vaccine could save lives and speed economic recovery. The United States is funding multiple efforts to develop vaccines. Developing a vaccine is a complicated process that is costly, typically requires 10 years or more, and has a low success rate, although efforts are underway to accelerate the process.

Chapter 7 - As the number of confirmed COVID-19 cases increases at an accelerating rate, interest has grown in developing a COVID-19 vaccine as an avenue for addressing the pandemic. Media reports indicate that a number of countries and companies are working on developing a vaccine. The National Institute of Allergy and Infectious Diseases (NIAID) and the biotechnology company Moderna, Inc., recently initiated the first clinical trials of a potential vaccine in the United States at a hospital in Seattle. However, developing a new vaccine and obtaining approval to market it can take a long time. This Sidebar discusses the licensure (i.e., approval) process for vaccines under the Public Health Service Act (PHS Act) and the federal Food, Drug, and Cosmetic Act (FD&C Act), as well as potential legal avenues for expediting that process to bring a new vaccine to market sooner.

Chapter 8 - Private companies, universities, and governmental entities are working to develop a vaccine for coronavirus disease 2019 (COVID-19). Vaccines are biological products regulated under the Public Health Service Act (PHSA) and the Federal Food, Drug, and Cosmetic Act (FD&C Act). New vaccines must generally be licensed by the U.S. Food & Drug Administration (FDA) before they can be marketed and used in the United States. To obtain licensure, the vaccine must be tested in human subjects through clinical trials. The clinical trials inform the dosing schedule and labeling that will be used for the approved vaccine. Sponsors use the data from clinical trials, along with other information, to prepare a biologics license application (BLA) to submit to FDA. FDA approves the BLA if it determines that the vaccine is safe, potent, and pure. Because the development and review process can be lengthy, the FD&C Act provides several avenues to accelerate this process for pharmaceutical products intended to treat or prevent serious diseases or conditions. FDA may grant fast track product and breakthrough-therapy designation at the sponsor's request for products that are intended to fill an unmet need or improve on existing therapies. Both designations entitle the sponsor to increased communication with FDA regarding the clinical trial design and data collected, as well as rolling review of the BLA. Products may also qualify for accelerated approval based on intermediate or surrogate endpoints likely to predict a clinical benefit. In addition, FDA may designate products for priority review. In certain emergency situations, FDA may temporarily authorize the use of unapproved products or approved products for unapproved uses through an emergency use authorization (EUA). For FDA to issue an EUA, the Secretary of Health and Human Services (HHS) must determine (1) that a qualifying emergency exists caused by a biological, chemical, radiological, or nuclear (BCRN) agent and (2) that the BCRN agent can cause a serious or life-threatening disease. The Secretary, through FDA, must also determine for each product that (3) it is reasonable to believe, based on the totality of the evidence available, that the product may treat or prevent the disease caused by the BCRN agent and that the known and potential benefits outweigh the known and potential risks, and (4) there are no approved, adequate, and available alternatives. If FDA issues an EUA, the product may be marketed and used for the authorized use while the emergency persists unless FDA revokes the EUA. FDA may also modify or waive good manufacturing practice and prescription requirements when issuing an EUA. FDA approval of a vaccine allows for its marketing, but does not guarantee that the vaccine will be widely available or affordable. Because patents grant inventors the exclusive rights in a patented invention, patents may influence COVID-19 vaccine affordability and access. Federal agencies and funding support many of the COVID-19 vaccine candidates in development, which may affect the allocation and scope of patent rights. The Bayh-Dole Act allows a federal contractor to obtain the patent on a federally funded invention, but the government retains a free license to use the invention and may "march in" to grant patent licenses to third-party manufacturers in limited circumstances. If federal support is provided through an "other transaction" agreement, however, the allocation of patent rights will depend on the terms of that contract. The federal government has several authorities that it could exercise should patent rights limit the affordability of or access to a COVID-19 vaccine. For vaccines developed with federal funding or support, the government may secure up-front guarantees on pricing or distribution via funding or purchasing contracts with vaccine developers. For vaccines protected by patents subject to the Bayh-Dole Act, the funding agency could seek to invoke march-in rights to enable other producers to manufacture the vaccine. For any U.S. patent, the federal government could use its "eminent domain" powers under 28 U.S.C. § 1498, which allows the government to make and use patented inventions without license—so long as the use is by or for the United States and compensation is provided to the patent holder. As U.S. patent rights are a creation of Congress, targeted legislation is another option, subject to the constraints of the U.S. Constitution and international treaties. A COVID-19 vaccine is likely to be subject to specialized rules limiting legal liability under the Public Readiness and Emergency Preparedness (PREP) Act. To encourage the expeditious development and deployment of medical countermeasures, the Secretary of HHS has declared COVID-19 to be a public health emergency and invoked the PREP Act to limit liability for losses relating to the use of covered medical countermeasures during the public health emergency. Under HHS's declaration, covered persons—including COVID-19 vaccine developers, manufacturers, distributors, and health care professionals who administer a vaccine—are generally immune from legal liability for losses relating to administration or use of an FDA-approved COVID-19 vaccine, except for willful misconduct resulting in death or serious physical injury. However, individuals who are injured or die as a result of receiving a COVID-19 vaccine may seek compensation through the Countermeasures Injury Compensation Program, a regulatory process administered by HHS.

Chapter 9 - Widespread immunization efforts have been linked to increased life expectancy and reduced illness. U.S. vaccination programs, headed by the Centers for Disease Control and Prevention (CDC) within the Department of Health and Human Services (HHS), have helped eradicate smallpox and nearly eradicate polio globally, and eliminate several infectious diseases domestically. With the Coronavirus Disease 2019 (COVID-19) pandemic now causing major health and economic impacts across the world, efforts are underway to make safe and effective vaccines available quickly to help curb spread of the virus. *Background.* Federal regulation of vaccine safety began with the Biologics Control Act of 1902, which was the first federal law to require premarket review of pharmaceutical products. Since the 1902 law was enacted, federal vaccine safety activities have expanded, with the aim of minimizing the possibility of adverse events following vaccination and detecting new adverse events as quickly as possible. Today, as covered in this chapter, federal efforts to ensure vaccine safety include the following activities:

- Premarket requirements: Clinical trials, or testing of investigational vaccines in human subjects, and U.S. Food and Drug Administration (FDA) licensure or authorization.

- Clinical recommendations: Recommendations for the clinical use of vaccines by the Advisory Committee on Immunization Practices (ACIP), and CDC clinical guidance and resources.
- Postmarket safety: Manufacturing requirements and ongoing safety monitoring of vaccines administered to patients.
- Federal research on vaccine safety: Ongoing research to inform a better scientific understanding of vaccine safety and comprehensive scientific reviews on the safety of vaccines in use.
- Vaccine injury compensation: In nonemergency circumstances, the National Vaccine Injury Compensation Program (VICP) provides compensation to eligible individuals found to have been injured by a covered vaccine. In emergency circumstances, like COVID-19, a separate Countermeasures Injury Compensation Program (CICP) may be used.
- Vaccine distribution: Programs and requirements to ensure safety controls in vaccine distribution programs, led by CDC.

COVID-19 Vaccine Safety Considerations. Safety considerations for COVID-19 vaccines in development are unique in many ways. FDA has never licensed a vaccine for a coronavirus, and much remains unknown about potential safety issues related to COVID-19 vaccines. Under Operation Warp Speed (OWS)—the Trump Administration's major medical countermeasure development initiative—COVID-19 vaccines are under an expedited development timeline. FDA may initially make the vaccine available under an Emergency Use Authorization (EUA) instead of its standard biologics licensing process—a first for the agency for a previously unapproved vaccine. In light of reported concerns from the public surrounding the safety and effectiveness of COVID-19 vaccines developed on an expedited timeline, FDA officials have sought to clarify that any vaccine candidate "will be reviewed according to the established legal and regulatory standards for medical products." If made available within the next several months, available safety and effectiveness data would be based on months of data collection rather than on years of data collection typically used in vaccine development. In addition, efforts are underway with regard to (1) clinical guidance and prioritization of individuals to receive the likely limited initial supply of COVID-19 vaccines; (2) strengthening safety monitoring systems to collect ongoing safety surveillance data on vaccines administered to the population; and (3) preparing for safety controls in vaccine distribution and patient administration, in addition to other activities. *Congressional Considerations.* Ever since the Biologics Control Act of 1902, Congress and the Administration (especially through FDA and CDC) have strived to ensure the safety of vaccines in the United States—from initial development to patient administration. Congress may consider how to best leverage existing requirements and programs to ensure that risk of harm from eventual COVID-19 vaccines is mitigated and minimized. OWS, FDA, CDC, and others are working to expedite the availability of COVID-19 vaccines and to prepare for a nationwide immunization campaign. Safety has been cited as a consideration in all of these efforts. Congress may consider how to best provide oversight and make legislative changes to ensure a safe and successful COVID-19 vaccination campaign. In addition, Congress may consider and evaluate the entire federal vaccine safety system and assess whether this system warrants any policy changes to help ensure ongoing safety of all recommended vaccines.

Chapter 10 - Vaccines are safe and effective. Because vaccines are given to millions of healthy people — including children — to prevent serious diseases, they're held to very high safety standards.

In this section, you'll learn more about vaccine safety — and get answers to common questions about vaccine side effects.

Chapter 11 - For more than 50 years, the United States has taken an interest in the eradication of vaccine-preventable diseases (VPDs) in children worldwide, as well as vaccine research and development, particularly since playing a vital role in the global campaign to eradicate smallpox in the 1960s. Since then, vaccinating children against VPDs has been a major U.S. foreign policy effort. Vaccinations are one of the most cost-effective ways to prevent infectious disease and associated morbidity and mortality. According to UNICEF, immunizations save around 3 million lives per year. As of 2019, VPDs continue to cause high levels of morbidity (illness) and mortality (death), and the World Health Organization (WHO) notes that the adoption of new vaccines by low- and middle-income countries (which often have the highest disease burdens) has been slower than in high-income countries. Receiving a vaccination during childhood can protect the recipient from VPDs, decrease the spread of related diseases, and improve child survival prospects (as children, particularly those under five years old, are more likely than adults to die from VPDs). Recently, a global resurgence of certain VPDs has caused concern among public health officials and drawn attention to the challenges of vaccine hesitancy and stigma. For example, polio continues to elude global eradication and remains endemic in three countries. In 2019 measles has seen a resurgence in some middle- and high-income countries due to a variety of factors, including reluctance among some individuals and religious communities to vaccinate their children. In April 2019, the WHO reported an increase in global measles cases compared to the same period in 2018, with the greatest surges in cases in the Americas, the Middle East, and Europe. A number of European countries are at risk of or have lost their measles eradication certificate from the WHO, raising questions about global consensus on the use of vaccines, participation in and support for the Global Alliance for Vaccines and Immunization (GAVI, now called GAVI, the Vaccine Alliance) and other global immunization efforts. Prompted in part by this global resurgence, the WHO has listed "vaccine hesitancy" as one of the 10 biggest global public health threats. The U.S. government is the second-leading government donor to global vaccination campaigns. Through annual appropriations to the Department of Health and Human Services (HHS) and the Department of State, Congress funds global immunization activities through the Centers for Disease Control and Prevention (CDC), the United States Agency for International Development (USAID), and GAVI. In recent years, annual appropriations by Congress for multilateral immunizations campaigns led by GAVI have averaged $290 million and $226 million for bilateral campaigns led by CDC. USAID works to support routine immunization overseas through health systems strengthening, and Global Polio Eradication Initiative Activities. The authorization, appropriation, and oversight of U.S. funding for global child vaccination is thus an ongoing area of concern for many in Congress. Other key issues for Congress include the extent of donor coordination and burden-sharing for such efforts, and the extent to which global child vaccination promotes U.S. foreign policy, development, and domestic health security (i.e., pandemic preparedness) goals.

Chapter 12 - According to the latest available data from the Centers for Disease Control and Protection (CDC), 7 states in the United States are currently in the midst of 10 separate measles outbreaks. With 880 total confirmed cases so far this year, 2019 now has the greatest number of reported cases of measles since 1994 and since measles was declared eliminated in the United States in 2000. These cases, the majority of which involves unvaccinated individuals, follows a number of notable measles outbreaks over the past several years, including an outbreak of 383 cases in 2014 among unvaccinated Amish communities in Ohio and another multi-state outbreak of 147 cases in 2015 linked to an amusement park in California. In addition to measles, for about every 5 years since 2006, outbreaks of other vaccine-preventable diseases, such as mumps, have also been reported in the United States. In light of these outbreaks and their association with unvaccinated individuals, this Sidebar provides an overview of the relevant state and federal authority to require vaccination for U.S. residents.

Chapter 13 - This chapter estimates the potentially large health and economic losses in the United States associated with influenza pandemics and discusses why the most commonly used vaccine production technologies are unlikely to mitigate these losses. We estimate the value of new vaccine technologies that would make vaccines available more quickly and likely improve their effectiveness in moderating the risks of pandemics. We discuss why private market incentives may be insufficient to develop new vaccine technologies or promote the uptake of existing, faster but more expensive technologies, despite their large expected value to society. And we argue that increased utilization of, and investment in, these new technologies—along with public-private partnerships, to spur innovation—may be valuable to decrease the impact of both pandemic and seasonal influenza. Every year, millions of Americans suffer from seasonal influenza, commonly known as "the flu," which is caused by influenza viruses. A new vaccine is formulated annually to decrease infections resulting from the small genetic changes that continually occur in the most prevalent viruses and make them less recognizable to the human immune system. There is, however, a 4 percent annual probability of pandemic influenza resulting from large and unpredictable genetic changes leading to an easily transmissible influenza virus for which much of the population would lack the residual immunity that results from prior virus exposures and vaccinations. The Council of Economic Advisors (CEA) finds that in a pandemic year, depending on the transmission efficiency and virulence of the particular pandemic virus, the economic damage would range from $413 billion to $3.79 trillion. Fatalities in the most serious scenario would exceed half a million people in the United States. Millions more would be sick, with between approximately 670,000 to 4.3 million requiring hospitalization. In a severe pandemic, healthy people might avoid work and normal social interactions in an attempt to avert illness by limiting contact with sick persons. By incapacitating a large fraction of the population, including individuals who work in critical infrastructure and defense sectors, pandemic influenza could threaten U.S. national security. Large-scale, immediate immunization is the most effective way to control the spread of influenza, but the predominant, currently licensed, vaccine manufacturing technology would not provide sufficient doses rapidly enough to mitigate a pandemic. Current influenza vaccine production focuses on providing vaccines for the seasonal flu and primarily relies on growing viruses in chicken eggs. Egg-based production can take six months or more to deliver substantial amounts of vaccines after a pathogenic, influenza virus is identified—too slowly to stave off the rapid spread of infections if an unexpected and highly contagious pandemic virus emerges. Egg-based production can also diminish vaccines' efficacy in protecting against influenza infection in both seasonal and pandemic years. Influenza viruses must be adapted to grow in chicken eggs, which can lead to modifications in their surface proteins (antigens) so that the vaccine prepared from them may not match the circulating influenza viruses well.

In addition, the length of time needed for egg-based production may impair vaccine efficacy in two ways: the virus selected for vaccine manufacture may no longer be the predominant circulating virus six months later; or, even if the selected virus remains the predominant circulating virus, it may mutate between the time it is identified and the time the vaccine is available six months later, making the vaccine less effective. During the severe 2017–18 influenza season, the overall effectiveness of the vaccine against the circulating viruses was 38 percent. The vaccine created for the last pandemic, which occurred in 2009–10, was 62 percent effective in protecting people under age 65 years and 43 percent effective for those age 65 and older—the age group at highest risk of medical complications and death from influenza. And in 2014–15, when there was a mismatch between the virus used for the vaccine and the predominant circulating virus, the vaccine was only 19 percent effective. Improving the speed of vaccine production and vaccine efficacy are both important goals to mitigate pandemic risks and may also decrease the costs of seasonal influenza. Our analysis shows that innovation to increase the speed of vaccine production is key. Improving vaccine efficacy alone will be of little value in a pandemic if, as is the case with current egg-based production, the vaccine only becomes available after a large number of infections have occurred. Improving efficacy only yields value after greater speed has been achieved. The CEA finds that technologies that could deliver sufficient doses of vaccine at the outset of an influenza pandemic could produce about a $730 billion benefit for Americans over the course of an average pandemic, primarily due to the prevention of loss of life and health. Combining this increase in production speed with a 30 percent increase over the vaccine effectiveness seen in the last pandemic (2009–10) would generate a larger benefit of about $953 billion— about one half the cost of an average pandemic. The benefits dissipate quickly, however, with each week of delay in the vaccine's availability, as the number of unexposed people to protect diminishes. The cost of a 1-week delay at the baseline vaccine effectiveness from the last pandemic is $41 billion per week, on average, for the first 12 weeks; falls to $20 billion per week for the next 12 weeks; and disappears entirely if the vaccine's availability is delayed by more than 39 weeks, because the outbreak would be over before the vaccine prevented new infections. Adding a 30 percent improvement to the vaccine effectiveness seen in the last pandemic makes the per-week cost of delay $53 billion over the first 12 weeks, on average, falling to $26 billion over the next 12 weeks. The expected value of having a vaccine available at the outset of a pandemic—that is, the savings discounted by the 4 percent annual probability of having a pandemic—is $29 billion, or $89.63 per American. Adding a 30 percent increase to the baseline pandemic vaccine's effectiveness to the faster production increases the expected value to $38 billion, or $117.07 per American. The expected per capita value from increasing the production speed for pandemic vaccines is over four times the current per-dose cost for egg-based vaccines. Newer technologies, like cell-based or recombinant vaccines, have the potential to cut production times and improve efficacy compared with egg-based vaccines and are currently priced below the expected per capita value of improved production speeds for pandemic vaccines. But these existing technologies have not yet been adopted on a large scale. Besides improving pandemic preparedness, new vaccine technologies may have an additional benefit of potentially improving vaccine efficacy for seasonal influenza. We estimate the economic benefits that these new technologies could generate for each seasonal influenza vaccine recipient, and find that the benefits are particularly compelling for older adults (65+) who are at high risk of influenza complications and death. We discuss why the private market has not embraced these newer vaccine production technologies and the lack of private incentives to develop and utilize improved vaccine production technologies that could better mitigate pandemic risk. First, there is a key misalignment between the social and private returns from medical research and development (R&D) and capital investment in pandemic vaccines. R&D and investment costs are only recouped by sales when the pandemic risk occurs. Part of the value of vaccines that can mitigate future pandemic risks, however, is their insurance value today that provides protection against possible damage. This insurance value accrues even if the pandemic does not occur in the future, and it implies that the social value of faster production and better vaccines is much larger than its private return to developers. This divergence leads to an underprovision in vaccine innovation because it does not get rewarded for its insurance value. Second, pandemics represent a risk with a small probability of occurring but with large and highly correlated losses across the population. The rarity of influenza pandemics and the fact that the last serious one in this country occurred a hundred years ago may lead consumers and insurers to underestimate the probability and potential impact of a future influenza pandemic. Moreover, the risk cannot be effectively pooled because everyone is at risk concurrently. Although vaccine innovation is not currently rewarded for its insurance value, public-private partnerships created under a 2006 statute have been key in the development of the newer vaccine production technologies that offer the prospect of improved seasonal influenza vaccines and the accelerated timelines needed for improved pandemic preparedness. Push incentives like public-private partnerships combined with pull incentives—such as the government's preferential purchase of vaccines produced domestically with newer, faster technologies—that may create more efficacious seasonal vaccines, especially for older people, can promote additional cost-effective innovation and lessen the impact of future pandemics.

Chapter 14 - *Influenza vaccine* can prevent *influenza (flu). Flu* is a contagious disease that spreads around the United States every year, usually between October and May. Anyone can get the flu, but it is more dangerous for some people. Infants and young children, people 65 years of age and older, pregnant women, and people with certain health conditions or a weakened immune system are at greatest risk of flu complications. Pneumonia, bronchitis, sinus infections and ear infections are examples of flu-related complications. If you have a medical condition, such as heart disease, cancer or diabetes, flu can make it worse. Flu can cause fever and chills, sore throat, muscle aches, fatigue, cough, headache, and runny or stuffy nose. Some people may have vomiting and diarrhea, though this is more common in children than adults. Each year *thousands of people in the United States die from flu*, and many more are hospitalized. Flu vaccine prevents millions of illnesses and flu-related visits to the doctor each year.

Chapter 15 - Foot-and-mouth disease (FMD) is a severe and highly contagious viral disease. The FMD virus affects cows, pigs, sheep, goats, deer, and other animals with divided, or split, hooves. Animals with FMD typically develop a fever and blisters on the tongue and lips, in and around the mouth, on the mammary glands, and around the hooves. Other signs of illness include depression, anorexia, excessive salivation, lameness, and reluctance to move or stand. Most affected adult animals will not die from FMD, but the disease leaves them weakened, resulting in reduced meat/milk production. Younger animals may not survive. As part of its overall mission to protect American agriculture, the United States Department of Agriculture's (USDA) Animal and Plant Health Inspection Service works to ensure the continued health of the nation's livestock and poultry healthy. USDA works to keep foreign animal diseases out of the country and to deal with outbreaks of serious animal diseases. If a foreign animal disease like FMD occurs in the U.S., USDA would be the lead Federal agency responding to the outbreak, working closely with state animal health agencies and other agencies. FMD is a worldwide concern as it can spread quickly and cause significant economic losses. A single detection of FMD could close international export markets for meat, dairy and other products, causing billions of dollars in lost trade for the United States. If FMD is found in the United States, USDA with its partners would need to act quickly to eradicate the disease and keep it from spreading throughout the country.

Chapter 16 - The ongoing opioid epidemic in the United States impacts lives on both a personal and national level. More than 10 million people abused opioids in 2017, with more than 47,000 opioid-related deaths — a nearly six-fold increase since 1999. Opioid vaccines could offer advantages over current treatment options.

In: Vaccines
Editor: Oliver Huerta

ISBN: 978-1-53619-059-5

Chapter 1

FROM THE FACTORY TO THE FRONTLINES: THE OPERATION WARP SPEED STRATEGY FOR DISTRIBUTING A COVID-19 VACCINE*

U.S. Department of Health and Human Services

WHAT THIS STRATEGY AIMS TO DO

This chapter to Congress details a strategy to achieve the principal purpose and objective of Operation Warp Speed (OWS): ensuring that every American who wants to receive a COVID-19 vaccine can receive one, by delivering safe and effective vaccine doses to the American people beginning January 2021.

The leadership of OWS has committed to being transparent with Congress, the media, and the American people. OWS has provided regular briefings on topics of interest to Congress and the media and will continue to provide updates and announcements as OWS reaches new milestones.

---

* This is an edited, reformatted and augmented version of U.S. Department of Health and Human Services Publication.

Congress has been a vital partner in the all-of-America response to the COVID-19 pandemic.

With support provided through emergency supplemental and flexible discretionary funding, OWS has now made strong progress toward a safe and effective COVID-19 vaccine, with multiple candidates in Phase 3 clinical trials.

Simultaneously, OWS and partners are developing a plan for delivering a safe and effective product to Americans as quickly and reliably as possible. Experts from the Department of Health and Human Services (HHS) are leading vaccine development, while experts from the Department of Defense (DoD) are partnering with the Centers for Disease Control and Prevention (CDC) and other parts of HHS to coordinate supply, production, and distribution of vaccines.

Successful implementation of the national COVID-19 vaccination program requires precise coordination across federal, state, local, tribal, and territorial governments and among many public and private partners. Cooperation on each of these fronts has already begun, as detailed throughout this strategy document.

OWS is harnessing the strength of existing vaccine delivery infrastructure while leveraging innovative strategies, new public-private partnerships, and robust engagement of state, local, tribal, and territorial health departments to ensure efficient, effective, and equitable access to COVID-19 vaccines.

Some variables that will impact the planning of this vaccination program are unknown until a vaccine is authorized or approved by the Food and Drug Administration (FDA), such as populations for whom a given vaccine is most appropriate, distribution and storage requirements, dosage requirements, and other variables. This document lays out a flexible strategy that can accommodate a range of scenarios.

Through the COVID-19 vaccination program, OWS seeks to achieve maximum uptake of the vaccine across all population groups. The eventual objective of the vaccination program is to leave the U.S. government and commercial infrastructure better able to respond to pandemics and public health crises in the future.

WHAT IS THE STRATEGY?

Once a vaccine has received approval or authorization from the FDA, the four key tasks to achieve the primary objective of ensuring vaccine access for every American who wants it are to:

- Continue engaging with state, tribal, territorial, and local partners, other stakeholders, and the public to communicate public health information, before and after distribution begins, around the vaccine and promote vaccine confidence and uptake.
- Distribute vaccines immediately upon granting of Emergency Use Authorization/Biologics License Application, using a transparently developed, phased allocation methodology.
- Ensure safe administration of the vaccine and availability of administration supplies.
- Monitor necessary data from the vaccination program through an information technology (IT) system capable of supporting and tracking distribution, administration, and other necessary data.

This chapter lays out the requirements for each of these tasks and how OWS has taken action and is planning future actions to execute on them.

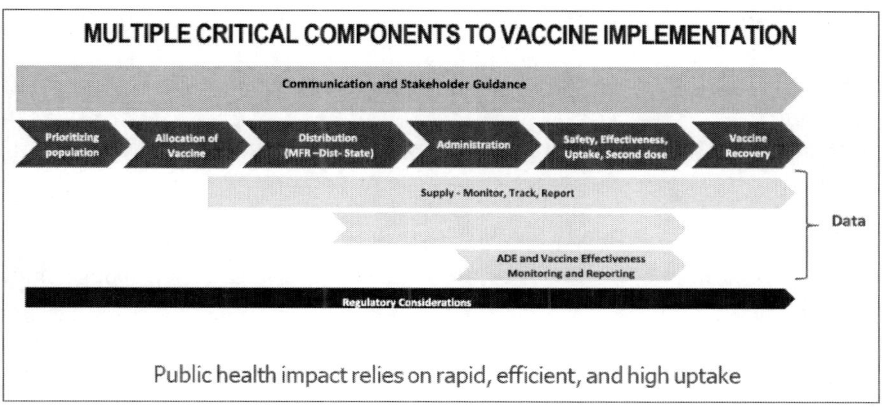

DISTRIBUTION

What is Required

A distribution plan must be able to deliver vaccines immediately upon FDA authorization or licensure to all possible administration endpoints, while remaining flexible enough to accommodate a variety of factors, including varying product requirements and manufacturing timelines and volumes. Any distribution effort must ensure safety of the products, maintain control and visibility, manage uptake and acceptance, ensure traceability of product, and maximize coverage, which requires a centralized solution as well as close local partnerships.

What We Are Doing

OWS is developing a cooperative plan for centralized distribution that will be executed in phases by the federal government, the 64 jurisdictions CDC works with (all 50 states, six localities, and territories and freely associated states), Tribes, industry partners, and other entities.

Distribution has three key components:

- Partnerships with state, local and tribal health departments, territories, Tribes, and federal entities to allocate and distribute vaccines, augmented by direct distribution to commercial partners.
- A centralized distributor contract with potential for back-up distributors for additional storage and handling requirements.
- A flexible, scalable, secure web-based IT vaccine tracking system for ongoing vaccine allocation, ordering, uptake, and management.

State, Tribal, and Local Partnerships

CDC is working with state, local and tribal health departments to hone existing plans for vaccine distribution and administration. CDC has worked for decades with these partners, including under cooperative agreements, to ensure public health systems are prepared with plans, trained personnel, strategic relationships and partnerships, data systems, and other resources needed for sustaining a successful routine immunization infrastructure, and these plans will be adapted for this vaccine program.

CDC awarded grants as part of the Coronavirus Aid, Relief, and Economic Security (CARES) Act and the Families First Coronavirus Response Act that can help immunization programs begin preparation for vaccine distribution and administration. The funding will be used to enhance capacity to support staffing, communication and stakeholder engagement, pandemic preparedness, and mass vaccination.

A multi-agency federal team has worked with five pilot jurisdictions—California, Florida, Minnesota, North Dakota, and Philadelphia—to utilize a basic plan for administration and adapt it to create jurisdiction-specific plans that will serve as models for other jurisdictions. Jurisdiction planning will cover coordination with federal facilities in their jurisdiction, coordination with national chain partners, vaccination of critical work forces, and reaching underserved populations.

Each jurisdiction will be required to develop a "microplan," based on their existing plans as well as outputs from the first five jurisdictions supported, with CDC providing technical assistance. These microplans will identify vaccination sites and necessary logistical considerations and lay out how the sites will be onboarded into the necessary IT system. The microplans will need to be flexible to allow adaptation as more information about the specific characteristics of the vaccines becomes available.

Under their cooperative agreements with CDC through which CARES Act awards were made, jurisdictions will then onboard providers to the IT system and identify and plan for the necessary vaccination workforce. Jurisdictions will also be responsible for laying specific groundwork for vaccinating high-risk and prioritized populations through various outreach efforts, including a work group or stakeholder groups, and forming a vaccination committee.

Jurisdictions will be expected to incorporate planning for distribution of vaccines to mem- bers of Tribes into their microplans. In addition, CDC and OWS are working with the Indian Health Service (IHS) to develop a plan for direct IHS distribution of vaccine to Tribes that desire that option.

Centralized Distribution

Centralized distribution allows the government full visibility, control, and ability to shift assets and use data to optimize vaccine uptake. On August 14, CDC announced its centralized distributor contract by executing an existing contract option with McKesson, which distributed the H1N1 vaccine during the H1N1 pandemic in 2009–2010. The current contract with McKesson, awarded as part of a competitive bidding process in 2016, includes an option for the distribution of vaccines in the event of a pandemic.

Once vaccines are allocated to a given jurisdiction or authorized partner, McKesson will deliver a specific amount of vaccine to a designated location. In many instances, delivery locations will be sites where vaccine will be administered. Alternatively, vaccines can be delivered to locations in jurisdictions to be further distributed to administration sites within health department networks. Vaccines can also be delivered to locations integrated into national retail pharmacy networks for distribution to individual pharmacies.

This system will be scalable to meet demand. Some vaccine with ultra-cold storage requirements may be shipped directly from the manufacturer to the administration sites, but all distribution will be managed by this centralized system.

If necessary, the McKesson contract can cover rapid distribution of doses of refrigerated (2–8° Celsius) and frozen (-20 °C) vaccines.

The COVID-19 pandemic has likely accelerated a trend towards different ways of engaging with the healthcare system, and successful delivery of this vaccine will need to incorporate new types of sites and approaches for vaccine delivery. For example, during H1N1, once vaccines became widely available pharmacies played an important role in the vaccine distribution; pharmacies' role is even more critical to vaccinations today and will be fully integrated into the distribution plan.

Ordering and Tracking Systems

Vaccine allocation and centralized distribution will utilize HHS's Vaccine Tracking System (VTrckS), which is a secure, web-based IT system that integrates the entire publicly funded vaccine supply chain from purchasing and ordering through distribution to participating state, local, and territorial health departments and healthcare providers.

VTrckS is being scaled for distribution of pandemic vaccines, to include the onboarding of new providers under each jurisdiction's microplan. For the COVID-19 vaccination program, additional providers, including private partners (e.g., pharmacy chains) and other federal entities (e.g., the Indian Health Service), will be onboarded to enable allocation to and ordering directly by these partners, in addition to the state, local, and territory allocations.

Through the linkage of a number of systems, information technology will also help direct people to where to get vaccinated using web-based "finder" systems.

A Potential Phased Structure

Phase 1

Upon FDA authorization or approval, initial vaccine doses will be distributed in a focused manner, with the goal of maximizing vaccine acceptance and public health protection while minimizing waste and inefficiency.

Although final decisions about prioritization will not be made until closer to implementation, select scenarios have been developed to assist with state and local planning. State and local health departments have been given specific scenarios to plan for during this stage, while scenario planning for distribution and administration plans specific to focused populations has begun at the federal level.

Phase 2

As the volume of available vaccine increases, distribution will expand, increasing access to the larger population. When larger quantities of vaccine become available, there will be two simultaneous objectives: 1) to provide widespread access to vaccination and achieve coverage across the United States population and 2) to ensure high uptake in target populations, particularly those who are at high risk for severe outcomes from COVID-19.

Phase 3

If the risk of COVID-19 persists such that there remains a public health need for an ongoing vaccination program, COVID-19 vaccines will ultimately be universally available and integrated into routine vaccination programs, run by both public and private partners.

Based on the timeline associated with FDA regulatory decision-making, increasing quantities of produced vaccines may be stockpiled as manufacturing proceeds before a regulatory decision has been made, which would mean that distribution may begin directly with Phase 2 or Phase 3.

Allocation

Allocations in the early phases will be based in part on methodology previously developed and reviewed by public health experts as part of pandemic planning. This methodology will be adjusted based on experience from COVID-19, real-time data on the virus and its impact on populations, performance of each vaccine, and the ongoing needs of the essential workforce.

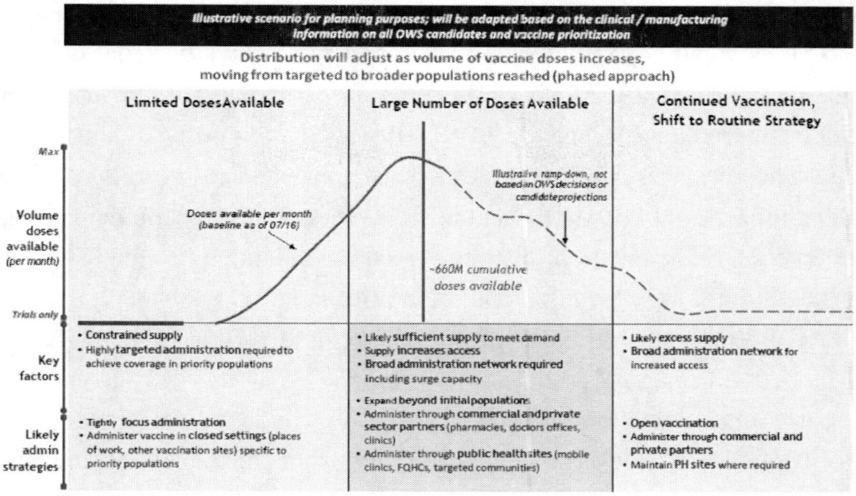

To develop and update populations to target in settings with limited doses of vaccine, the National Institutes of Health (NIH) and CDC requested that the National Academies of Sciences, Engineering, and Medicine and the National Academy of Medicine (NAM) develop an overarching framework to assist policymakers in the U.S. and global health communities in planning for equitable allocation of vaccines against COVID-19.

NAM established a committee to consider the criteria that should be used to set priorities for equitable distribution of potential vaccine and released a discussion draft of a preliminary allocation framework on September 1. The findings from the NAM committee will be shared with the CDC's Advisory Committee on Immunization Practices (ACIP), to help inform the committee's deliberations related to vaccine priority groups and ensuring equity in vaccination in the United States.

ACIP will review evidence on COVID-19 epidemiology and burden, vaccine safety, vaccine efficacy, evidence quality, and implementation issues to inform recommendations for COVID-19 vaccine policy, including priority groups for vaccination, which are submitted to the CDC director for adoption. ACIP meetings are open to the public, and committee records are required to be made available to the public, ensuring transparency and visibility for this recommendation-making process.

ACIP formed a COVID-19 Vaccine Work Group to help inform its evidence-based approaches to COVID-19 vaccination policy, including the initial vaccine prioritization strategy to be presented to the full ACIP for deliberation at public ACIP meetings, development of recommendations, and eventual presentation of these recommendations to the CDC for consideration in determining population prioritization.

ACIP embarked on early planning for these efforts. The framework developed during, and the lessons learned from, the H1N1 influenza vaccine implementation are being used to guide COVID-19 vaccine prioritization. CDC learned several lessons from the H1N1 response and vaccine distribution, including the real possibility of uncertainties in the pharmaceutical manufacturing process, which requires the distribution plan to anticipate delays and respond to changing circumstances. Further, demand is likely to vary regionally and in diverse populations within a given geographic area. Nimble delivery and allocation strategies will be essential.

Administration

What is required: Successful administration requires identifying prioritized populations and working cooperatively with state, local and tribal public health departments and other key partners to ensure individuals in targeted groups safely receive vaccines when limited doses initially become available.

What we are doing: Through collaborative planning with states and private sector provider partners such as pharmacies, vaccine administration sites will be selected to optimize access to vaccines throughout the distribution process.

Administration tasks within each distribution phase will include:

- Delivery of vaccine to sites, with the goal of no upfront costs to providers and no out- of-pocket cost to the vaccine recipient.
- Ensuring administration sites, as covered in the jurisdiction's microplans, have the capabilities for storing, handling, and administering vaccine products with specific distribution and administration requirements.
- Supporting reliable distribution of ancillary supplies that may be necessary for vaccine administration.
- Engagement of traditional and non-traditional administration sites and approaches in vaccination planning to allow for flexibility to accommodate vaccine requirements.

Delivery and Cost

The federal government is procuring hundreds of millions of doses of safe and effective vaccines, and has contracted with McKesson for purposes of vaccine distribution, such that no American will be charged for either the COVID-19 vaccine or its distribution. Various plans, supported by the CARES Act and the Families First Coronavirus Response Act, are under development with the objective of ensuring no one will be charged any out–of-pocket expenses for the administration of the vaccine either. The objective is to ensure no one desiring vaccination will face an economic barrier to receiving one.

Section 3203 of the CARES Act (P.L. 116-136) requires health insurance issuers and plans to cover any ACIP-recommended COVID-19 preventive service, including vaccines, without cost- sharing within 15 days of such recommendation to the CDC. Once a licensed COVID-19 vaccine is recommended by ACIP, and the recommendation is adopted by the CDC Director, required coverage for vaccines as preventative services for Medicaid Early and Periodic Screening, Diagnostic and Treatment beneficiaries and the Affordable Care Act provisions for most private insurance coverage and for the Medicaid expansion populations will also apply.

Ancillary Supplies

Supporting and securing an adequate quantity of ancillary supplies needed for administration has been a collaborative, interagency effort. OWS has aimed to procure and assemble 6.6 million ancillary supply kits, including pediatric, adult, and mixed-use kits, which would support the vaccination of up to 660 million doses of vaccine. These kits will include needles, syringes, alcohol pads, vaccination cards, and limited PPE for vaccinators.

HHS's Biomedical Advanced Research and Development Authority (BARDA) has awarded four large task orders for needles and syringes. BARDA will support additional solicitations, in coordination with the Strategic National Stockpile, to maximize the availability of needles and syringes toward the end of 2020. BARDA and the DoD Joint Program Executive Office for Chemical, and Biological, Radiological, and Nuclear Defense (JPEO-CBRND) have awarded three agreements to increase needle and syringe capacity in the U.S. for the future, some of which will be available in time to support the COVID-19 vaccination in early 2021. BARDA and the JPEOCBRND have also awarded agreements with two domestic manufacturers of vials to increase capacity necessary to support multiple vaccine candidates.

Administration Sites

Administration site options will vary depending on the nature of the vaccine and the phase of the vaccination program. During Phase 1, administration sites may be more limited to settings that can optimize reaching the target population while meeting the early requirements for storage and handling of vaccine product. During Phase 2, an expanded administration network would, for instance, likely include adult and pediatric healthcare providers and pharmacies. These considerations will be part of planning done by the jurisdictions discussed in the Distribution section.

As part of efforts to make administration sites easily accessible, the program will make maximum use of all healthcare professionals licensed to administer vaccines, including allied health professionals such as pharmacists.

HHS is also committed to ensuring rural populations can receive the vaccine, and has decades of experience working with public health partners addressing the needs of hard-to-reach populations. CDC will work with local communities, governments, and other partners to identify the best places and times to reach this population and utilize strategic distribution points via community health centers, schools, workplaces, mobile clinics, and pharmacies.

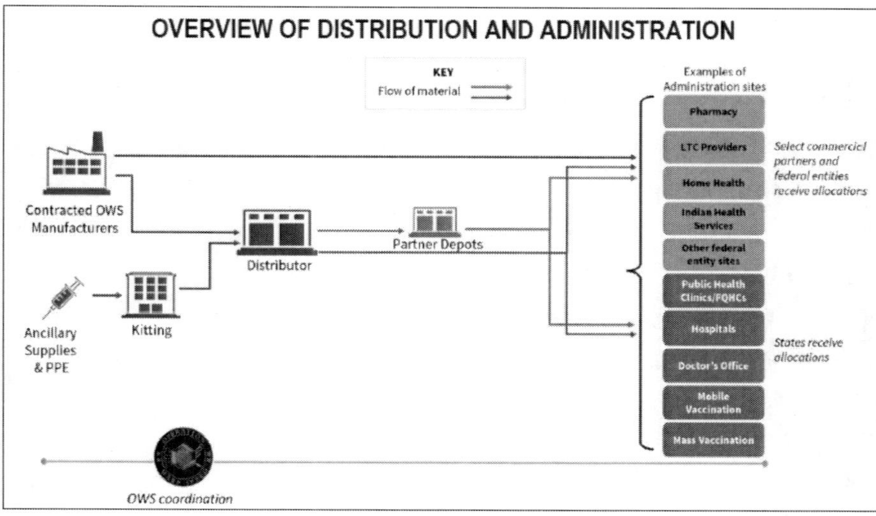

Monitoring

What is Required

The vaccination program requires extensive data monitoring infrastructure, including appropriate IT architecture, to incorporate claims and payment processes, to identify when a person needs a potential second dose, to monitor outcomes and adverse events, and to account for products the U.S. government is spending billions of dollars to research, develop, and produce. Data will need to be available both federally and at the state, local, and tribal level to ensure efficient management of the vaccination program.

What We Are Doing

OWS will construct and integrate an IT architecture that achieves this objective, building off of existing IT infrastructure and filling gaps with new IT solutions.

CDC has already been working to improve the data infrastructure needed to better track vaccines, vaccination, and related information. The COVID-19 vaccination program requires significant enhancement of the IT that will support enhancements and data exchange that are critical for a multi-dose candidate to ensure proper administration of a potential second dose.

Immunization Information Systems used by state, territory, and city entities that deliver public vaccinations will be central to this IT infrastructure. Major pharmaceutical retailers have proven and reliable dispensing record systems, while healthcare systems, hospitals, and private providers employ Electronic Health Record systems to store, monitor, and track patient information. Points of administration with undeveloped infrastructure—such as ad hoc mobile clinics and other rapidly mobilized mass vaccination sites—will be provided with free access and training for purpose-built web-based applications to support vaccine data administration and tracking, with an array of options available to make these accessible.

Together, this data will be reported into a common IT infrastructure that will support analysis and reporting. The IT infrastructure will support partners with a broad range of tools for record-keeping, data on who is being vaccinated, and reminders for second doses.

In all cases, administration records will be aggregated, anonymized, and de-identified to protect personally identifiable, private health information to the maximum extent possible.

Before a vaccine is authorized for use, evidence of its safety and efficacy is limited to the results from clinical trials, where patients are selected carefully and followed up very closely under controlled conditions. Because some technologies have limited previous data on safety in humans, the long-term safety of these vaccines will be carefully assessed using pharmacovigilance surveillance and Phase 4 (post-licensure) clinical trials.

The key objective of pharmacovigilance is to determine each vaccine's performance in real-life scenarios, to study efficacy, and to discover any infrequent and rare side effects not identified in clinical trials. OWS will also use pharmacovigilance analytics, which serves as one of the instruments for the continuous monitoring of pharmacovigilance data. Robust analytical tools will be used to leverage large amounts of data and the benefits of using such data across the value chain, including regulatory obligations. Pharmacovigilance provides timely information about the safety of each vaccine to patients, healthcare professionals, and the public, contributing to the protection of patients and the promotion of public health.

ENGAGEMENT

What is Required

To support vaccine distribution, administration, and monitoring, as well as promote vaccine uptake, vaccine confidence, and reporting of adverse events, a successful vaccination program requires engaging a nationwide network of partners. Working with established partners—especially those that are trusted sources for target audiences—is critical to advancing public understanding of, access to, and acceptance of eventual vaccines.

What We Are Doing

To build partnerships as part of the vaccination program and deliver an effective communications strategy, OWS is engaging public, nonprofit, and private partners, while leveraging the government's longstanding relationships with state health departments, tribal nations and organizations, healthcare systems, the vaccine industry, health insurance issuers and plans, and non-traditional partners.

Partnerships

State, local and tribal health departments have conducted pandemic vaccination planning with immunization and preparedness funding from CDC for over a decade. Rapidly updating these vaccination response plans for COVID-19 will ensure readiness for timely administration of COVID-19 vaccines.

This work builds on existing successful partnerships: Each year, CDC safely distributes more than 80 million doses of vaccines to approximately 40,000 public and private health providers across the country, in addition to the tens of millions of other vaccines distributed through other channels. During the 2009 H1N1 pandemic, more than 70,000 provider sites participated in the expanded vaccination program. This represents strong baseline capacity and partnerships for distribution and administration.

HHS's Office of Intergovernmental and External Affairs has established communication channels with almost 30 private sector organizations representing hospitals, physicians, nurses, nursing homes, community health centers, health insurance issuers and plans, drug stores, influencers, foundations, patients, and seniors' groups to provide regular updates on the work of OWS, including the distribution program.

HHS has also been holding regular calls with intergovernmental partners at the state, local, tribal, and territorial levels, with robust dialogue on how the federal government will successfully partner with them on the vaccination program.

Further, work has begun with organizations representing minority populations and vulnerable communities, with consultation already occurring with more than 150 organizations dedicated to addressing health disparities. Faith-based and other trusted community organizations can also be critical in addressing vaccine hesitancy, and HHS's Center for Faith and Opportunity Initiatives is working with minority-serving faith and community groups to enlist their help in educating Americans and encouraging participation in the vaccination program.

Communications

Strategic communications and public messaging are critical to ensure maximum acceptance of vaccines, requiring a saturation of messaging across the national media.

An information campaign led by HHS's public affairs department—developed using human- centered design, extensive public and stakeholder engagement, and research on message development and delivery—will focus on vaccine safety and efficacy, and target key populations and communities to ensure maximum vaccine acceptance.

CDC and other HHS components are working collaboratively within OWS to ensure that consistent and accurate information is at the foundation of the communications effort. The plan will also help inform the American people about the OWS strategy of delivering faster results while still following the same processes for safety and effectiveness that Americans expect with any other vaccine.

Identifying the right messages to promote vaccine confidence, countering misinformation, and targeting outreach to vulnerable and at-risk populations will be necessary to achieve high coverage. CDC will build on its existing relationships with local public health partners and health departments to effectively implement communications, and CDC is also working to develop innovative approaches to improve vaccine uptake among hard-to-reach critical populations.

Understanding that public confidence in vaccines is necessary for vaccine uptake and acceptance, CDC will make use of its strategic framework, Vaccinate with Confidence, which it has used successfully to strengthen public trust in vaccines and prevent vaccine-preventable disease outbreaks. This framework emphasizes three key priorities: protect communities, empower families, and stop myths. Within this framework, CDC is already working with local partners and using trusted messengers to establish new partnerships and contain the spread of misinformation.

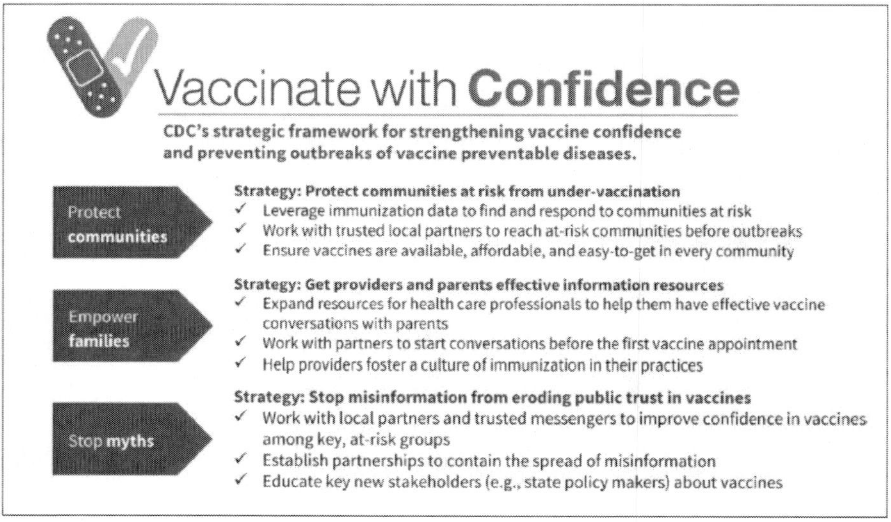

In: Vaccines
Editor: Oliver Huerta
ISBN: 978-1-53619-059-5

Chapter 2

EXPLAINING OPERATION WARP SPEED*

U.S. Department of Health and Human Services

WHAT'S THE GOAL?

Operation Warp Speed's goal is to produce and deliver 300 million doses of safe and effective vaccines with the initial doses available by January 2021, as part of a broader strategy to accelerate the development, manufacturing, and distribution of COVID-19 vaccines, therapeutics, and diagnostics (collectively known as countermeasures).

HOW WILL THE GOAL BE ACCOMPLISHED?

By investing in and coordinating countermeasure development, OWS will allow countermeasures such as a vaccine to be delivered to patients more rapidly while adhering to standards for safety and efficacy.

* This is an edited, reformatted and augmented version of U.S. Department of Health and Human Services Publication.

WHO'S WORKING ON OPERATION WARP SPEED?

OWS is a partnership among components of the Department of Health and Human Services (HHS), including the Centers for Disease Control and Prevention (CDC), the National Institutes of Health (NIH), and the Biomedical Advanced Research and Development Authority (BARDA), and the Department of Defense (DoD). OWS engages with private firms and other federal agencies, including the Department of Agriculture, the Department of Energy, and the Department of Veterans Affairs. It will coordinate existing HHS-wide efforts, including the NIH's Accelerating COVID-19 Therapeutic Interventions and Vaccines (ACTIV) partnership, NIH's Rapid Acceleration of Diagnostics (RADx) initiative, and work by BARDA.

WHAT'S THE PLAN AND WHAT'S HAPPENED SO FAR?

Development

To accelerate development while maintaining standards for safety and efficacy, OWS has been selecting the most promising countermeasure candidates and providing coordinated government support.

Protocols for the demonstration of safety and efficacy are being aligned, which will allow these harmonized clinical trials to proceed more quickly, and the protocols for the trials will be overseen by the federal government (NIH), as opposed to traditional public-private partnerships, in which pharmaceutical companies decide on their own protocols. Rather than eliminating steps from traditional development timelines, steps will proceed simultaneously, such as starting manufacturing of vaccines and therapeutics at industrial scale well before the demonstration of efficacy and safety as happens normally. This increases the financial risk, but not the product risk.

Select actions to support OWS vaccine and therapeutic development so far include:

- *March 30:* HHS announced $456 million in funds for Johnson & Johnson's (Janssen) candidate vaccine. Phase 1 clinical trials began in Belgium on July 24th and in the U.S on July 27th. Janssen's large-scale Phase 3 clinical trial began on September 22, 2020, making them the fourth OWS candidate to enter Phase 3 clinical trials in the United States. Up to 60,000 volunteers will be enrolled in the trial at up to nearly 215 clinical research sites in the United States and internationally.
- *April 16:* HHS made up to $483 million in support available for Moderna's candidate vaccine, which began Phase 1 trials on March 16 and received a fast-track designation from FDA. This agreement was expanded on July 26 to include an additional $472 million to support late-stage clinical development, including the expanded Phase 3 study of the company's mRNA vaccine, which began on July 27th.
- *May 21:* HHS announced up to $1.2 billion in support for AstraZeneca's candidate vaccine, developed in conjunction with the University of Oxford. The agreement is to make available at least 300 million doses of the vaccine for the United States, with the first doses delivered as early as October 2020, if the product successfully receives FDA EUA or licensure. AstraZeneca's large-scale Phase 3 clinical trial began on August 31, 2020.
- *July 7:* HHS announced $450 million in funds to support the large-scale manufacturing of Regeneron's COVID-19 investigational anti-viral antibody treatment, REGN-COV2. This agreement is the first of a number of OWS awards to support potential therapeutics all the way through to manufacturing. As part of the manufacturing demonstration project, doses of the medicine will be packaged and ready to ship immediately if clinical trials are successful and FDA grants EUA or licensure.

- *July 7:* HHS announced $1.6 billion in funds to support the large-scale manufacturing of Novavax's vaccine candidate. By funding Novavax's manufacturing effort, the federal government will own the 100 million doses expected to result from the demonstration project.
- *July 22:* HHS announced up to $1.95 billion in funds to Pfizer for the large-scale manufacturing and nationwide distribution of 100 million doses of their vaccine candidate. The federal government will own the 100 million doses of vaccine initially produced as a result of this agreement, and Pfizer will deliver the doses in the United States if the product successfully receives FDA EUA or licensure, as outlined in FDA guidance, after completing demonstration of safety and efficacy in a large Phase 3 clinical trial, which began July 27th.
- *July 31:* HHS announced approximately $2 billion in funds to support the advanced development, including clinical trials and large scale manufacturing, of Sanofi and GlaxoSmithKline's (GSK) investigational adjuvanted vaccine. By funding the manufacturing effort, the federal government will own the approximately 100 million doses expected to result from the demonstration project. The adjuvanted vaccine doses could be used in clinical trials or, if the FDA authorizes use, as outlined in agency guidance, the doses would be distributed as part of a COVID-19 vaccination campaign.
- *August 5:* HHS announced approximately $1 billion in funds to support the large-scale manufacturing and delivery of Johnson & Johnson's (Janssen) investigational vaccine candidate. Under the terms of the agreement, the U.S. Government will own the resulting 100 million doses of vaccine, and will have the option to acquire more. The company's investigational vaccine relies on Janssen's recombinant adenovirus technology, AdVac, a technology used to develop and manufacture Janssen's Ebola vaccine with BARDA support; that vaccine received European Commission approval and was used in the Democratic Republic of

the Congo (DRC) and Rwanda during the 2018-2020 Ebola outbreak that began in the DRC.

- *August 11:* HHS announced up to $1.5 billion in funds to support the large-scale manufacturing and delivery of Moderna's investigational vaccine candidate. Under the terms of the agreement, the U.S. Government will own the resulting 100 million doses of vaccine, and will have the option to acquire more. The vaccine, called mRNA-1273, has been co-developed by Moderna and scientists from the National Institute of Allergy and Infectious Diseases (NIAID), part of the National Institutes of Health. NIAID has continued to support the vaccine's development including nonclinical studies and clinical trials. Additionally, BARDA has supported phase 2/3 clinical trials, vaccine manufacturing scale up and other development activities for this vaccine. The Phase 3 clinical trial, which began July 27, is the first government-funded Phase 3 clinical trial for a COVID-19 vaccine in the United States.
- *August 23:* As part of the agency's efforts to combat COVID-19, the FDA issued an emergency use authorization (EUA) for investigational convalescent plasma. Based on available scientific evidence, the FDA determined convalescent plasma may be effective in lessening the severity or shortening the length of COVID-19 illness in hospitalized patients, and that the known and potential benefits of the product outweigh the known and potential risks. The EUA authorizes the distribution of convalescent plasma in the U.S. as well as its administration by health care providers, as appropriate, to treat suspected or confirmed cases of COVID-19. Click here to learn more about EUAs.
- *October 9:* HHS announced an agreement with AstraZeneca for late-stage development and large-scale manufacturing of the company's COVID-19 investigational product AZD7442, a cocktail of two monoclonal antibodies, that may help treat or prevent COVID-19. The goal of AstraZeneca's partnership with the U.S. Government is to develop a monoclonal antibody cocktail

that can help prevent infection. An effective monoclonal antibody that can prevent COVID-19, particularly one that is long-lasting and delivered by intramuscular injection, may be of particular use in certain groups. This includes people who have compromised immune function, those who are over 80 years old, and people undergoing medical treatments that preclude them from receiving a COVID-19 vaccine.

As announced on May 15, the vaccine development plan is as follows, subject to change as work proceeds:

- *Fourteen* promising candidates have been chosen from the 100+ vaccine candidates currently in development—some of them already in clinical trials with U.S. government support.
- *The 14* vaccine candidates are being narrowed down to about seven candidates, representing the most promising candidates from a range of technology options (nucleic acid, viral vector, protein subunit), which will go through further testing in early-stage clinical trials.
- *Large-scale* randomized trials for the demonstration of safety and efficacy will proceed for the most promising candidates.

Manufacturing

The federal government is making investments in the necessary manufacturing capacity at its own risk, giving firms the confidence to invest aggressively in development which will allow faster distribution of an eventual vaccine. Manufacturing capacity for selected candidates will be advanced while they are still in development, rather than scaled up after approval or authorization. Manufacturing capacity developed will be used for whatever vaccine is eventually successful, if possible given the nature of the successful product, regardless of which firms have developed the capacity.

Select actions to support OWS manufacturing efforts so far include:

- The *May 21, April 16,* and *March 30* HHS agreements with AstraZeneca, Moderna, and Johnson & Johnson respectively include investments in manufacturing capabilities.
- *June 1:* HHS announced a task order with Emergent BioSolutions to advance domestic manufacturing capabilities and capacity for a potential COVID-19 vaccine as well as therapeutics, worth approximately $628 million, using Emergent's BARDA-supported Center for Innovation in Advanced Department and Manufacturing.
- *July 27:* HHS announced a task order with Texas A&M University and FUJIFILM to advance domestic manufacturing capabilities and capacity for a potential COVID-19 vaccine, worth approximately $265 million, using another BARDA-supported CIADM.
- *August 4:* Grand River Aseptic Manufacturing Inc., (GRAM) Grand Rapids, Michigan, was awarded a $160 million firm-fixed-price contract for domestic aseptic fill and finish manufacturing capacity for critical vaccines and therapeutics in response to the COVID-19 pandemic.
- *October 13:* HHS announced a $31 million agreement with Cytiva to expand the company's manufacturing capacity for products that are essential in producing COVID-19 vaccines, such as liquid and dry powder cell culture media, cell culture buffers, mixer bags, and XDR bioreactors. Cytiva is a major manufacturer of pharmaceutical consumables and hardware products and the primary supplier to many of the companies currently working with the U.S. government to develop COVID-19 vaccines. This capacity expansion will help Cytiva respond to the demand for COVID-19 vaccine consumables and hardware products without impacting on current manufacturing output.

Distribution

OWS and our private partners are developing a plan for delivering a safe and effective product to Americans as quickly and reliably as possible. Experts from HHS are leading vaccine development, while experts from DoD are partnering with the CDC and other parts of HHS to coordinate supply, production, and distribution of vaccines.

Select actions to support OWS distribution efforts include:

May

May 12: DoD and HHS announced a $138 million contract with ApiJect for more than 100 million prefilled syringes for distribution across the United States by year-end 2020, as well as the development of manufacturing capacity for the ultimate production goal of over 500 million prefilled syringes in 2021.

June

- *June 9:* HHS and DoD announced a joint effort to increase domestic manufacturing capacity for vials that may be needed for vaccines and treatments.
- *June 11:* HHS announced $204 million in funds to Corning to expand the domestic manufacturing capacity to produce approximately 164 million Valor Glass vials per year if needed. Valor Glass provides chemical durability to minimize particulate contamination. The specialized glass allows for rapid filling and capping methods that can increase manufacturing throughput by as much as 50 percent compared with conventional filling lines, which in turn can reduce the overall manufacturing time for vaccines and therapies.

- *June 11:* HHS announced $143 million to SiO2 Materials Science to ramp up capacity to produce the company's glass-coated plastic container, which can be used for drugs and vaccines. The new lines provide the capacity to produce an additional 120 million vials per year if needed.

August

- *August 14:* HHS and DoD announced that McKesson Corporation will be a central distributor of future COVID-19 vaccines and related supplies needed to administer the pandemic vaccinations. The CDC is executing an existing contract option with McKesson to support vaccine distribution. The company also distributed the H1N1 vaccine during the H1N1 pandemic in 2009-2010. The current contract with McKesson, awarded as part of a competitive bidding process in 2016, includes an option for the distribution of vaccines in the event of a pandemic. Detailed planning is underway to ensure rapid distribution as soon as the FDA authorizes one or more vaccines. Once these decisions are made, McKesson will work under CDC's guidance to ship COVID-19 vaccines to administration sites.

September

- *September 16*: HHS and DoD released two documents outlining the Trump Administration's detailed strategy to deliver safe and effective COVID-19 vaccine doses to the American people as quickly and reliably as possible. The documents, developed by HHS in coordination with DoD and the Centers for Disease Control and Prevention (CDC), provide a strategic distribution overview along with an interim playbook for state, tribal, territorial, and local public health programs and their partners on how to plan and operationalize a vaccination response to COVID-19 within their respective jurisdictions.

WHO'S LEADING OPERATION WARP SPEED?

HHS Secretary Alex Azar and Defense Secretary Mark Esper oversee OWS, with Dr. Moncef Slaoui designated as chief advisor and General Gustave F. Perna confirmed as the chief operating officer. To allow these OWS leaders to focus on operational work, in the near future the program will be announcing separate points of contact, with deep expertise and involvement in the program, for communication with Congress and the public.

WHAT ARE YOU DOING TO MAKE THESE PRODUCTS AFFORDABLE FOR AMERICANS?

The Administration is committed to providing free or low-cost COVID-19 countermeasures to the American people as fast as possible. Any vaccine or therapeutic doses purchased with US taxpayer dollars will be given to the American people at no cost.

HOW IS OPERATION WARP SPEED BEING FUNDED?

Congress has directed almost $10 billion to this effort through supplemental funding, including the CARES Act. Congress has also appropriated other flexible funding. The almost $10 billion specifically directed includes more than $6.5 billion designated for countermeasure development through BARDA and $3 billion for NIH research.

In: Vaccines
Editor: Oliver Huerta

ISBN: 978-1-53619-059-5

Chapter 3

TRUMP ADMINISTRATION EXPANDS MANUFACTURING CAPACITY WITH CYTIVA FOR COMPONENTS OF COVID-19 VACCINES*

U.S. Department of Health and Human Services

To meet the Trump Administration's Operation Warp Speed goals, the U.S. Department of Health and Human Services (HHS) and Department of Defense (DoD) today announced an agreement with Cytiva, headquartered in Massachusetts, to expand the company's manufacturing capacity for products that are essential in producing COVID-19 vaccines.

The Biomedical Advanced Research and Development Authority (BARDA), part of the HHS Office of the Assistant Secretary for Preparedness and Response, collaborated with the DoD Joint Program Executive Office for Chemical, Biological, Radiological and Nuclear Defense and Army Contracting Command, to provide approximately $31 million to Cytiva for vaccine-related consumable products, such as liquid

* This is an edited, reformatted and augmented version of U.S. Department of Health and Human Services Publication.

and dry powder cell culture media, cell culture buffers, mixer bags, and XDR bioreactors.

> "As part of Operation Warp Speed, we are expanding U.S.-based manufacturing of the products that are essential in the development and manufacturing of COVID-19 vaccines," said HHS Secretary Alex Azar. "By expanding capacity now, not only do we help deliver these products as quickly as possible, but we also return manufacturing to America, boosting the economy and preparing us for future crises."

Under the agreement, the company will expand manufacturing capacity in the company's Massachusetts facilities and create duplicate capabilities in Cytiva's Utah facilities to be complete in less than 12 months. Currently, the company only manufactures consumables in Massachusetts.

Cytiva is a major manufacturer of pharmaceutical consumables and hardware products and the primary supplier to many of the companies currently working with the U.S. government to develop COVID-19 vaccines. This capacity expansion will help Cytiva respond to the demand for COVID-19 vaccine consumables and hardware products without impacting on current manufacturing output.

The agreement with Cytiva is the latest to increase manufacturing capacity in the United States to aid in developing, manufacturing, and administering COVID-19 vaccines and therapeutics.

To date, the federal government has obligated a total of more than $1.1 billion to purchase needles, syringes, vials and supply kits, and to expand the capacity to manufacture these ancillary supplies and the fill-finish manufacturing capacity in the United States for COVID-19 vaccines and therapeutics. HHS and DOD are working with Becton Dickinson, Corning Pharmaceutical Technologies, Goldbelt Security, Marathon Medical, Retractable Technologies Inc., SiO2, ApiJect, Smiths Medical, and Thermo Fisher Scientific. BARDA also is working with its Centers for Innovation in Advanced Development and Manufacturing in Maryland and Texas to expand vaccine manufacturing capacity for federal vaccine development partners.

About Operation Warp Speed (OWS)

OWS is a partnership among components of the Department of Health and Human Services and the Department of Defense, engaging with private firms and other federal agencies, and coordinating among existing HHS-wide efforts to accelerate the development, manufacturing, and distribution of COVID-19 vaccines, therapeutics, and diagnostics.

About HHS, ASPR, and BARDA

HHS works to enhance and protect the health and well-being of all Americans, providing for effective health and human services and fostering advances in medicine, public health, and social services. The mission of ASPR is to save lives and protect Americans from 21st century health security threats. Within ASPR, BARDA invests in the innovation, advanced research and development, acquisition, and manufacturing of medical countermeasures – vaccines, drugs, therapeutics, diagnostic tools, and non-pharmaceutical products needed to combat health security threats. To date, 55 BARDA-supported products have achieved FDA approval, licensure or clearance. For more on BARDA's portfolio for COVID-19 diagnostics, vaccines and treatments and about partnering with BARDA, visit medicalcountermeasures.gov. To learn more about federal support for the all-of-America COVID-19 response, visit coronavirus.gov.

About the JPEO-CBRND

The Joint Program Executive Office for Chemical, Biological, Radiological and Nuclear Defense (JPEO-CBRND) protects the Joint Force by providing medical countermeasures and defense equipment against chemical, biological, radiological and nuclear (CBRN) threats. JPEO-CBRND's goal is to enable the Joint Force to fight and win unencumbered by a CBRN environment. JPEO-CBRND facilitates the rapid response, advanced development, manufacturing and acquisition of medical solutions, such as vaccines, therapeutics, and diagnostics, to combat CBRN and emerging threats such as COVID-19. To learn more about JPEO-CBRND's COVID-19 response, visit https://www.jpeocbrnd.osd.mil/coronavirus or follow JPEO-CBRND on social media at @JPEOCBRND.

In: Vaccines
Editor: Oliver Huerta
ISBN: 978-1-53619-059-5

Chapter 4

DEVELOPMENT AND REGULATION OF MEDICAL COUNTERMEASURES FOR COVID-19 (VACCINES, DIAGNOSTICS, AND TREATMENTS): FREQUENTLY ASKED QUESTIONS*

Agata Dabrowska, Frank Gottron, Amanda K. Sarata and Kavya Sekar

SUMMARY

In recent months, the Coronavirus Disease 2019 (COVID-19) pandemic has spread globally, with the United States now reporting the highest number of cases of any country in the world.

Currently, there are few treatment options available to lessen the health impact of the disease and no vaccines or other prophylactic treatments to curb the spread of the virus.

* This is an edited, reformatted and augmented version of Congressional Research Service Publication No. R46427, dated June 25, 2020.

The biomedical community has been working to develop new therapies or vaccines, and to repurpose already approved therapeutics, that could prevent COVID-19 infections or lessen severe outcomes in patients. In addition, efforts have been underway to develop new diagnostic tools (i.e., testing) to help better identify and isolate positive cases, thereby reducing the spread of the disease. To this end, Congress has appropriated funds for research and development into new *medical countermeasures* (MCMs) in several recent supplemental appropriations acts. MCMs are medical products that may be used to treat, prevent, or diagnose conditions associated with emerging infectious diseases or chemical, biological, radiological, or nuclear (CBRN) agents. MCMs include biologics (e.g., vaccines, monoclonal antibodies), drugs (e.g., antimicrobials, antivirals), and medical devices (e.g., diagnostic tests).

This chapter answers frequently asked questions about current efforts related to research and development of medical countermeasures, their regulation, and related policy issues. Although several efforts are underway, medical product research, development, and approval is a difficult and high-risk endeavor that takes years in typical circumstances. In response to COVID-19, this process has been expedited, including through several federal programs and mechanisms covered in this chapter. However, expedited medical product development can carry certain risks, such as a more limited safety profile for new products upon approval.

INTRODUCTION

In recent months, the Coronavirus Disease 2019 (COVID-19) pandemic has spread globally, with the United States now reporting the highest number of cases of any country in the world.

Currently, there are few treatment options available to lessen the health impact of the disease and no vaccines or other prophylactic treatments to curb the spread of the virus. Treatment of severe COVID-19 cases can require significant health care resources, such as ventilators for patients with serious respiratory complications. A portion of severe cases are fatal.

The biomedical community has been working to develop new therapies or vaccines, and to repurpose already approved therapeutics, that could prevent COVID-19 infections or lessen severe outcomes in patients. In addition, efforts have been underway to develop new diagnostic tools (i.e., testing) to help better identify and isolate positive cases, thereby reducing the spread of the disease. To this end, Congress has appropriated funds for research and development into new medical countermeasures (MCMs) in several recent supplemental appropriations acts.

On May 15, the Trump Administration announced Operation Warp Speed, the major federal effort to accelerate and coordinate the development, manufacturing, and distribution of MCMs. The public-private partnership involves several federal agencies (including those covered in this chapter), as well as private firms. A key feature of the initiative is greater federal involvement and coordination in research, development, and manufacturing for selected MCM candidates than is typical for most U.S. pharmaceutical research and development (R&D).

This chapter summarizes current efforts related to research and development of medical countermeasures (including studying novel uses of already approved MCMs), their regulation, and related policy issues. Although several efforts are underway, medical product research, development, and approval is a difficult and high-risk endeavor that takes years in typical circumstances. In response to COVID-19, this process has been expedited, including through several federal programs and mechanisms covered in this chapter. However, expedited medical product development can carry certain risks, such as a more limited safety profile for new products upon approval. Particularly in the context of a pandemic, regulators are faced with the challenge of weighing the benefits and risks in introducing any new product into the market on a rapid timeline. This chapter focuses on therapeutics, vaccines, and diagnostics for COVID-19 and generally does not discuss other types of medical devices relevant to the treatment of COVID-19 (e.g., ventilators, personal protective equipment). This chapter also does not discuss MCM affordability, coverage, or supply chain issues.

BACKGROUND

What are MCMs?

MCMs are medical products that may be used to treat, prevent, or diagnose conditions associated with emerging infectious diseases or chemical, biological, radiological, or nuclear (CBRN) agents. MCMs include biologics (e.g., vaccines, monoclonal antibodies),[1] drugs (e.g., antimicrobials, antivirals), and medical devices (e.g., diagnostic tests).[2]

How Are Medical Products Like MCMs Typically Developed?

Developing any new medical product typically requires several stages of research:

- basic research to understand the fundamental mechanisms of a disease;
- identification of a potential product (i.e., a drug);
- preclinical testing in the laboratory, often using animals, tissue samples, and/or computer models;
- testing in several stages (typically three phases) of human clinical trials in progressively larger groups of human subjects to assess products for safety and effectiveness.

---

[1] Monoclonal antibodies are preparations of a specific type of antibody designed to bind to a single target. See NIH, "Monoclonal antibodies crucial to fighting emerging infectious diseases, say NIH officials," March 8, 2018, https://www.nih.gov/news-events/news-releases/monoclonal-antibodies-crucial-fighting-emerging-infectious-diseases-say-nih-officials.

[2] Food and Drug Administration (FDA), "What Are Medical Countermeasures?," accessed April 15, 2020, https://www.fda.gov/emergency-preparedness-and-response/about-mcmi/what-are-medical-countermeasures. Personal protective equipment is also a type of medical device and MCM; however, a discussion of these products is outside the scope of this chapter.

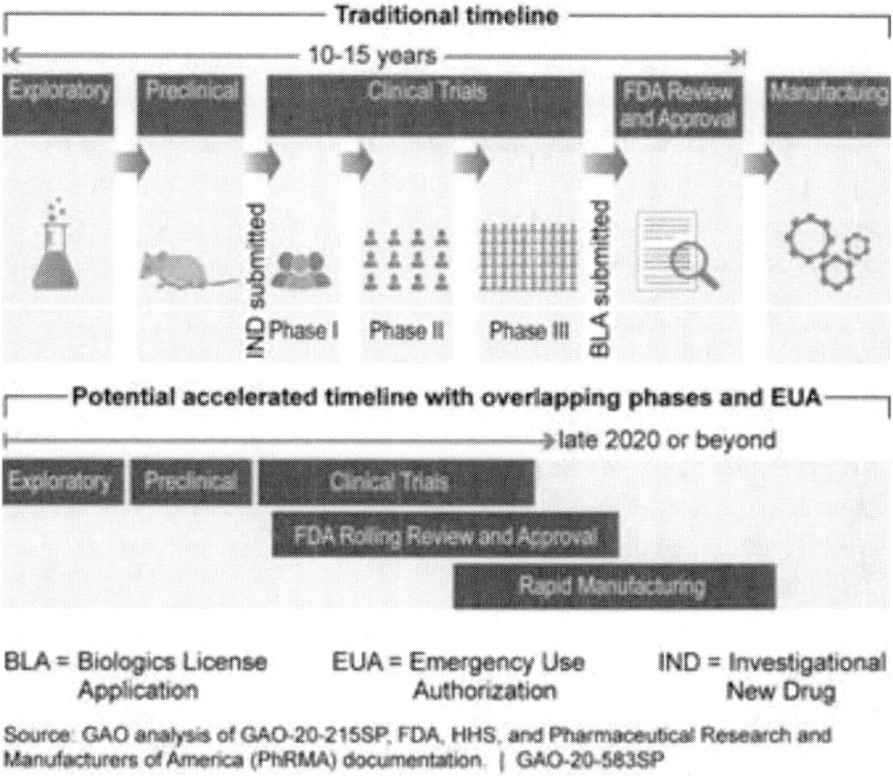

Source: Government Accountability Office (GAO), "The Reward and Risk of Expediting COVID-19 Testing and Vaccine Development," May 28, 2020, https://blog.gao.gov/2020/05/28/the-reward-and-risk-of-expediting-covid-19-testing-and-vaccine-development/.

Figure 1.Traditional Pharmaceutical R&D Timeline Versus an Accelerated Timeline.

In addition, companies must develop the manufacturing capabilities to produce a new product at scale. In most cases, medical products must be approved by the U.S. Food and Drug Administration (FDA) before being marketed in the United States. In typical circumstances, the development and approval of new drugs takes an average of 10-15 years from discovery to approval.[3] This process may be abbreviated in the case of an already approved therapeutic whereby safety has been established, but clinical testing is still needed to evaluate its effectiveness for a new use. This is

[3] CRS Infographic IG10013, The Pharmaceutical Drug Development Process.

sometimes referred to as drug repurposing. Additional safety studies may be needed if the route of administration or dosage of the therapeutic for the new use differs from that previously approved.

To make products available for the COVID-19 pandemic, the federal government is aiming to accelerate and coordinate various elements of the process, as shown in the Government Accountability Office (GAO) graphic below (see *Figure 1*).

In typical circumstances, the public sector generally finances much of the basic research and some preclinical testing and clinical research of new pharmaceutical products—such as through research supported by the National Institutes of Health (NIH)—mostly in the early stage of R&D, such as Phase 1 clinical trials.[4] The private sector tends to support much of the later-stage R&D of new medical products, such as late-stage and large-scale Phase 3 clinical trials, and the development of manufacturing capabilities.[5]

The federal government has recognized that countermeasures to some public health threats, such as emerging infectious diseases or bioterrorism agents, may have fewer market incentives than other pharmaceutical products, such as those treating chronic diseases. Manufacturers generally lack a profit incentive to develop products or capabilities in anticipation of a potential pandemic disease. As a result, the federal government has invested in agencies and programs that support the development of new MCMs. For example, the Biomedical Advanced Research and Development Authority (BARDA) can specifically support later-stage R&D and the manufacturing capabilities of new MCMs. Other incentives, such as regulatory exclusivity and tax incentives, can also support the development of new products.[6]

---

[4] Gillian K. Gresham, Stephan Ehrhardt, and Jill L. Meinhert, "Characteristics and Trends of Clinical Trials Funded by the National Institutes of Health Between 2005 and 2015," *Clinical Trials*, vol. 15, no. 1 (2018), pp. 65-74.

[5] National Academies of Sciences, Engineering, and Medicine, *Making Medicines Affordable: A National Imperative*, 2018, pp. 31-70.

[6] The sponsor of an new drug application (NDA) or biologics license application (BLA) for a new MCM may receive, upon approval, a period of exclusivity during which FDA may not approve an NDA or BLA from another sponsor for a certain number of years. For example,

Which Federal Agencies Are Usually Involved in MCM Development?

Several federal agencies, some of which are listed below, support medical and health R&D, while the FDA regulates the marketing of medical products in the United States. These agencies can contribute to and facilitate the development of new medical products, particularly in the event of an infectious disease threat.

The *National Institutes of Health (NIH)* within the Department of Health and Human Services (HHS) is the primary federal agency that supports medical and health research. NIH funds much of the basic biomedical science research in the United States, and it supports some development of new medical products.[7] One NIH institute, the National Institute of Allergy and Infectious Diseases (NIAID), aids in the response to new infectious disease threats as a part of its mission— supporting both basic scientific research and the development of new MCMs.[8]

The *Centers for Disease Control and Prevention (CDC)* within HHS generally supports public health and laboratory research related to new infectious disease threats. In the event of emerging infectious disease outbreaks, CDC has been the first to develop a diagnostic testing kit for use in U.S. public health laboratories—a model followed during the H1N1 influenza pandemic, the 2016 Zika outbreak, and now during the COVID-19 pandemic.[9] Aside from diagnostic test development, the agency supports a limited amount of MCM R&D; for example, past clinical trials for pre-exposure prophylaxis (PrEP) for HIV infections.[10] CDC also

---

provided that statutory criteria are met, a drug that contains a new chemical entity is eligible for five years of data exclusivity.

[7] CRS Report R41705, The National Institutes of Health (NIH): Background and Congressional Issues.

[8] National Institute of Allergy and Infectious Diseases (NIAID), "NIAID Strategic Plan 2017," https://www.niaid.nih.gov/sites/default/files/NIAIDStrategicPlan2017.pdf.

[9] Centers for Disease Control and Prevention (CDC), "The 2009 H1N1 Pandemic: Summary Highlights, April 2009- April 2010," 2010, https://www.cdc.gov/h1n1flu/cdcresponse.htm.

[10] CDC, "CDC U.S. Extended PrEP Safety Trial: Quick Facts on Trial Design," July 2010, https://www.cdc.gov/ nchhstp/newsroom/docs/US-PrEP-Study-7-15-10-508.pdf.

supports postmarket surveillance (i.e., data collection) on the safety and effectiveness of certain MCMs on the market, such as for vaccines.[11]

The *Biomedical Advanced Research and Development Authority (BARDA)* under the HHS Office of the Assistant Secretary for Preparedness and Response (ASPR) supports MCM development for use against emerging infectious diseases; pandemic influenza; and chemical, biological, radiological, and nuclear threat agents. Its efforts focus on supporting the transition from basic research to advanced development, clinical testing, FDA approval, and acquisition of some MCMs into the Strategic National Stockpile (SNS).[12]

FDA within HHS regulates the safety, effectiveness, and quality of MCMs through premarket review and postmarket requirements (e.g., adverse event reporting). FDA provides guidance, regulatory advice, and technical assistance to entities developing MCMs. The agency also conducts intramural and funds extramural regulatory science research to support the development of tools, standards, and approaches for assessing and developing MCMs.[13] In addition, FDA has created the Coronavirus Treatment Acceleration Program (CTAP), which seeks to accelerate clinical testing of potential therapeutics and move new treatments to patients as quickly as possible.[14]

The *Department of Defense (DOD)* operates several medical research and MCM development efforts, including through the Congressionally Directed Medical Research Program (CDMRP), the U.S. Army Medical Research and Development Command (USAMRDC), and the Defense

---

[11] CDC, "Vaccine Safety Monitoring," https://www.cdc.gov/vaccinesafety/ensuringsafety/monitoring/index.html.

[12] The Strategic National Stockpile (SNS) refers to the supply of medicine and medical supplies maintained by the U.S. government to respond to a public health emergency severe enough to deplete local supplies (e.g., hurricane, infectious disease outbreak, or terrorist attack). The SNS includes antibiotics, intravenous fluids, and other medical supplies such as PPE and ventilators, as well as certain medicines, such as anthrax and smallpox vaccines and treatments that may not be otherwise available for public use. For additional information, see CRS In Focus IF11574, *National Stockpiles: Background and Issues for Congress*, by G. James Herrera and Frank Gottron.

[13] FDA, "MCM Regulatory Science," https://www.fda.gov/emergency-preparedness-and-response/medical- countermeasures-initiative-mcmi/mcm-regulatory-science.

[14] FDA, "Coronavirus Treatment Acceleration Program (CTAP)," https://www.fda.gov /drugs/coronavirus-covid-19-drugs/coronavirus-treatment-acceleration-program-ctap.

Advanced Research Projects Agency (DARPA). For example, DARPA's Pandemic Prevention Platform program is focused on developing a platform that would aid in the rapid development of new MCMs in response to the identification of any known or unknown infectious threat.[15]

CDC, NIH, and FDA participate in the *Public Health Emergency Medical Countermeasures Enterprise (PHEMCE)*, along with DOD, the U.S. Department of Veterans Affairs (VA), the Department of Homeland Security (DHS), and the U.S. Department of Agriculture (USDA). The PHEMCE, under the leadership of ASPR, facilitates interagency coordination and strategy for the development, regulation, and availability of medical countermeasures in preparation for public health emergencies such as infectious disease outbreaks. As required by Public Health Service Act (PHSA) Section 2811,[16] the PHEMCE assesses and updates a strategy plan annually for MCM preparedness.[17]

RESEARCH AND DEVELOPMENT (R&D)

What Mechanisms Are Available for Agencies to Accelerate MCM R&D?

Several federal agencies have mechanisms to support rapid MCM R&D in the context of an infectious disease threat. Typically, agencies' grant-making, contract, and procurement processes can take several months when conducted pursuant to laws and regulations. However, several agencies have other transaction (OT) authority—additional authorities that provide flexibility and allow for expedited research funding and product procurement—particularly during a public health emergency.

---

[15] Defense Advanced Research Projects Agency (DARPA), "Pandemic Prevention Platform," https://www.darpa.mil/ program/pandemic-prevention-platform.

[16] 42 U.S.C. §300hh-10.

[17] The Assistant Secretary for Preparedness and Response (ASPR), "2017-2018 PHEMCE Strategy and Implementation Plan," 2017, https://www.phe.gov/Preparedness/mcm/phemce/Pages/strategy.aspx.

In addition, several agencies have existing research efforts or partnerships that can be mobilized to address emerging infectious disease threats.

NIH supports both intramural research in NIH-operated facilities and extramural research conducted by scientists at research institutions (i.e., universities, medical centers, and nonprofits). During a public health emergency, NIH has authority to award supplemental extramural research funding to existing research projects and to expedite the review process for new research proposals.[18] NIH also has several OT authorities that allow for expedited and flexible funding of new projects. In particular, NIH has OT authority for projects involving "high impact cutting- edge research that fosters scientific creativity and increases fundamental biological understanding leading to the prevention, diagnosis, or treatment of diseases and disorders, or research urgently required to respond to a public health threat."[19]

NIH intramural researchers can shift efforts to address a new public health threat, such as the current work by the NIAID Vaccine Research Center on COVID-19 vaccines.[20] NIAID was able to redirect existing intramural research efforts related to other coronaviruses to the virus causing COVID-19.[21] In addition, NIH can leverage private funding through the Foundation for the NIH[22] to support MCM development, such as announced on April 17, 2020, for the Accelerating COVID-19 Therapeutic Interventions and Vaccines (ACTIV) partnership aimed at accelerating the development of new vaccines and therapeutic candidates.[23]

---

[18] Public Health Service Act (PHSA) §494.

[19] 42 U.S.C. §282(n)(1)(C).

[20] NIH, "NIH Clinical Trial of Investigational Vaccine for COVID-19 Begins," press release, March 16, 2020, https://www.nih.gov/news-events/news-releases/nih-clinical-trial-investigational-vaccine-covid-19-begins.

[21] NIH, "New Coronavirus Stable for Hours on Surfaces," press release, March 17, 2020, https://www.nih.gov/news- events/news-releases/new-coronavirus-stable-hours-surfaces.

[22] The Foundation for the NIH is a not-for-profit organization established by Congress in 1990 to raise private funds in support of the NIH's mission and facilitate public-private partnerships. See CRS Report R46109, *Agency-Related Nonprofit Research Foundations and Corporations*.

[23] NIH, "NIH to Launch Public-Private Partnership to Speed COVID-19 Vaccine and Treatment Options," press release, April 17, 2020, https://www.nih.gov/news-events/news-releases/nih-launch-public-private-partnership-speed- covid-19-vaccine-treatment-options.

BARDA supports MCM development through funding, technical assistance, and other core services. Funding support includes contracts with product developers (e.g., pharmaceutical and biotechnology companies) for advanced development, including preclinical and clinical testing and manufacturing scale-up. COVID-19-related supplemental appropriations have increased the number of promising vaccine and therapeutic candidates that BARDA can support. Prior to the COVID-19 pandemic, BARDA used its OT authority to form partnerships with several companies to develop MCMs against threats such as pandemic influenza and Ebola.[24] In February, BARDA used the OT authority flexibility to redirect these efforts to speed the development of COVID-19 countermeasures.[25] BARDA's core services program can provide technical and regulatory assistance for countermeasure developers. These services include the Centers for Innovation in Advanced Development and Manufacturing, which is a public-private partnership that provides infrastructure for domestic production of MCMs; the Fill Finish Manufacturing Network, which assists MCM developers with final drug product manufacturing (e.g., vial filling); and the Clinical Studies Network which provides clinical study services from designing clinical protocols to managing clinical trial sites.[26]

---

[24] Department of Health and Human Services (HHS), "HHS, Janssen Research & Development join forces on innovative influenza products," press release, September 15, 2017, https://www.phe.gov/Preparedness/news/Pages/ janssen-flu.aspx.

[25] The Biomedical Advanced Research and Development Authority (BARDA), "HHS, Regeneron Collaborate to Develop 2019-nCoV Treatment," press release, February 4, 2020, https://www.hhs.gov/about/news/2020/02/04/hhs- regeneron-collaborate-to-develop-2019-ncov-treatment.html; and BARDA, "HHS, Janssen Collaborate To Develop Coronavirus Therapeutics," press release, February 18, 2020, https://www.hhs.gov/about/news/2020/02/18/hhs-janssen-collaborate-to-develop-coronavirus-therapeutics.html.

26 HHS Public Health Emergency, "Core Services," accessed June 23, 2020, https://www.medicalcountermeasures.gov/ barda/core-services.aspx. See also, "Department of Health and Human Services' Centers for Innovation in Advanced Development and Manufacturing," https://www.medicalcountermeasures.gov/barda/core-services/ciadm/.

What Is Operation Warp Speed and How Does It Differ from Typical R&D?

Operation Warp Speed is a new national program to "accelerate the development, manufacturing, and distribution of COVID-19 vaccines, therapeutics, and diagnostics."[27] The program is intended to coordinate MCM efforts "between components of HHS, including CDC, FDA, NIH, and BARDA; the Department of Defense; private firms; and other federal agencies." Its stated goal is to accelerate selected MCM testing while developing manufacturing infrastructure to allow mass distribution faster than would be possible otherwise (see *Figure 1*). Not all government-supported countermeasures will participate in Operation Warp Speed.

Aside from Operation Warp Speed, How Is the Federal Government Supporting the Development of MCMs for COVID-19?

BARDA has used supplemental appropriations to support preclinical and clinical testing of more than 20 diagnostic, vaccine, and therapeutic candidates.[28] In addition, BARDA created the CoronaWatch portal to serve as a single point of entry that enables potential medical countermeasure developers to connect with the most appropriate potential federal funding source.[29]

NIH is supporting both extramural and intramural research related to COVID-19 and the development of MCMs. NIH, particularly NIAID, has issued several funding opportunity announcements for emergency research funding related to COVID-19, including for the development of new diagnostic tests, therapeutic candidates, and vaccine candidates. NIH

---

[27] HHS, "Trump Administration Announces Framework and Leadership for 'Operation Warp Speed,'" press release, May 15, 2020, https://www.hhs.gov/about/news/2020/05/15/trump-administration-announces-framework-and- leadership-for-operation-warp-speed.html.

[28] HHS Public Health Emergency, https://www.medicalcountermeasures.gov/newsroom/.

[29] HHS Public Health Emergency, "Request a USG CoronaWatch Meeting," https://www.medicalcountermeasures.gov/Request-BARDA-TechWatch-Meeting/.

supports basic scientific research on the virus and disease that will help inform the development of new products.[30] NIH can support both basic and laboratory research, as well as clinical research with humans, such as for clinical testing of new MCMs.

NIH has announced two major research initiatives related to COVID-19. Announced on April 17, 2020, Accelerating COVID-19 Therapeutic Interventions and Vaccines (ACTIV) is a public- private partnership with several companies and federal agencies that aims to accelerate research and development on new vaccines and therapeutics by prioritizing vaccine and drug candidates, streamlining clinical trials, coordinating regulatory processes, and leveraging the assets of partners for new products.[31] The Rapid Acceleration of Diagnostics (RADx) initiative announced on April 29 is a prize competition that aims to incentivize the development of new diagnostics for COVID-19.[32]

DOD has reported research efforts into new vaccines and treatments that complement those of NIH and BARDA.[33]

FDA is working with MCM developers to provide regulatory advice and technical assistance with respect to development programs and testing.[34]

---

[30] NIH, "Notice of Special Interest (NOSI) regarding the Availability of Emergency Competitive Revisions for Research on Severe Acute Respiratory Syndrome Coronavirus 2 (SARS-CoV-2) and Coronavirus Disease 2019 (COVID-19)," March 25, 2020, https://grants.nih.gov/grants/guide/notice-files/NOT-AI-20-034.html.

[31] NIH, "NIH to Launch Public-Private Partnership to Speed COVID-19 Vaccine and Treatment Options," press release, April 17, 2020, https://www.nih.gov/news-events/news-releases/nih-launch-public-private-partnership-speed- covid-19-vaccine-treatment-options.

[32] NIH, "NIH Mobilizes National Innovation Initiative for COVID-19 Diagnostics," press release, April 29, 2020, https://www.nih.gov/news-events/news-releases/nih-mobilizes-national-innovation-initiative-covid-19-diagnostics.

[33] Department of Defense (DOD), "Defense Department Press Briefing Investigating and Developing Vaccine Candidates Against COVID-19," March 5, 2020, https://www.defense.gov/Newsroom/Transcripts/Transcript/Article/2104736/defense-department-press-briefing-investigating-and-developing-vaccine-candidat/.

[34] FDA, "MCM Regulatory Science," https://www.fda.gov/emergency-preparedness-and-response/medical-countermeasures-initiative-mcmi/mcm-regulatory-science. FDA, "Coronavirus Treatment Acceleration Program (CTAP)," https://www.fda.gov/drugs/coronavirus-covid-19-drugs/coronavirus-treatment-acceleration-program-ctap.

What Is the State of MCM Development in the COVID-19 Response?

Currently, no FDA-approved MCMs are available to treat COVID-19. Federal agencies, pharmaceutical and biotech companies, nongovernmental organizations, and global regulators have been working to develop MCMs for COVID-19. Examples of such efforts are provided below.

Therapeutics

Researchers have initiated studies examining unapproved drug candidates, as well as unapproved uses of already approved drugs. NIH has issued COVID-19 treatment guidelines, which identify several therapeutic options currently under investigation,[35] and the federal clinical trials database maintained by the National Library of Medicine at NIH lists more than 1,000 clinical trials for COVID-19.

With respect to already approved drugs, on March 28, 2020, FDA issued the first emergency use authorization (EUA) for a COVID-19 therapeutic, authorizing the emergency use of hydroxychloroquine and chloroquine, two FDA-approved anti-malarial drugs. The EUA specifically authorized the use of hydroxychloroquine and chloroquine donated to the SNS by drug manufacturers and distributed to states to treat patients hospitalized with COVID-19 for whom a clinical trial is not available or participation is not feasible.[36] According to the EUA letter that has since been revoked, FDA determined that based on the totality of scientific evidence, it was reasonable to believe that these drugs may be effective in treating COVID-19, and that when used in accordance with the conditions of the EUA, the known and potential benefits outweigh the known and potential risks. Some stakeholders—including several former FDA officials— expressed concern regarding the EUA, stating that the available data on the safety and effectiveness of these drugs for treatment of COVID-19 was largely anecdotal and that expanding access may

---

[35] NIH, "COVID-19 Treatment Guidelines," accessed June 17, 2020, https://covid19 treatmentguidelines.nih.gov/ therapeutic-options-under-investigation/.

[36] FDA, Letter of Authorization, March 28, 2020, https://www.fda.gov/media/136534/download.

jeopardize research into the drugs.[37] On April 24, 2020, FDA issued a drug safety communication warning against the use of these drugs for treatment of COVID-19 outside of the hospital setting or a clinical trial due to risk of heart rhythm problems.[38] On June 15, 2020, FDA revoked its EUA, determining that the statutory standard for EUA issuance was no longer met.[39] More specifically, FDA determined that based on emerging scientific data, hydroxychloroquine and chloroquine are unlikely to be effective in treating COVID-19, and that in light of serious cardiac adverse events and other potential serious side effects, the known and potential benefits of the drugs no longer outweigh the known and potential risks for this use. NIH updated its treatment guidelines to recommend against the use of hydroxychloroquine and chloroquine for the treatment of COVID-19, except in a clinical trial.[40]

Researchers are investigating the potential of other approved drugs. For example, the Randomised Evaluation of COVID-19 Therapy (RECOVERY) trial at the University of Oxford in the United Kingdom is evaluating a range of potential treatments, including the HIV drug lopinavir-ritonavir, the steroid dexamethasone, and the antibiotic azithromycin.[41] Early results reported from the trial found that low-dose dexamethasone reduced deaths by one-third in ventilated patients with COVID-19.[42] Domestically, FDA has partnered with the Critical Path

---

[37] C. Piller, "Former FDA leaders decry emergency authorization of malaria drugs for coronavirus," Science, April 7, 2020, https://www.sciencemag.org/news/2020/04/former-fda-leaders-decry-emergency-authorization-malaria-drugs- coronavirus.

[38] FDA, "FDA cautions against use of hydroxychloroquine or chloroquine for COVID-19 outside of the hospital setting or a clinical trial due to risk of heart rhythm problems," April 24, 2020, https://www.fda.gov/drugs/drug-safety-and- availability/fda-cautions-against-use-hydroxychloroquine-or-chloroquine-covid-19-outside-hospital-setting-or.

[39] FDA, "Coronavirus (COVID-19) Update: FDA Revokes Emergency Use Authorization for Chloroquine and Hydroxychloroquine," June 15, 2020, https://www.fda.gov/news-events/press-announcements/coronavirus-covid-19-update-fda-revokes-emergency-use-authorization-chloroquine-and.

[40] NIH, "COVID-19 Treatment Guidelines," as updated June 16, 2020, https://www.covid 19treatmentguidelines.nih.gov/whats-new/.

[41] RECOVERY, Randomised Evaluation of COVID-19 Therapy, accessed June 17, 2020, https://www.recoverytrial.net/.

[42] University of Oxford, "Dexamethasone reduces death in hospitalised patients with severe respiratory complications of COVID-19," June 16, 2020, http://www.ox.ac.uk/news/2020-06-16-dexamethasone-reduces-death-hospitalised-patients-severe-respiratory-complicati ons.

Institute (C-Path) and NIH's National Center for Advancing Translational Sciences (NCATS) on the CURE Drug Repurposing Collaboratory (CDRC), which includes a COVID-19 pilot project.[43] The CDRC aims to capture real-world clinical outcome data (e.g., data on off-label use captured by electronic medical records) to advance drug repurposing and inform future clinical trials for diseases of unmet medical need.

With respect to unapproved drug candidates, some therapeutics are further along in clinical testing (e.g., Gilead's antiviral drug remdesivir) than others. Gilead initiated two Phase 3 clinical studies evaluating the safety and effectiveness of its experimental drug in adults diagnosed with COVID-19.[44] In addition, on February 21, 2020, NIAID launched a randomized, double-blind, placebo-controlled trial of remdesivir as a potential treatment for hospitalized adult patients diagnosed with COVID-19.[45] NIH reported early results on April 29, 2020, finding that based on a preliminary analysis of the trial data, hospitalized patients with severe COVID-19 who received remdesivir recovered faster than similar patients who received placebo.[46] Other clinical studies of remdesivir are being carried out internationally. On the basis of data from the NIAID trial (NCT04280705) and a Gilead-sponsored Phase 3 trial (NCT04292899), on May 1, 2020, FDA granted EUA for remdesivir, determining that it is reasonable to believe that the known and potential benefits of the drug outweigh the known and potential risks for treatment of patients hospitalized with severe COVID-19.[47]

Two investigational blood-derived therapies also are being studied for the treatment of COVID- 19: convalescent plasma and hyperimmune

---

[43] FDA, "Coronavirus (COVID-19) Update: Daily Roundup," news release, June 23, 2020, https://www.fda.gov/news-events/press-announcements/coronavirus-covid-19-update-daily-roundup-june-23-2020. See also, Critical Path Institute, CURE Drug Repurposing Collaboratory, https://c-path.org/programs/cdrc/.

[44] Gilead, Remdesivir Clinical Trials, NCT04292730 and NCT04292899, https://www.gilead.com/purpose/advancing-global-health/covid-19/remdesivir-clinical-trials.

[45] NLM, Clinicaltrials.gov, NCT04280705, accessed April 15, 2020, https://clinicaltrials.gov/ct2/show/NCT04280705.

[46] NIH, "NIH clinical trial shows Remdesivir accelerates recovery from advanced COVID-19," April 29, 2020, https://www.nih.gov/news-events/news-releases/nih-clinical-trial-shows-remdesivir-accelerates-recovery-advanced- covid-19.

[47] FDA, Letter of Authorization to Gilead Sciences, Inc., May 1, 2020, https://www.fda.gov/media/137564/download.

globulin.[48] *Convalescent plasma* refers to blood plasma collected from an individual who has recovered (i.e., "convalesced") from a disease, and thus presumably has developed antibodies against the virus that causes the disease—in this case SARS-CoV-2—that is then administered to a patient actively sick with COVID-19 for treatment. A related therapy is *hyperimmune globulin*, a manufactured biological product containing concentrated antibodies collected from convalescent plasma. Although convalescent plasma units vary in antibody specificities and levels based on the plasma donor, hyperimmune globulin preparations are typically standardized.[49] FDA has announced the availability of an expanded access protocol for convalescent plasma for patients across the United States—limited to those with severe or life-threatening COVID-19, or those judged by the treating provider to be at high risk of progression to severe or life-threatening disease.[50] More than 2,000 sites and over 8,000 physicians have signed on to participate in the expanded access protocol, with the Mayo Clinic acting as the Institutional Review Board (IRB).[51] Plasma transfusions are generally safe; however, they are not without risk and can cause allergic reactions and other side effects in some patients. Data are limited regarding the safety and effectiveness of convalescent plasma in treating COVID-19, but anecdotal evidence suggests the treatment may be safe and effective for some patients.[52]

---

[48] FDA, "Coronavirus (COVID-19) Update: FDA Coordinates National Effort to Develop Blood-Related Therapies for COVID-19," April 3, 2020, https://www.fda.gov/news-events/press-announcements/coronavirus-covid-19-update-fda-coordinates-national-effort-develop-blood-related-therapies-covid-19. FDA, "Investigational COVID-19 Convalescent Plasma," April 2020, updated May 1, 2020, https://www.fda.gov/media/136798/download.

[49] J. D. Roback and J. Guarner, "Convalescent Plasma to Treat COVID-19 Possibilities and Challenges," *JAMA* (March 27, 2020).

[50] Ibid.

[51] FDA, "Coronavirus (COVID-19) Update: FDA Encourages Recovered Patients to Donate Plasma for Development of Blood-Related Therapies," April 16, 2020, https://www.fda.gov/news-events/press-announcements/coronavirus-covid-19-update-fda-encourages-recovered-patients-donate-plasma-development-blood.

[52] FDA, "Investigational COVID-19 Convalescent Plasma - Emergency INDs Frequently Asked Questions," April 3, 2020, https://www.fda.gov/media/136470/download. JD Roback and J Guarner, "Convalescent Plasma to Treat COVID-19 Possibilities and Challenges," *JAMA* (March 27, 2020). A Joseph, "Everything we know about coronavirus immunity and antibodies—and plenty we still don't," *STAT News*, April 20, 2020, https://www.statnews.com/2020/04/20/everything-we-know-about-coronavirus-immunity-and-

The antibody-based therapies mentioned above have many different antibodies in them, only some of which might be effective against COVID-19. At least 50 companies and academic laboratories are trying to identify and isolate antibodies that specifically bind parts of the coronavirus and stop the infection process.[53] Once isolated, these monoclonal antibodies can be mass produced. This approach has led to successful treatments for diseases as diverse as cancer and Ebola. Some groups are also testing whether monoclonal antibodies can confer temporary immunity from COVID-19 infection so that they could be used prophylactically until the development of a safe and effective vaccine.

Vaccines

Researchers and product developers are testing numerous types of vaccines—both in the laboratory and in some early-stage testing in humans. As of June 12, 2020, at least 120 experimental vaccines are known to be in development around the world.[54] The experimental vaccines rely on different platforms, or technologies, that aim to induce an immune response to protect against COVID-19 virus infection. Some rely on technology that has traditionally been used in vaccines to date, such as inactivated viruses or preparations of proteins involved in the immune response.[55] Others involve novel approaches such as viral vectors, where an existing virus is weakened so it cannot cause disease and is genetically engineered to produce COVID-19 proteins—an approach used for the recently approved Ebola vaccine.[56]

---

antibodies-and-plenty-we-still-dont/. See also CRS Report R46375, *The U.S. Blood Supply and the COVID-19 Response: In Brief*, by Jared S. Sussman and Agata Dabrowska.

[53] Jon Cohen, "The Race is on for Antibodies that Stop the New Coronavirus," *Science,* May 5, 2020, https://www.sciencemag.org/news/2020/05/race-antibodies-stop-new-coronavirus.

[54] Jonathan Corum and Carl Zimmer, "Coronavirus Vaccine Tracker," *New York Times*, June 12, 2020, https://www.nytimes.com/interactive/2020/science/coronavirus-vac cine-tracker.html.

[55] Jon Cohen, "With Record-Setting Speed, Vaccinemakers Take Their First Shots at the New Coronavirus," *Science*, March 31, 2020, https://www.sciencemag.org/news/2020/03/record-setting-speed-vaccine-makers-take-their-first- shots-new-coronavirus; and Fatima Amanat and Florian Krammer, "SARS-CoV-2 Vaccines: Status Report," *Cell*, vol. 52 (April 14, 2020), pp. 583-589, https://www.cell.com/immunity/pdf/S1074-7613(20)30120-5.pdf.

[56] Ewen Callaway, "The Race for Coronavirus Vaccines: A Graphical Guide," *Nature*, April 28, 2020, https://www.nature.com/articles/d41586-020-01221-y.

Some of the proposed vaccine technologies have never been used before in FDA-licensed vaccines, such as the nucleic-acid based vaccines. For example, the NIAID-supported Moderna vaccine uses messenger RNA (mRNA) as a genetic platform to induce cells to produce a protein involved in the immune response against the virus.[57] The new mRNA and DNA-based vaccines build on epidemic preparedness efforts by DARPA[58] and groups such as the Coalition for Epidemic Preparedness (CEPI)[59] that have worked to develop flexible vaccine platforms that could be used to quickly develop a new vaccine in the event of an epidemic, regardless of the specific pathogen.[60] These vaccines have also built on efforts to develop vaccines for other coronaviruses such as SARS-CoV-1 and MERS-CoV.[61]

As of early June 2020, several vaccines are in various stages of clinical trials in several countries, including the United States, Germany, China, and the United Kingdom.[62] Several Phase 1 trials have been completed, with various vaccines moving onto Phase 2, Phase 3, or combined Phase 2/3 phases. Scientists and product developers are planning innovative clinical trial designs and coordination or harmonization of multiple trials with the goal of expediting the development process for COVID-19 vaccines, such as through the efforts by NIH's ACTIV program.[63] As a

---

[57] NIH, "NIH Clinical Trial of Investigational Vaccine for COVID-19 Begins," March 16, 2020, https://www.nih.gov/ news-events/news-releases/nih-clinical-trial-investigational-vaccine-covid-19-begins.

[58] Moderna, "DARPA Awards Moderna Therapeutics a Grant for up to $25 Million to Develop Messenger RNA Therapeutics™," press release, October 2, 2013, https://investors.modernatx.com/news-releases/news-release-details/darpa-awards-moderna-therapeutics-grant-25-million-develop.

[59] The Coalition for Epidemic Preparedness (CEPI) is a public-private global partnership that finances vaccine development for emerging infectious diseases. See https://cepi.net /about/whoweare/.

[60] Tung Thanh Le, Zacharias Andreadakis, and Arun Kumar, "The COVID-19 Vaccine Development Landscape," *Nature Reviews Drug Discovery*, April 9, 2020.

[61] NIH, "NIH Clinical Trial of Investigational Vaccine for COVID-19 Begins," press release, March 16, 2020, https://www.nih.gov/news-events/news-releases/nih-clinical-trial-investigational-vaccine-covid-19-begins.

[62] Jonathan Corum and Carl Zimmer, "Coronavirus Vaccine Tracker," *New York Times*, June 12, 2020, https://www.nytimes.com/interactive/2020/science/coronavirus-vaccine-tracker.html.

[63] Jocelyn Kaiser, "To Streamline Coronavirus Vaccine and Drug Efforts, NIH and Firms Join Forces," *Science*, April 17, 2020, https://www.sciencemag.org/news/2020/04/tame-testing-chaos-nih-and-firms-join-forces-streamline- coronavirus-vaccine-and-drug; and Lawrence Corey, John R. Mascola, and Anthony S. Fauci, et al., "A Strategic Approach to COVID-19

part of Operation Warp Speed, the Trump Administration has selected five companies with candidate vaccines for investment, and those companies have received more than $2 billion from the Administration.[64] Moving forward, a challenge for large-scale vaccine trials is the shifting geography of the pandemic. Locations affected by the virus are changing; therefore, planning a clinical trial in a given location is difficult.[65]

Vaccine development is usually a long, complex, and risky process—most existing vaccines took 10 to 30 years to go from the beginning of clinical trials to licensure. Most vaccines fail in preclinical and clinical trials; less than 1 in 15 vaccine candidates that enter Phase 2 clinical trials gain FDA licensure.[66] The claims that a COVID-19 vaccine will be available within one year would represent the fastest development time of any vaccine to date.[67] The Trump Administration has announced intentions to accelerate the development of AstraZeneca's vaccine, with the first doses available in October.[68] Some experts express skepticism that this timeline is feasible, given that many vaccines have faced unexpected challenges during development.[69] Other experts posit that a COVID-19 vaccine should be easier to develop than vaccines for other diseases, such as HIV and Hepatitis C, which have posed greater challenges in development in part because a respiratory virus may be easier to develop a

---

Vaccine R&D," *Science*, May 29, 2020, pp. 948-50, https://science.sciencemag.org/content/368/6494/948/tab-figures-data.

[64] Noah Weiland and David E. Sanger, "Trump Administration Selects Five Coronavirus Vaccine Candidates as Finalists," *The New York Times*, June 9, 2020, https://www.nytimes.com/2020/06/03/us/politics/coronavirus-vaccine- trump-moderna.html.

[65] Jon Cohen, "'It's Really Complicated.' United States and Others Wrestle with Putting COVID-19 Vaccines to the Test," *Science*, June 12, 2020.

[66] R. Gordon Douglas and Vijay B. Samant, "The Vaccine Industry," in *Plotkin's Vaccines*, 7th ed. (Elsevier, 2017), pp. 41-50.

[67] Tung Thanh Le, Zacharias Andreadakis, and Arun Kumar, "The COVID-19 Vaccine Development Landscape," *Nature Reviews Drug Discovery*, April 9, 2020.

[68] HHS, "Trump Administration's Operation Warp Speed Accelerates AstraZeneca COVID-19 Vaccine to be Available Beginning in October," press release, May 21, 2020, https://www.hhs.gov/about/news/2020/05/21/trump-administration-accelerates-astrazeneca-covid-19-vaccine-to-be-available-beginning-in-october.html.

[69] Holden and Thorp, "Underpromise, Overdeliver," *Science*, March 27, 2020, https://science.sciencemag.org/content/ 367/6485/1405; and Jon Cohen, "Doubts Greet $1.2 Billion Bet by United States on a Coronavirus Vaccine by October," *Science*, May 22, 2020, https://www.sciencemag.org/news/2020/05/doubts-greet-12-billion-bet-united-states-coronavirus-vaccine-october.

vaccine for than for blood-borne viruses.[70] Scientists continue to learn about the biology of COVID-19 and robust data on the efficacy of any vaccine candidate in protecting against COVID-19 is likely months away.[71]

Still unknown is whether vaccination or antibodies raised in response to infection with SARS- CoV-2 will confer immunity at all, and if so, to what extent. Current estimates for potential duration of immunity come from other coronaviruses, which suggest that immunity may wane after one or more years.[72] Despite anecdotal reports of reinfection with the virus, it is uncertain whether patients reporting reinfection may have simply never cleared the virus, despite negative diagnostic test results. The accuracy of results of diagnostic testing where the virus is at or close to the limit of detection is not robust. Additionally, positive test results after an initial resolution of symptoms may indicate the presence of inactive virus leftover from the original infection, rather than a new unique active infection.

Diagnostics

Generally, coronavirus diagnostics (in vitro diagnostics, or IVDs) may be molecular, serological, or antigen tests. Tests are characterized by their methods—molecular tests are based on nucleic acid amplification techniques—as well as by the substance they directly identify—antigens, antibodies, or viral nucleic acid. To date, development of COVID-19 tests has been largely focused on molecular tests—specifically on a test using Polymerase Chain Reaction (PCR)—and serology tests—those tests that identify the presence of antibodies to the SARS-CoV-2 virus. PCR is a

---

[70] Jon Cohen, "With Record-Setting Speed, Vaccinemakers Take Their First Shots at the New Coronavirus," *Science*, March 31, 2020, https://www.sciencemag.org/news/2020/03/record-setting-speed-vaccine-makers-take-their-first- shots-new-coronavirus.

[71] Jon Cohen, "'It's Really Complicated.' United States and Others Wrestle with Putting COVID-19 Vaccines to the Test," *Science*, June 12, 2020, https://www.sciencemag.org/news/2020/06/it-s-really-complicated-united-states-and-others-wrestle-putting-covid-19-vaccines-test.

[72] Daniel M. Altmann, Daniel C. Douek, and Rosemary J. Boyton, "What Policy Makers Need to Know About COVID-19 Protective Immunity," *The Lancet*, April 27, 2020, https://thelancet.com/journals/lancet/article/PIIS0140- 6736(20)30985-5/fulltext, and Fatima Amanat and Florian Krammer, "SARS-CoV-2 Vaccines: Status Report," *Cell*, vol. 52 (April 14, 2020), pp. 583-589, https://www.cell.com/immunity/pdf/S1074-7613(20)30120-5.pdf.

fairly time-intensive and expensive technique, and for this reason, other techniques have been employed and are being researched, including loop-mediated isothermal amplification (which, unlike PCR, does not require temperature cycling), CRISPR-based tests, and, most recently, next generation sequencing (NGS)-based tests. Loop-mediated isothermal amplification, for example, was used in diagnostics during the outbreak of SARS, and it was found to be faster, less expensive, and simpler than other molecular methods, while maintaining comparable sensitivity and specificity.[73] The FDA-EUA-authorized Abbott IDNow test uses this technique. Although the test has encountered some accuracy issues in its roll-out, and FDA now requires negative results to be considered to be presumptive negatives until they are confirmed using an authorized high sensitivity molecular test, the test is used at the point of care and helps with access issues in certain cases.[74]

CRISPR-based systems are typically used to edit genetic sequences, but they are also an effective tool for identifying a specific genetic sequence.[75] Such systems rely on a combination of (1) an enzyme that cuts DNA (a nuclease) and (2) a guiding piece of genetic material (guide RNA) to target a location in a genome for cleavage. Cleaving the genetic material releases a signal that is detectable by simple methods. Diagnostics using CRISPR can provide for "high sensitivity (can detect as few as 10 gene copies), specificity, portability, easy read-out (e.g., colorimetric with paper strips), speed (~ 45 min), and low cost (few dollars per sample)."[76] Researchers recently published details of a CRISPR-based test, the SARS-CoV-2 DETECTR test, clinical validation of which the authors report is

---

[73] The National Academies Press, "Rapid Expert Consultation on SARS-CoV-2 Laboratory Testing for the COVID-19 Pandemic," April 8, 2020 https://www.nap.edu/catalog/25775/rapid-expert-consultation-on-sars-cov-2-laboratory-testing-for-the-covid-19-pandemic-april-8-2020.

[74] FDA, "Abbott IDNow COVID-19 EUA Letter of Authorization," updated June 1, 2020, https://www.fda.gov/media/ 136522/download.

[75] See CRS Report R44824, *Advanced Gene Editing: CRISPR-Cas9*, by Marcy E. Gallo et al., for more information.

[76] The National Academies Press, "Rapid Expert Consultation on SARS-CoV-2 Laboratory Testing for the COVID-19 Pandemic," April 8, 2020 https://www.nap.edu/catalog/25775/rapid-expert-consultation-on-sars-cov-2-laboratory-testing-for-the-covid-19-pandemic-april-8-2020.

ongoing in response to FDA guidance for COVID-19 diagnostics.[77] In addition, FDA granted its first EUA for a CRISPR-based test in early May, for a test called Sherlock CRISPR SARS-CoV-2 Kit.[78] This test is for use only in clinical laboratories certified to perform high complexity testing per the Clinical Laboratory Improvement Amendments of 1988 (CLIA) regulations (not for use at the point of care),[79] returns results in one hour, and requires no specialized instruments.

Because CRISPR-based tests do not necessarily require specialized laboratory equipment and use inexpensive components in addition to leveraging a fast and portable read-out, they have the potential to be used as a point-of-care test.[80] Specifically, the DETECTR test "can be performed with portable heat blocks, readily available reagents, and disposable lateral flow strips."[81] In addition, this test uses different reagents than those used in PCR tests, and it might eventually be able to be used without RNA extraction, both of which might ease certain supply chain stressors. Finally, test manufacturers are developing tests that use next-generation sequencing techniques— also referred to as *massively parallel sequencing*—that are both highly accurate and may be used to monitor changes in the virus's genetic code over time, because they sequence the partial or complete viral genome as part of the testing. FDA recently authorized the first COVID-19 diagnostic that uses next-generation sequencing technology.[82] In addition, this type of testing

---

[77] J. P. Broughton et al., "CRISPR–Cas12-based detection of SARS-CoV-2," *Nature Biotechnology*, April 16, 2020, https://www.nature.com/articles/s41587-020-0513-4.

[78] FDA, "Sherlock CRISPR SARS-Cov-2 Kit Letter of Authorization," May 6, 2020, https://www.fda.gov/media/137747/download.

[79] Point-of-care testing may be defined as follows, "Point-of-care testing means that results are delivered to patients in the patient care settings, like hospitals, urgent care centers and emergency rooms, instead of samples being sent to a laboratory." See https://www.fda.gov/news-events/press-announcements/coronavirus-covid-19-update-fda-issues-first-emergency-use-authorization-point-care-diagnostic.

[80] Science Magazine, "CRISPR Gene Editing May Help Scale Up Coronavirus Testing," April 23, 2020, https://www.scientificamerican.com/article/crispr-gene-editing-may-help-scale-up-coronavirus-testing/.

[81] 360dx.com, "UCSF, Mammoth Bio Develop Rapid Coronavirus Diagnostic Using CRISPR-Cas12 Method," April 16, 2020, https://www.360dx.com/gene-silencinggene-editing/ucsf-mammoth-bio-develop-rapid-coronavirus- diagnostic-using-crispr-cas12#.XqiK4GhKg4k.

[82] FDA, "Coronavirus (COVID-19) Update: FDA Authorizes First Next Generation Sequence Test for Diagnosing COVID-19," https://www.fda.gov/news-events/press-announcements/

platform is being investigated as a way to support the high-volume testing capacity that many expect to be needed as employers and schools undertake large-scale screening initiatives.

In addition to research into different molecular techniques for carrying out testing, manufacturers and clinical laboratories are working to develop testing components and tests that may be used in decentralized settings, including near-patient settings, such as urgent care centers and emergency rooms, and in the home. In particular, FDA has authorized a kit for at-home specimen collection developed by EverlyWell[83] and has authorized modifications to existing EUAs to accommodate the use of at-home collection kits. For example, LabCorp developed a home sample collection kit, and FDA reissued the EUA for LabCorp's PCR test to allow for use of samples self-collected by patients at home.[84] In addition, the use of different sample types is also under investigation— specifically saliva, which would offer benefits including ease of sample collection and a reduction in supply shortages (e.g., a shortage of swabs used by current tests to collect samples from the nose and throat). FDA has authorized a Rutgers University PCR-based laboratory-developed test (LDT) to permit testing of saliva samples self-collected by patients at home.[85] FDA has not granted EUA to any complete at-home tests, but many are under development, and the agency has stated that it expects to authorize this type of test in the future.[86]

---

coronavirus-covid-19-update-fda-authorizes-first-next-generation-sequence-test-diagnosing-covid-19.

[83] FDA, "Everlywell COVID-19 Test Home Collection Kit Letter of Authorization," May 15, 2020, https://www.fda.gov/media/138144/download.

[84] FDA, "Coronavirus (COVID-19) Update: FDA Authorizes First Test for Patient At-Home Sample Collection," https://www.fda.gov/news-events/press-announcements/coronavirus-covid-19-update-fda-authorizes-first-test-patient- home-sample-collection.

[85] FDA, "Coronavirus (COVID-19) Update: FDA Authorizes First Diagnostic Test Using At-Home Collection of Saliva Specimens," https://www.fda.gov/news-events/press-announcements/coronavirus-covid-19-update-fda-authorizes-first-diagnostic-test-using-home-collection-saliva.

[86] FDA, "FAQs on Diagnostic Testing for SARS-CoV-2," https://www.fda.gov/medical-devices/emergency-situations- medical-devices/faqs-diagnostic-testing-sars-cov-2.

REGULATION AND APPROVAL

How Are MCMs Regulated?

FDA—under the Federal Food, Drug, and Cosmetic Act (FFDCA) and the PHSA—regulates the safety and effectiveness of MCMs domestically. The statutory and regulatory requirements governing MCMs vary depending on whether a product meets the definition of a drug, biologic, or medical device.

Drugs and Biologics

Drugs are "articles intended for use in the diagnosis, cure, mitigation, treatment, or prevention of disease"[87] and generally include biologics such as monoclonal antibodies and vaccines.[88] While drugs are typically chemically synthesized, small molecule compounds with well-defined structures, biologics are relatively large and complex molecules derived from living organisms or made in living systems. An MCM that meets the definition of a drug, including a biologic, must receive approval or licensure from FDA prior to marketing.[89] Except under limited circumstances, to support approval or licensure, FDA requires a sponsor (typically the drug manufacturer) to submit data from clinical trials—formally designed, conducted, and analyzed studies in which the investigational drug or biologic is administered to human subjects to provide evidence of a drug's safety and effectiveness, or in the case of a biologic, safety, purity, and potency.[90] The requirements regarding approval

---

[87] FFDCA §201(g)(1) [21 U.S.C. §321(g)(1)].

[88] PHSA §351(i)(1) [21 U.S.C. §262(i)(1)] defines a biologic as "a virus, therapeutic serum, toxin, antitoxin, vaccine, blood, blood component or derivative, allergenic product, protein, or analogous product, or arsphenamine or derivative of arsphenamine (or any other trivalent organic arsenic compound), applicable to the prevention, treatment, or cure of a disease or condition of human beings." For additional information, see CRS Report R44620, *Biologics and Biosimilars: Background and Key Issues*, by Agata Dabrowska.

[89] FFDCA §505(a) [21 U.S.C. §355(a)]; PHSA §351(a) [42 U.S.C. §262(a)].

[90] PHSA 351(a)(2)(C) [42 U.S.C. §262(a)(2)(C)]. While FDA approves drugs that are *safe and effective*, the equivalent terminology for biologics is *safe, pure, and potent*. In an April 2015 FDA guidance document, *Scientific Considerations in Demonstrating Biosimilarity to a Reference Product*, the agency states that the standard for licensure of a biologic as potent

and submission of clinical trial data generally apply regardless of whether the drug is a new molecular entity (i.e., contains a new active ingredient not previously approved by FDA) or whether the drug has been approved by FDA for one use and is to be repurposed for a new use.

Before beginning clinical testing, a sponsor must file with FDA an investigational new drug application (IND), which is a request for permission to administer an investigational drug or biologic to humans prior to approval or licensure.[91] An IND must include information about the investigational drug or biologic and its chemistry, manufacturing, and controls; the proposed clinical study design; completed animal test data; and the lead investigator's qualifications, among other things.[92] The investigator also must provide assurance that an Institutional Review Board (IRB) will provide initial and continuous review and approval of each of the studies in the clinical investigation to ensure that participants are aware of the drug's investigative status and that any risk of harm will be necessary, explained, and minimized.[93] FDA has 30 days to review an IND, after which a manufacturer may begin clinical testing if FDA has not objected and imposed a clinical hold. Clinical trials are typically conducted in three phases. Phase 1 clinical trials assess safety—and for biologics, safety and immunogenicity[94]—in a small number of volunteers. Phase 2 trials assess dosing and side effects and may enroll hundreds of volunteers. Phase 3 trials assess effectiveness and continue to monitor safety and typically enroll hundreds to thousands of volunteers.[95]

---

has long been interpreted to include effectiveness (under 21 C.F.R. §600.3(s)). In guidance, FDA often uses the terms *safety and effectiveness* and *safety, purity, and potency* interchangeably.

[91] FFDCA §505(i) [21 U.S.C. §355(i)]; PHSA §351(a)(3) [21 U.S.C. §262(a)(3)]. 21 C.F.R. Part 312.

[92] 21 C.F.R. §312.23.

[93] 21 C.F.R. §312.23(a)(1)(iv) and 21 C.F.R. Part 56.

[94] *Immunogenicity* refers to an immune response to a therapeutic that may have the potential to affect product safety and effectiveness. One FDA guidance document specifically defines immunogenicity (for the purpose of the guidance) as "the propensity of a therapeutic protein product to generate immune responses to itself and to related proteins or to induce immunologically related adverse clinical events." See *Immunogenicity Assessment for Therapeutic Protein Products*, August 2014, https://www.fda.gov/media/85017/download.

[95] FDA, "Vaccine Product Approval Process," https://www.fda.gov/vaccines-blood-biologics/development-approval- process-cber/vaccine-product-approval-process.

Once a sponsor completes clinical trials, it submits the results of those investigations, along with other information, to FDA in a new drug application (NDA) or a biologics license application (BLA).[96] While drugs are approved via an NDA under the FFDCA, biologics—including vaccines—are licensed for marketing via a BLA under the PHSA. The requirements and review pathways for NDAs and BLAs are generally similar, and biologics are subject to various FFDCA provisions. In reviewing an NDA or BLA, FDA considers whether the drug is safe and effective—or whether the biologic is safe, pure, and potent—for its *intended use*; whether the proposed labeling is appropriate; and whether the methods and controls used to manufacture the product are adequate to preserve its identity, strength, quality, and purity.[97]

Diagnostics

In vitro diagnostic devices (IVDs) are devices used in the laboratory analysis of human samples. IVDs include commercial test kits, laboratory-developed tests (LDTs), and instruments used in testing, among other things. LDTs are a class of IVD that is designed, manufactured, and used within a single laboratory. LDTs are often used to test for conditions or diseases that are either rapidly changing (e.g., new strains of known infectious diseases) or that are the subject of rapidly advancing scientific research (e.g., genomic testing for cancer).[98] Traditionally, LDTs have been regulated by FDA differently than commercial test kits. IVDs may be used in a variety of settings, including a clinical laboratory, a physician's office, or in the home. IVDs used in the clinical management of patients fall under the definition of medical "device" in the FFDCA[99] and therefore

---

[96] FFDCA §505(b) [21 U.S.C. §355(b)] and 21 C.F.R. §314.50.

[97] For additional information, see CRS Report R41983, *How FDA Approves Drugs and Regulates Their Safety and Effectiveness*, by Agata Dabrowska and Susan Thaul.

[98] For more information, see CRS In Focus IF11389, *FDA Regulation of Laboratory-Developed Tests (LDTs)*, by Amanda K. Sarata.

[99] The term "device" is statutorily defined as "an instrument, apparatus, implement, machine, contrivance, implant, *in vitro reagent*, or other similar or related article, including any component, part, or accessory" (emphasis added) that is "intended for use in the diagnosis of disease or other conditions, or in the cure, mitigation, treatment, or prevention of disease, in man or other animals, or is intended to affect the structure or any function of the body of man or other animals." FFDCA §201(h); 21 U.S.C. §321.

are subject to regulation by FDA. As with other medical devices, the application of FDA regulatory requirements to IVDs depends on the IVD's risk classification according to its intended use.

Medical devices are grouped into three classes: Class I (low risk, generally no premarket review required); Class II (usually requires premarket notification and may require special controls, such as specific labelling); and Class III (usually requires premarket approval prior to marketing).

Generally, Class II devices require 510(k) clearance demonstrating that a device is substantially equivalent to a device already on the market (i.e., a predicate device). A 510(k) application typically does not require submission of clinical data. Generally, Class III devices require a premarket approval application (PMA), with some exceptions. FDA issues an approval order when a PMA demonstrates reasonable assurance that a device is safe and effective for its intended use(s). Effectiveness must be based on well-controlled investigations, which generally means clinical trial data. Unless specifically excluded by regulation, all devices must meet general controls, which include premarket and postmarket requirements; for example, registration, labeling, and compliance with current good manufacturing practices (CGMPs) as set forth in FDA's quality system regulations (QSRs).[100]

IVDs are defined in regulation as a specific subset of medical devices that include "reagents, instruments, and systems intended for use in the diagnosis of disease or other conditions ... in order to cure, mitigate, treat, or prevent disease ... [s]uch products are intended for use in the collection, preparation, and examination of specimens taken from the human body."[101] As indicated by this definition, an IVD may be either a complete test or a component of a test. In either case, an IVD comes under FDA's regulatory purview. Regulated test components include both non-diagnostic ingredients, called general purpose reagents (GPRs), and the active ingredient(s) in a diagnostic test, referred to as the analyte specific reagent

---

[100] For more information, see CRS In Focus IF11083, *Medical Product Regulation: Drugs, Biologics, and Devices*, by Agata Dabrowska and Victoria R. Green.

[101] 21 C.F.R. §809.3(a); Definitions.

(ASR). LDTs, as opposed to commercially manufactured and distributed test kits, have traditionally been exempt from FDA's premarket review requirements.

In some limited cases, IVDs may fall under the statutory definition of a biological product. In those cases, the IVD would be subject to the requirements of the PHSA for the licensure of biological products.[102] Such IVDs include, for example, blood donor screening tests for infectious agents (HIV, hepatitis B and C).

What FDA Pathways Are Available to Expedite Availability of MCMs?

Because clinical testing and the FDA review process typically take several years, FDA and Congress have established mechanisms to (1) expedite the premarket development and review processes for new products coming onto the market, and (2) expand access to products that are still under investigation.[103] As used in this section, the term *drugs* generally includes biologics, unless noted otherwise.

Expedited Development and Review Programs for MCMs

FDA uses several formal mechanisms to expedite the development and review processes for drugs that address unmet medical need in the treatment of a serious or life-threatening condition. These four programs are fast track product designation, breakthrough therapy designation, accelerated approval, and priority review.[104] An already approved drug being studied for a new use (e.g., a drug approved for the treatment of HIV being studied for COVID-19) may be eligible for one of these expedited programs provided the applicable statutory criteria are met, and drugs may be designated to more than one program. Separately, there is a breakthrough device designation for medical devices.

---

[102] PHSA §351 [42 U.S.C. §262]; Regulation of Biological Products.

[103] CRS In Focus IF11379, Medical Product Innovation and Regulation: Benefits and Risks.

[104] FFDCA §506 [21 U.S.C. §356]. FDA, "Guidance for Industry Expedited Programs for Serious Conditions – Drugs and Biologics," May 2014, https://www.fda.gov/media/86377/download.

Breakthrough therapy and fast track product designation are both intended to streamline the drug development process, but the qualifying criteria and features of these programs differ. To qualify for *fast track product designation*, a drug must be intended to treat a serious condition and nonclinical or clinical data must demonstrate the drug's potential to address an unmet medical need.[105] A drug (but not a biologic) also may qualify for fast track if it has been designated as a qualified infectious disease product (QIDP).[106] The sponsor of a fast track-designated drug is eligible for frequent interactions with the FDA review team, priority review, and rolling review (i.e., FDA reviews portions of an NDA or BLA before a complete application is submitted).[107] To qualify for *breakthrough designation*, a drug must be intended to treat a serious condition, and preliminary clinical evidence must indicate that the drug may demonstrate substantial improvement on a clinically significant endpoint(s) over available therapies. Features of breakthrough therapy designation include rolling review; intensive FDA guidance on designing an efficient drug development program; involvement of "senior managers and experienced review and regulatory health project management staff in a proactive, collaborative, cross-disciplinary review" to expedite the development and review of a breakthrough therapy; and eligibility for other expedited programs. An interested sponsor must submit to FDA a request for fast track product or breakthrough therapy designation; a request may be submitted either with the IND or any time after,[108] as further specified in FDA guidance.[109]

The *accelerated approval* pathway allows a drug to be approved based on its effect on a surrogate endpoint (e.g., a laboratory measurement) that predicts the effectiveness of a new treatment, or on a clinical endpoint that can be measured earlier than irreversible morbidity or mortality.

---

[105] FFDCA §506(b) [21 U.S.C. §356(b)].

[106] A qualified infectious disease product (QIDP) is an antibacterial or antifungal drug for human use that is intended to treat serious or life-threatening infections. FFDCA §505E(g) [21 U.S.C. §355E(g)].

[107] FFDCA §506(a) [21 U.S.C. §356(a)].

[108] FFDCA §506(a)(2) & (b)(2) [21 U.S.C. §356(a)(2) & (b)(2)].

[109] FDA, "Guidance for Industry Expedited Programs for Serious Conditions – Drugs and Biologics," May 2014, https://www.fda.gov/media/86377/download.

Postmarketing confirmatory studies generally must be completed to demonstrate actual effectiveness.[110] To qualify for accelerated approval, a drug must (1) treat a serious condition, (2) generally provide a meaningful advantage over available therapies, and (3) demonstrate an effect on an endpoint that is reasonably likely to predict clinical benefit.

A *priority review* designation means FDA's goal is to take action on an application within six months of its filing, in contrast to 10 months for standard review. An NDA or BLA may qualify for priority review designation if, for example, it is for a drug that treats a serious condition and that, if approved, would provide a significant improvement in safety or effectiveness. An NDA or BLA also may qualify for priority review if submitted with a priority review voucher[111] or if the drug (but not biologic) is designated as a QIDP.

The 21st Century Cures Act (P.L. 114-255) and the FDA Reauthorization Act of 2017 (P.L. 115- 52) established a new *breakthrough device* category allowing FDA to expedite development and prioritize review of devices that (1) provide more effective diagnosis or treatment of a life- threatening or irreversibly debilitating condition, and (2) represent breakthrough technologies for which no approved alternatives exist, offer significant advantages over existing alternatives, or are in the best interest of patients.[112] The Breakthrough Device Program, a voluntary program, expedites development, assessment, and review of breakthrough devices as they go through premarket approval, 510(k) clearance, or marketing authorization via the de novo classification process.

---

[110] FFDCA §506(c) [21 U.S.C. §356(c)].

[111] Currently, three priority review voucher programs are authorized in the FFDCA: (1) the tropical disease priority review program, (2) the rare pediatric disease priority review program, and (3) the material threat MCM priority review voucher program. Under each of these programs, the sponsor of an NDA or BLA that meets the statutory requirements of the specific program is eligible to receive, upon approval, a transferable voucher, and the sponsor may either use that voucher for the priority review of another application or sell it to another sponsor to use.

[112] FFDCA §515B [21 U.S.C. §360e-3].

Enabling Access to Investigational MCMs

In general, a drug, biologic, or medical device may be provided to patients only if FDA has approved, licensed, or cleared its marketing application or authorized its use in a clinical trial under an IND or Investigational Device Exemption (IDE). In certain circumstances, however, patients may access investigational MCMs outside this framework through expanded access (i.e., compassionate use) programs and through emergency use authorization (EUA).

Expanded Access

Individuals who are not eligible for participation in a clinical trial (e.g., because they do not meet the study criteria, or because the trial is not enrolling new patients) may request, through their physician, access to an investigational product through an expanded access protocol,[113] provided that an IND or IDE is submitted to FDA and

- the physician determines (1) that the patient has no comparable or satisfactory alternative, and (2) that the probable risk from the investigational product is not greater than the probable risk from the disease or condition; and
- FDA determines (1) there is sufficient evidence of safety and effectiveness and (2) that provision of the investigational product will not interfere with "the initiation, conduct, or completion of clinical investigations to support marketing approval."[114]

A physician also may request an emergency IND (eIND) for an individual patient.[115] The provision of an investigational product in a clinical trial is intended to generate evidence of safety and effectiveness to support marketing approval. In contrast, expanded access protocols are not primarily intended to be used to obtain safety and effectiveness data; instead, they are intended to provide investigational therapies to patients

---

[113] FFDCA §561(b) [21 U.S.C. §360bbb(b)].
[114] FFDCA §561(b)(3) [21 U.S.C. §360bbb(b)(3)].
[115] 21 C.F.R. §312.310.

who have exhausted all other options.[116] FDA approves the majority of expanded access requests it receives.[117]

For FDA to grant permission, a manufacturer must have agreed to provide the investigational product. Manufacturers are not always willing to provide an investigational product outside of a clinical trial for various reasons, including supply constraints, liability concerns, and lack of clarity regarding how FDA may use adverse event or outcome data when considering approval in the future.

Due to perceived limitations with FDA's expanded access program, in 2018, the Right to Try (RTT) Act (P.L. 115-176) was enacted. The RTT Act created a pathway for eligible patients to access an eligible investigational drug (but not a device) without FDA's authorization. The manufacturer must still agree to provide the drug. An *eligible patient* is a patient who has (1) been diagnosed with a life-threatening disease or condition; (2) exhausted approved treatment options and is unable to participate in a clinical trial involving the eligible investigational drug; and (3) provided written informed consent to the treating physician regarding the eligible investigational drug.[118] An *eligible investigational drug* is an investigational drug that meets the following criteria: (1) a Phase 1 clinical trial has been completed; (2) the drug has not been approved or licensed by FDA for any use; (3) an NDA or BLA has been filed, or the drug is under investigation in a clinical trial, as specified; and (4) the active development or production of the drug is ongoing, and FDA has not placed a clinical hold on the trial.[119] FDA does not approve or review RTT Act requests and, with limited exceptions, FDA may not use a clinical outcome associated with the use of an eligible investigational drug to delay or adversely affect its review or approval.[120] Given interest in generating safety and effectiveness data and resource and supply constraints, the RTT pathway is

---

[116] FDA, Guidance for Industry, *Expanded Access to Investigational Drugs for Treatment Use - Questions and Answers*, p. 3, June 2016, https://www.fda.gov/media/85675/download.

[117] FDA, "Expanded Access (compassionate use) submission data," updated March 16, 2020, https://www.fda.gov/news-events/expanded-access/expanded-access-compassionate-use-submission-data.

[118] FFDCA §561B(a)(1) [21 U.S.C. §360bbb-0a(a)(1)].

[119] FFDCA §561B(a)(2) [21 U.S.C. §360bbb-0a(a)(2)].

[120] FFDCA §561B(c) [21 U.S.C. §360bbb-0a(c)].

unlikely to be used to provide access to COVID-19 investigational therapies.

Emergency Use Authorization (EUA)

FDA may enable access to unapproved MCMs by granting EUA, if the HHS Secretary declares that circumstances exist to justify the emergency use of an unapproved product or an unapproved use of an approved medical product.[121] This emergency declaration by the HHS Secretary is authorized under FFDCA Section 564, is distinct from the Public Health Emergency (PHE) declaration made pursuant to PHSA Section 319, and may be made in the absence of a PHE declaration made pursuant to PHSA Section 319.[122] The HHS Secretary's declaration must be based on one of four determinations; for example, a determination that there is an actual or significant potential for a public health emergency that affects or has significant potential to affect national security or the health and security of U.S. citizens living abroad.[123] Following the HHS Secretary's declaration, FDA, in consultation with ASPR, NIH, and CDC, may issue an EUA authorizing the emergency use of a specific drug, device, or biologic, provided that the following criteria are met:

- the agent that is the subject of the EUA can cause a serious or life-threatening disease or condition;
- based on the totality of the available scientific evidence, it is reasonable to believe that the product may be effective in diagnosing, treating, or preventing such disease or condition, and that the known and potential benefits of the product outweigh its known and potential risks; and

---

[121] FFDCA §564 [21 U.S.C. §360bbb-3]. For additional information, see CRS In Focus IF10745, *Emergency Use Authorization and FDA's Related Authorities*.

[122] For example, on August 5, 2014, the HHS Secretary declared, pursuant to FFDCA Section 564, that circumstances exist justifying the authorization of emergency use of in vitro diagnostics for detection of Ebola virus. The HHS Secretary's declaration was made in the absence of a PHE declaration under PHSA Section 319. Instead, the HHS Secretary's declaration was made on the basis of a determination by the Secretary of the Department of Homeland Security that the Ebola virus presents a material threat against the U.S. population sufficient to affect national security.

[123] FFDCA §564(b)(1) [21 U.S.C. §360bbb-3(b)(1)].

- there is no adequate, approved, or available alternative to the product.[124]

FDA must impose certain conditions as part of an EUA to the extent practicable (e.g., distributing certain information to health care providers and patients) and may impose additional discretionary conditions where appropriate.[125] FDA may waive or limit current good manufacturing practices (e.g., storage and handling) and prescription dispensing requirements for products authorized under EUA. FDA also may establish conditions on advertisements and other promotional printed matter that relates to the emergency use of a product. An EUA remains in effect for the duration of the emergency declaration made by the HHS Secretary under FFDCA Section 564, unless revoked at an earlier date.

On February 4, 2020, the HHS Secretary determined that there is a public health emergency that has a significant potential to affect national security or the health and security of U.S. citizens living abroad, and that involves COVID-2019.[126] On the basis of this determination, the HHS Secretary subsequently declared that circumstances exist justifying the authorization of emergency use of unapproved in vitro diagnostics for the detection and/or diagnosis of COVID- 19; personal respiratory protective devices; medical devices, including alternative products used as medical devices; and therapeutics. Pursuant to these declarations, FDA subsequently issued numerous EUAs authorizing the emergency use of specific diagnostics, drugs, and other medical devices during the COVID-19 outbreak.[127]

---

[124] FFDCA §564(c) [21 U.S.C. §360bbb-3(c)]. These criteria are explained in more detail in the FDA guidance *Emergency Use Authorization of Medical Products and Related Authorities*, January 2017, p. 7, https://www.fda.gov/ media/97321/download.

[125] FFDCA §564(e) [21 U.S.C. §360bbb-3(e)].

[126] 85 *Federal Register* 13907, publication date March 10, 2020, effective date February 4, 2020.

[127] FDA "Emergency Use Authorizations," accessed April 15, 2020, https://www.fda.gov/ medical-devices/emergency- situations-medical-devices/emergency-use-authorizations.

AVAILABILITY

How are MCMs in Development for COVID-19 Available to U.S. Patients?

In the absence of approved MCMs for COVID-19, patients can access investigational, unapproved MCMs in several ways, including through EUA, by participating in clinical trials, and through expanded access programs. In addition, FDA-approved drugs may be prescribed off- label (i.e., for unapproved uses) by physicians for treatment of COVID-19.

Emergency Use Authorization (EUA)

Patients hospitalized with severe COVID-19 may obtain access to products granted EUA. For therapeutics, as of the date of this chapter, remdesivir is the only drug subject to an EUA.[128] Hydroxychloroquine and chloroquine were subject to an EUA that has since been revoked by FDA. However, physicians may still prescribe these drugs off-label for individual patients. To date, FDA has not granted EUA to any COVID-19 vaccines. However, numerous clinical trials are underway, and some experts and industry members think that if a vaccine shows adequate results from the first trials, it may be made available to certain populations (such as health care workers) before clinical trials are completed via an EUA.[129]

Diagnostics are available for clinical use through authorized marketing pursuant to an EUA during the COVID-19 emergency. EUAs have been granted for more than 100 molecular diagnostics (both commercial test kits and LDTs), as well as for several serology tests and one antigen test.[130] The

[128] FDA, Letter of Authorization to Gilead Sciences, Inc., May 1, 2020, https://www.fda.gov/media/137564/download.

[129] Jon Cohen, "With Record-Setting Speed, Vaccinemakers Take Their First Shots at the New Coronavirus," *Science*, March 31, 2020, https://www.sciencemag.org/news/2020/03/record-setting-speed-vaccine-makers-take-their-first- shots-new-coronavirus.

[130] A COVID-19 serology test identifies antibodies to the SARS-CoV-2 virus, usually in an individual blood sample. Antibodies are proteins generated by the immune system in response to an antigen, or foreign substance. An antigen may be a pathogenic virus or bacteria, for example, or generally any substance that is recognized by the immune system as both foreign and harmful. An antigen test uses antibodies to a specific antigen (e.g.,

EUA tests include several that may be used at the point of care, including for example, the Abbott IDNow molecular test. In addition, Quidel's antigen test is authorized for use in point-of-care settings. Thus far, no serology test has been authorized for use in point-of-care settings. The vast majority of EUAs have been granted for tests that must be carried out in a centralized clinical laboratory environment (i.e., higher complexity tests).

Through guidance, FDA has taken steps to liberalize the EUA process to expand access to tests.[131] Specifically, the agency has allowed, in specified cases, tests to be marketed and clinically used prior to being granted EUA but after validation and notification to FDA. In addition, the FDA initially allowed serology tests to be made available and marketed without EUA. While these policies have improved access, they have also resulted in access to diagnostics with less robust performance characteristics in some cases.

Expanded Access

Patients may enroll in one of various clinical trials studying the safety and effectiveness of new drugs and vaccines for COVID-19. If participation in a clinical trial is not feasible—because the trial is not enrolling new subjects or because the patient does not meet criteria for enrollment— patients may be able to receive the experimental drug through an expanded access program. In the case of convalescent plasma, for example, patients may access the Mayo Clinic-led expanded access protocol, which has more than 2,000 sites and over 8,000 physician investigators participating.[132] The federal clinical trials database maintained by the National Library of Medicine at NIH lists several expanded access programs for COVID-19 treatments, and it is likely not an

---

SARS-CoV-2 virus) to identify the virus in a patient's sample. A COVD-19 serology test may determine prior infection, whereas an antigen test may determine an active infection, because the serology test identifies a product of the immune response whose generation lags infection, whereas the antigen test directly identifies the actual virus.

[131] See, generally, FDA, "Policy for Coronavirus Disease-2019 Tests During the Public Health Emergency (Revised)," May 11, 2020, https://www.fda.gov/media/135659/download.

[132] FDA, "Coronavirus (COVID-19) Update: FDA Encourages Recovered Patients to Donate Plasma for Development of Blood-Related Therapies," April 16, 2020, https://www.fda.gov/news-events/press-announcements/coronavirus- covid-19-update-fda-encourages-recovered-patients-donate-plasma-development-blood.

exhaustive list.[133] In cases where access to a clinical trial or the expanded access protocol is not available, a physician may request an eIND for an individual patient for a specific investigational drug.

POSTMARKET SURVEILLANCE

In light of efforts to expedite access to MCMs for COVID-19, questions have been raised about postmarket monitoring of adverse events and the continued collection of safety and effectiveness data. While premarket studies are designed to identify common safety risks associated with a drug or biologic, they may not identify all long-term or rare adverse events. As such, FDA may request that sponsors conduct additional studies once a drug or biologic is on the market to further provide information about its risks, benefits, and optimal use.[134] These studies may be particularly useful when one of the expedited pathways is used because it allows for the marketing and benefits of a product to be realized sooner, while at the same time allowing for a fuller safety and effectiveness profile to be developed. FDA also may require a sponsor to conduct a postapproval study or clinical trial to assess a known serious risk or in response to signals of serious risk related to use of the drug or biologic.[135]

FDA has several systems for monitoring medical product safety following approval or licensure. For example, drug and biologic manufacturers must report all serious and unexpected adverse events to the FDA Adverse Event Reporting System (FAERS) within 15 days of becoming aware of them, and they must report other adverse events in mandated periodic reports to the agency.[136] The reports are made publicly

---

[133] NLM, "Clinical Trials," accessed April 15, 2020, https://clinicaltrials.gov/ct2/results?cond=COVID-19&age_v=& gndr=&type=Expn&rslt=&Search=Apply.

[134] 21 C.F.R. §312.85. FFDCA §506(c)(2) [21 U.S.C. §356(c)(2)].

[135] PHSA §351(a)(2)(D) [42 U.S.C. §262(a)(2)(D)] and FFDCA §505(o)(3) [21 U.S.C. §355(o)(3)].

[136] 21 C.F.R. §314.80(c) and 21 C.F.R. §600.80(c). FDA Adverse Event Reporting System (FAERS) Public Dashboard, https://www.fda.gov/drugs/questions-and-answers-fdas-adverse-event-reporting-system-faers/fda-adverse-event-reporting-system-faers-public-

available through the FAERS public dashboard. For vaccines, adverse events must be reported to the Vaccine Adverse Event Reporting System (VAERS), which is co-sponsored by FDA and CDC. For medical devices, manufacturers must report device- related deaths, serious injuries, and malfunctions within 30 days of becoming aware of them; medical device reports (MDRs) are stored in the FDA's Manufacturer and User Facility Device Experience (MAUDE) database. Under typical circumstances, patients and health care providers are encouraged, but not required, to report adverse events to FDA through MedWatch.[137]

However, FDA may impose, as part of an EUA, conditions for monitoring and reporting adverse events associated with the emergency use of a product, including mandatory reporting by health care providers.[138] For example, the EUAs for hydroxychloroquine and chloroquine and for remdesivir require health care facilities and providers who administer the drugs to track and report any serious adverse events to FDA through MedWatch.[139] Similarly, EUAs for diagnostics require, as a condition of authorization, the manufacturer or laboratory granted the EUA to track adverse events (specifically false results) and report them to FDA. Adverse events also may be reported to the HHS Safety Reporting Portal (SRP), which is intended to streamline the process of reporting product safety issues to both FDA and NIH.[140]

FDA conducts active postmarket surveillance through its Sentinel System, which uses data obtained from electronic health records, patient registries, and other sources to provide information about the safety of a drug, medical device, vaccine, or biologic. FDA's Sentinel System is involved in several COVID-19-related activities, including "monitoring the use of drugs, describing the course of illness among hospitalized patients,

---

dashboard. Safety reporting is required during clinical testing and in expanded access programs (21 C.F.R. §312.32).

[137] FDA, "MedWatch: The FDA Safety Information and Adverse Event Reporting Program," https://www.fda.gov/ safety/medwatch-fda-safety-information-and-adverse-event-reporting-program.

[138] FFDCA §564(e).

[139] FDA, Letter of Authorization to Gilead Sciences, Inc., May 1, 2020, https://www.fda. gov/ media/137564/download. FDA, Letter of Authorization to BARDA, March 28, 2020, https://www.fda.gov/media/136534/download.

[140] HHS, The Safety Reporting Portal, https://www.safetyreporting.hhs.gov/SRP2/en/Home.aspx.

and evaluating the treatment impact of therapies actively being used under real-world conditions."[141] One component of Sentinel is the Post-Licensure Rapid Immunization Safety Monitoring (PRISM) program— established in 2009 as part of vaccine safety surveillance during the H1N1 influenza pandemic— which uses electronic health records from insurance providers and state immunization registries to monitor adverse events following vaccination.[142] FDA uses safety information and data generated from FAERS, VAERS, Sentinel, and other sources to inform regulatory action.

Ongoing surveillance and research may be particularly important when drugs or diagnostics are made available via EUA or expanded access, as the standard of evidence for authorizing early access to investigational products is different than that required for FDA clearance, approval, or licensure. EUA issuance, for example, is based on FDA's determination that the totality of the available scientific evidence suggests that a product may be effective in diagnosing, treating, or preventing a disease or condition and that the known and potential benefits of the product outweigh its known and potential risks. This determination is different from the standard required for FDA approval of a drug or biologic, which is based on *substantial evidence* of effectiveness derived from adequate and well-controlled studies.[143] Following issuance of the March 2020 EUA for hydroxychloroquine and chloroquine, and based on analysis of case reports in FAERS, the published medical literature, and poison control centers data, in April 2020, FDA published a Drug Safety Communication cautioning against use of these drugs outside the hospital or clinical trial setting due to risk of heart rhythm problems.[144] Data obtained by FDA

---

[141] Sentinel, FDA Sentinel System's Coronavirus (COVID-19) Activities, https://sentinelinitiative.org/drugs/fda- sentinel-system-coronavirus-covid-19-activities.

[142] PRISM is the vaccine component of FDA's Sentinel Initiative. The Sentinel system was implemented as an "Active Post-Market Risk Identification and Analysis program" under FFDCA §505(k)(3), as amended by §905 of the FDA Amendments Act, P.L. 110-85.

[143] FDA, "Understanding the Regulatory Terminology of Potential Preventions and Treatments for COVID-19," https://www.fda.gov/consumers/consumer-updates/understanding-regulatory-terminology-potential-preventions-and- treatments-covid-19.

[144] FDA, "FDA cautions against use of hydroxychloroquine or chloroquine for COVID-19 outside of the hospital setting or a clinical trial due to risk of heart rhythm problems," April 24, 2020, https://www.fda.gov/drugs/drug-safety- and-availability/fda-cautions-against-use-hydroxychloroquine-or-chloroquine-covid-19-outside-hospital-setting-or.

further led the agency to revoke the EUA in June 2020.[145] Diagnostic EUAs require manufacturers, laboratories, and authorized laboratories carrying out testing to "collect information on the performance of their product," and, more specifically, false positives, false negatives, and other deviations from a test's performance characteristics—all of which must be reported to FDA. In addition, in some cases, FDA will require a post-authorization clinical evaluation study as a condition of the authorization, with a requirement to update labelling based on the results of the study.[146]

FUNDING

What Funding is Available for COVID-19 MCM Development and Approval?

Recently enacted supplemental appropriations have included funding for several accounts that can be used to support the development and approval of COVID-19 MCMs, or to support scientific research that can aid in MCM development (as summarized in *Table 1*). The table below shows funding that can be used for MCM R&D or approval activities as provided in the three coronavirus supplemental appropriations acts:[147]

- Division A, Coronavirus Preparedness and Response Supplemental Appropriations Act, 2020 (P.L. 116-123), enacted on March 6, 2020.
- Division B, Coronavirus Aid, Relief, and Economic Security Act (P.L. 116-136), enacted on March 27, 2020.

---

[145] FDA, "Coronavirus (COVID-19) Update: FDA Revokes Emergency Use Authorization for Chloroquine and Hydroxychloroquine," June 15, 2020, https://www.fda.gov/news-events/press-announcements/coronavirus-covid-19-update-fda-revokes-emergency-use-authorization-chloroquine-and.

[146] See for example FDA, "Cue COVID-19 Test: Letter of Authorization," https://www.fda.gov/media/138823/download.

[147] The second supplemental appropriations measure, The Families First Coronavirus Response Act (P.L. 116-127) did not include available funding for MCM R&D.

- Division B, Paycheck Protection Program and Health Care Enhancement Act (P.L. 116-139), enacted on April 24, 2020.

Table 1 shows accounts from which funding can be used by FDA, NIH, DOD Defense Health Research, and components within the HHS Office of the Secretary (including BARDA). In some cases, funds are appropriated to those accounts; in others, transfers or set-asides to relevant agencies or accounts are either directed or allowed. (This transfer authority in several instances is either "not more than" or "not less than" a specified amount.) Funds to be transferred are shown in the account to which they were appropriated, not in the account to which they are to be transferred.

The purpose of the funds indicates their allowed uses as specified in the respective appropriations acts. Additional contextual information is included where appropriate. The period of availability is either the date after which funds are no longer available for obligation, or "until expended."

In some cases, funds are provided to accounts that are mostly for activities related to MCMs, such as funding for FDA, DOD Defense Health Program, or NIH accounts. In other cases, funds appropriated to the listed account may be allocated to MCM R&D-related activities at the discretion of the funded agency. For example, funds have been appropriated to the Public Health and Social Services Emergency Fund (PHSSEF) for a broad array of HHS emergency preparedness and response activities related to COVID-19, particularly those conducted by ASPR, where BARDA is based. The HHS Secretary generally has broad discretion to allocate the PHSSEF account amounts listed below to BARDA, except where set-asides or transfers are specified.

Table 1. Funding for MCM R&D in Coronavirus supplemental appropriations (Accounts with specific funding available for MCM R&D)

Account	Amount	Purpose	Availability
Coronavirus Preparedness and Response Supplemental Appropriations Act, 2020 (P.L. 116-123)[a]			
FDA—Salaries and Expenses	$61 million	"to prevent, prepare for, and respond to coronavirus, domestically or internationally, including the development of necessary medical countermeasures and vaccines, advanced manufacturing for medical products, the monitoring of medical product supply chains, and related administrative activities."	Until expended
NIH—NIAID	$836 million (less specified transfer of not less than $10 million)[b]	"to prevent, prepare for, and respond to coronavirus, domestically or internationally."	September 30, 2024
HHS Office of the Secretary (OS)—Public Health and Social Services Emergency Fund (PHSSEF; parent account for BARDA)	$3.1 billion and $300 million in contingent appropriations (less specified transfers of not more than $102 million)[c]	"to prevent, prepare for, and respond to coronavirus, domestically or internationally, including the development of necessary countermeasures and vaccines, prioritizing platform- based technologies with U.S.-based manufacturing	September 30, 2024

Table 1. (Continued)

Account	Amount	Purpose	Availability
		capabilities, and the purchase of vaccines, therapeutics, diagnostics, necessary medical supplies, medical surge capacity, and related administrative activities." The HHS Secretary may direct funding from this account to BARDA.	
CDC—CDC-Wide Activities and Program Support—Transfer to Infectious Disease Rapid Response Reserve Fund (IRRRDF)	Transfer of not less than $300 million	"to prevent, prepare for, and respond to coronavirus, domestically or internationally." Funding from IDRRRF is transferrable to NIH and PHSSEF accounts by the CDC Director pursuant to 42 U.S.C. §247d-4a.	September 30, 2022
Coronavirus Aid, Relief, and Economic Security Act (CARES Act) (P.L. 116-136)[d]			
DOD—Defense Health Program	$415 million	"Research, development, test and evaluation to prevent, prepare for, and respond to coronavirus, domestically or internationally."	September 30, 2021
FDA—Salaries and Expenses	$80 million	"to prevent, prepare for, and respond to coronavirus, domestically or internationally, including funds for the development of necessary medical countermeasures and vaccines, advanced	Until expended

Account	Amount	Purpose	Availability
		manufacturing for medical products, the monitoring of medical product supply chains, and related administrative activities."	
NIH—National Heart, Lung, and Blood Institute (NHLBI)	$103 million	"to prevent, prepare for, and respond to coronavirus, domestically or internationally."	September 30, 2024
NIH—NIAID	$706 million	"to prevent, prepare for, and respond to coronavirus, domestically or internationally." Not less than $156 million of the total is for "the study of, construction of, demolition of, renovation of, and acquisition of equipment for, vaccine and infectious diseases research facilities of or used by NIH, including the acquisition of real property."	September 30, 2024
NIH—National Institute of Biomedical Imaging and Bioengineering (NIBIB)	$60 million	"to prevent, prepare for, and respond to coronavirus, domestically or internationally."	September 30, 2024
NIH—National Library of Medicine (NLM)	$10 million	"to prevent, prepare for, and respond to coronavirus, domestically or internationally."	September 30, 2024
National Center for Advancing Translational Sciences (NCATS)	$36 million	"to prevent, prepare for, and respond to coronavirus, domestically or internationally."	September 30, 2024

Table 1. (Continued)

Account	**Amount**	**Purpose**	**Availability**
NIH—Office of the Director	$30 million	"to prevent, prepare for, and respond to coronavirus, domestically or internationally."	September 30, 2024
OS—PHSSEF (parent account for BARDA)[e]	$27 billion including the BARDA set-aside below (less other specified set- asides or transfers of roughly $16.5 billion)[g]	"to prevent, prepare for, and respond to coronavirus, domestically or internationally, including the development of necessary countermeasures and vaccines, prioritizing platform- based technologies with U.S.-based manufacturing capabilities, the purchase of vaccines, therapeutics, diagnostics, necessary medical supplies, as well as medical surge capacity, addressing blood supply chain, workforce modernization, telehealth access and infrastructure, initial advanced manufacturing, novel dispensing, enhancements to the U.S. Commissioned Corps, and other preparedness and response activities." The HHS Secretary may direct funding from this account to BARDA.	September 30, 2024
Set-aside to BARDA (non-	*Set-aside of not less than*	*"for necessary expenses of*	*As above*

Account	Amount	Purpose	Availability
add)	*$3.5 billion*	*manufacturing, production, and purchase, at the discretion of the Secretary, of vaccines, therapeutics, diagnostics, and small molecule active pharmaceutical ingredients, including the development, translation, and demonstration at scale of innovations in manufacturing platforms."*	
CDC—CDC-Wide Activities and Program Support- Transfer to IRRRDF	Transfer of $300 million	"to prevent, prepare for, and respond to coronavirus, domestically or internationally." Funding from IDRRRF is transferrable to NIH and PHSSEF accounts by the CDC Director pursuant to 42 U.S.C. §247d-4a.	September 30, 2024
Paycheck Protection Program and Health Care Enhancement Act (P.L. 116-139)[h]			
OS—PHSSEF[i]	$25 billion including transfers below (less other specified set-asides or transfers of not less than $13.8 billion)[i]	"to prevent, prepare for, and respond to coronavirus, domestically or internationally, for necessary expenses to research, develop, validate, manufacture, purchase, administer, and expand capacity for COVID–19 tests to effectively monitor and suppress COVID–19, including tests for both active infection and prior exposure, including molecular, antigen, and	Until expended

Table 1. (Continued)

Account	Amount	Purpose	Availability
		serological tests, the manufacturing, procurement and distribution of tests, testing equipment and testing supplies, including personal protective equipment needed for administering tests, the development and validation of rapid, molecular point-of-care tests, and other tests, support for workforce, epidemiology, to scale up academic, commercial, public health, and hospital laboratories, to conduct surveillance and contact tracing, support development of COVID–19 testing plans, and other related activities related to COVID–19 testing."	
Transfer to NIH National Cancer Institute (non-add)	*Transfer of not less than $306 million*	*"to develop, validate, improve, and implement serological testing and associated technologies."*	*As above*
Transfer to NIH NIBIB (non-add)	*Transfer of not less than $500 million*	*"to accelerate research, development, and implementation of point of care and other rapid testing related to coronavirus."*	*As above*
Transfer to NIH Office of the Director (non- add)	*Transfer of not less than $1 billion*	*"to develop, validate, improve, and implement testing and associated*	*As above*

Account	Amount	Purpose	Availability
		technologies; to accelerate research, development, and implementation of point of care and other rapid testing; and for partnerships with governmental and non-governmental entities to research, develop, and implement the activities outlined in this proviso."	
Set-aside to BARDA (non-add)	*Transfer of not less than $1 billion*	*"for necessary expenses of advanced research, development, manufacturing, production, and purchase of diagnostic, serologic, or other COVID–19 tests or related supplies, and other activities related to COVID–19 testing at the discretion of the Secretary."*	*As above*
Transfer to FDA (non- add)	*Transfer of $22 million*	*"to support activities associated with diagnostic, serological, antigen, and other tests, and related administrative activities."*	*As above*

Notes: Funding in other accounts not included in this table could potentially be used for activities related to MCM R&D, such as funding for Global Health, National Science Foundation and others. However, such funding is excluded from this presentation because MCM R&D is not a primary purpose of these accounts. Amounts shown rounded to first decimal place. The second supplemental appropriations measure, The Families First Coronavirus Response Act (P.L. 116-127) did not include available funding for MCM R&D.

Acronyms: FDA= Food and Drug Administration; NIH= National Institutes of Health; NIAID= National Institute of Allergy and Infectious Diseases; HHS= Department of Health and Human Services; BARDA= Biomedical Advanced Research and Development Authority; DOD= Department of Defense.

[a] HHS may transfer nearly all the funds appropriated to it in Title III, Division A, of P.L. 116-123 among accounts at CDC, NIH, or PHSSEF, provided the transfers are made to prevent, prepare for, and respond to the COVID-19 pandemic, domestically or internationally (see §304). HHS is to notify the House and the Senate appropriations committees 10 days in advance of such a transfer.

[b] Transfer to the National Institute of Environmental Health Sciences (NIEHS) for "worker-based training to prevent and reduce exposure of hospital employees, emergency first responders, and other workers who are at risk of exposure to coronavirus through their work duties."

[c] Transfers specified are $100 million to the Health Resources and Services Administration (HRSA) and up to $2 million to the HHS Office of Inspector General (OIG).

[d] HHS may transfer nearly all the funds appropriated to it in Title VIII, Division B, of P.L. 116-136 among accounts at CDC, PHSSEF, NIH, Administration for Children and Families (ACF), and the Administration for Community Living (ACL), provided the transfers are made to prevent, prepare for, and respond to the COVID-19 pandemic, domestically or internationally (see §18111). HHS is to notify the House and the Senate appropriations committees 10 days in advance of such a transfer.

[e] Not more than $4 million per Title VIII, Division B, Section 8113, is to be transferred to the HHS Office of the Inspector General (OIG) from the $127.29 billion total appropriated to PHSSEF for oversight of all activities supported with funds appropriated to HHS to prevent, prepare for, and respond to the COVID- 19 pandemic.

[f] Transfers specified are not more than $16 billion for the Strategic National Stockpile; not less than $250 million for grants or cooperative agreements with existing grantees or sub-grantees of the Hospital Preparedness Program; not more than $289 million to other federal agencies for care of persons under federal quarantine; and $1.5 million for a National Academies of Science, Engineering, and Medicine (NASEM) study on the security of the U.S. medical supply chain.

[g] HHS may transfer certain funds appropriated to it in Title I, Division B, of P.L. 116-139 among accounts at CDC, NIH, PHSSEF, and FDA, provided the transfers are made to prevent, prepare for, and respond to the COVID-19 pandemic (see §102). HHS is to notify the House and the Senate appropriations committees 10 days in advance of such a transfer.

[h] Not more than $6 million per Title I, Division B, Section 103, of P.L. 116-139 is to be transferred to the HHS Office of the Inspector General (OIG) from the $127.29 billion total appropriated to PHSSEF for oversight of all activities supported with funds appropriated to HHS to prevent, prepare for, and respond to the COVID-19 pandemic.

[i] Other specified transfers include not less than $11 billion for grants and cooperative agreements with states, localities, territories, tribes, and other jurisdictions/entities; not less than $1 billion to CDC-wide activities and program support; $600 million to HRSA for community health centers; $225 million for rural health clinics; and $1 billion for the cost of testing for the uninsured.

In: Vaccines
Editor: Oliver Huerta

ISBN: 978-1-53619-059-5

Chapter 5

TESTING, TESTING, (PHASE) 1-2-3: LEGAL CONSIDERATIONS FOR CLINICAL TRIALS OF POTENTIAL COVID-19 VACCINES*

Erin H. Ward

In the race to develop a Coronavirus Disease 2019 (COVID-19) vaccine, several pharmaceutical companies, governments, and educational institutions around the world have begun testing their potential COVID-19 vaccines in clinical trials. Clinical trials are used to assess whether a new pharmaceutical product, such as a vaccine, is safe for humans and effective in achieving its intended purpose. Companies must generally test new pharmaceutical products on humans through clinical trials to obtain U.S. Food and Drug Administration (FDA) approval to market the product. But using human subjects to test these novel products exposes them to unknown health and safety risks, raising ethical considerations for FDA and for the sponsors and Institutional Review Boards (IRBs) overseeing the

* This is an edited, reformatted and augmented version of Congressional Research Service Publication No. LSB10483, dated June 2, 2020.

investigations. These stakeholders—sponsors, IRBs, and FDA—aim to balance the need to ensure that the product is safe and effective against the desire to bring the product to market quickly, tensions that are heightened during a worldwide pandemic. Existing law requires FDA and IRBs to weigh these considerations when evaluating proposed clinical trial designs for COVID-19 vaccines.

This Sidebar describes the legal and regulatory framework that governs clinical trials for pharmaceutical products, such as vaccines, and some avenues researchers and Congress may consider for accelerating that process during the COVID-19 pandemic. (For ease of reference, this Sidebar uses the term *drugs* includes both traditional drugs and biological products, including vaccines.)

Clinical Trials of Investigational New Drugs

Sponsors use clinical trials to generate the data needed to obtain FDA approval to market their products. Because clinical trials expose human subjects to unapproved pharmaceutical products, they risk causing unanticipated serious adverse side effects in the participants. To manage these risks, the Federal Food, Drug, and Cosmetic Act (FD&C Act) and FDA regulations have imposed procedural requirements on clinical trials, such as advance and ongoing scientific and ethical review, to help protect the participants by minimizing risks, requiring informed consent, and ensuring that the studies collect the data needed to determine whether to approve the product.

Using Clinical Trials to Collect Substantial Evidence

Sponsors must submit "substantial evidence" to FDA that their products are safe and effective (or safe, potent, and pure) to obtain FDA approval. Section 505(d) of the FD&C Act defines substantial evidence to mean adequately and well-controlled investigations on the basis of which qualified scientific experts could fairly and responsible conclude that the product has the purported effect. FDA assesses both the quality and quantity of the data provided when determining whether a product meets this standard.

Quality refers to the strength of the evidence and the amount of certainty it provides as to the product's safety and effectiveness—i.e., whether the investigation is "adequate" and "well-controlled." The quality of the evidence depends on how the clinical trial is designed and how the study is conducted. Under FDA regulations, the design must allow for a valid comparison of the product to a control, such as a placebo, an existing therapy, or no treatment. FDA also evaluates whether the study's method for selecting participants and assigning them to groups is adequate to ensure that meaningful data are collected. The methodology must also include a well-defined and reliable means of assessing the participants' responses and explain the analytical and statistical methods used to assess the results. Finally, sponsors must provide a clear statement of the investigation's objectives and take adequate measures to minimize bias in the study. FDA may, however, waive any of these criteria for a specific investigation if the sponsor can show that the criteria is not reasonably applicable to the study and an alternative approach yields substantial evidence of effectiveness. FDA guidance further clarifies how sponsors should select their clinical trial design, endpoints, and statistical methods.

As for quantity, FDA generally requires that sponsors complete two "adequate and well-controlled clinical investigations" to meet the substantial evidence standard. FDA notes in its guidance that two studies, particularly those that are designed and conducted differently, reduces the likelihood of a design flaw, bias, or other issue or anomaly that could result in erroneous conclusions. However, under the Food and Drug Modernization Act of 1997, FDA may allow sponsors to rely on one large multi-center adequate and well-controlled clinical investigation supported by another form of additional data, such as data regarding the effectiveness of other drugs in the same pharmacological class. In deciding whether to allow a sponsor to rely on a single study, FDA states that it considers, among other factors, the seriousness of the disease, whether there is an unmet medical need, and whether additional trials would be ethical and practicable.

Given the flexibility afforded sponsors in designing and conducting their clinical trials, FDA uses written guidance and individual meetings to help sponsors ensure that their investigations will generate the substantial evidence needed for approval. Sponsors that obtain fast track product or breakthrough therapy designation for their products are entitled to additional assistance from and communication with FDA staff to craft efficient and effective clinical trial designs.

SUBMITTING AN INVESTIGATIONAL NEW DRUG APPLICATION TO FDA

New drugs and biological products that are being tested in clinical trials are referred to as investigational new drugs. Section 505(i) of the FD&C Act, Section 351(a)(3) of the Public Health Service Act, and their implementing regulations allow investigational new drugs to be used for research before they are approved. To conduct clinical trials of investigational new drugs, the company developing the product (i.e., sponsor) must generally receive FDA approval for the investigation and comply with regulatory requirements for human subjects research.

Sponsors obtain FDA approval to test an investigational new drug on human subjects through an investigational new drug application (IND). The IND gives FDA an opportunity to ensure that the study will protect the safety and rights of its human subjects and gather scientific data that adequately shows the product's safety and effectiveness. The sponsor may begin its clinical trials 30 days after submitting an IND unless FDA notifies the sponsor that it is either (1) authorizing the IND and the study can begin immediately or (2) imposing a clinical hold due to concerns about the study. If FDA imposes a clinical hold, the study cannot begin (or resume, for ongoing investigations) pending further notification.

FDA regulations prescribe the information that sponsors must include in an IND. The IND must contain information about the product, such as the substance and formulation; existing data on use in animals or humans if available; and anticipated risks and side effects. The IND also contains a general investigational plan, which explains why the sponsor is undertaking the study and includes, among other things, the indications being studied, the sponsor's approach to evaluating the product, the kinds of clinical trials being conducted, the anticipated number of participants, and any anticipated risks. Along with the general investigational plan, the IND must include specific protocols for each clinical trial phase.

The sponsor must also generally certify that an institutional review board (IRB) will provide initial and continuing review of each study, including the proposed protocols and any subsequent changes to the study. FDA may, however, waive any IRB requirements, including the requirement of IRB review itself.

INSTITUTIONAL REVIEW BOARD REVIEW AND APPROVAL

An IRB is a group convened by an institution to review and approve biomedical research involving humans. IRBs evaluate the initial clinical study design and protocols, along with any changes implemented during the investigation, in an effort to ensure that the rights and well-being of the human subjects are protected. To that end, IRBs assess whether risks to the participants are minimized and reasonable in relation to the anticipated benefits, both to the participants directly and from the knowledge expected to be gained through the study. IRBs also aim to ensure that the researchers will obtain adequate informed consent from all participants (unless an exemption applies) and that selection of the participants will be equitable. IRBs may also require (as appropriate) that the research plan provide for monitoring of the collected data to protect the participants' safety and privacy. To the extent the study may include participants from populations that may be vulnerable to coercion or undue influence (e.g., children, prisoners), IRBs must ensure that sufficient safeguards are in place to protect these populations in participant selection and during the clinical trials.

IRBs review clinical trial plans and protocols from various standpoints, including ensuring that the study complies with legal, ethical, and professional standards; is scientifically sound; and is free from illicit discrimination. Accordingly, to ensure adequate and independent review, IRBs must have at least five members from multiple backgrounds, including at least one member with a scientific background and at least one with a nonscientific background. At least one member must be independent from the institution running the clinical trials, and the IRB members cannot have any financial or other conflicting interests in the project. IRB review must comply with any other requirements relating to IRBs and human subject research found in Parts 50 and 56 of Chapter 21 of the Code of Federal Regulation.

Clinical Trial Phases

Clinical trials for a new pharmaceutical product generally proceed in three phases, transitioning from smaller trials focused on initial safety early on to larger trials assessing safety and effectiveness to inform approval and labeling. The size, duration, and specific purpose of each clinical trial phase varies from product to product depending on such factors as the type of product (e.g., a vaccine, treatment, or preventative medication), how the product works, and the relevant underlying patient population.

However, as defined by FDA regulations, a clinical investigation generally proceeds as follows:

- *Phase 1 Trials.* Phase 1 trials are the first time the product is introduced in human subjects. These carefully controlled trials typically involve 20 to 80 patients or volunteer subjects, though the exact numbers may vary depending on the product. Phase 1 trials generally assess how the product acts in the body and evaluate initial safety (i.e., side effects). They may also be used to determine the dosing levels to use in phase 2 (e.g., the maximum safe dose or what dose is required to have an effect). Depending on the product, phase 1 trials may also provide some initial indication as to whether the product may be effective. In the case of vaccines specifically, phase 1 trials also assess their ability to provoke an immune response in the body (i.e., immunogenicity).

- *Phase 2 Trials.* Phase 2 trials continue to assess safety but also evaluate the product's effectiveness and common short-term side effects or other risks associated with the product. Phase 2 trials are also used to determine the optimal dose of the product. For vaccines, phase 2 assesses how much of the vaccine to administer and on what dosing schedule (e.g., whether a boost is needed to maximize its effectiveness or whether the vaccine must be administered on a regular schedule to maintain immunity). As with phase 1 studies, phase 2 studies are carefully controlled. However, phase 2 involves a larger (though still relatively limited) number of volunteer subjects—generally no more than a few hundred participants.
- *Phase 3 Trials.* Phase 3 trials involve an expanded number of participants—from several hundred to thousands—and are used to assess the product's safety and effectiveness across a wide range of patient categories through controlled and uncontrolled studies. These trials are intended to present a clearer picture of expected risks and benefits under real-world conditions. The information obtained from phase 3 trials also forms the basis for the product's labeling.

Sponsors must generally complete all three phases to obtain FDA approval unless they obtain accelerated approval, in which case FDA requires post-approval trials to confirm the expected clinical benefit. FDA may also require, at its discretion, additional clinical trials after approval (i.e., phase 4 trials) for any approved product to continue assessing the product's safety and effectiveness once on the market.

CONSIDERATIONS FOR CONGRESS

The current legal framework seeks to balance various competing interests, which may be amplified in the current crisis. The FD&C Act and implementing regulations provide standards and factors to consider but otherwise give FDA and IRBs discretion to evaluate investigational plans and clinical trial protocols for investigational new drugs. FDA may also waive requirements relating to IRB review and clinical trial design. To the extent Congress may seek to direct how FDA and IRBs exercise that discretion with respect to any potential COVID-19 vaccine, Congress could consider implementing legislation that provides more specific direction on how to approach clinical trials either specifically for the current COVID-19 pandemic or in epidemic, pandemic, or other emergency situations more generally. For example, courts have determined that Congress can cabin FDA's discretion by imposing mandatory (e.g., "shall") rather than permissive (e.g., "may") language in a statute.

In light of the multiple companies involved in developing potential COVID-19 vaccines, Congress could also consider facilitating the coordination of any clinical trials or appointing a neutral scientific body to consider the ethical and scientific considerations and generate guidelines or a master protocol. The World Health Organization (WHO) employed this approach to facilitate development of an Ebola vaccine following the 2014 to 2016 Ebola epidemic. Congress could also direct or fund increased global collaboration between regulators to promote information sharing, which could potentially result in more streamlined clinical investigations with fewer participants being exposed to investigational vaccines.

Congress could also consider providing additional funding or other resources to facilitate the clinical trials themselves or any research directed toward understanding the SARS-CoV-2 virus or COVID-19 disease to allow for improved risk minimization in future clinical trials.

In: Vaccines
Editor: Oliver Huerta

ISBN: 978-1-53619-059-5

Chapter 6

COVID-19 VACCINE DEVELOPMENT*

United States Government Accountability Office

WHY THIS MATTERS

SARS-CoV-2 causes COVID-19, and developing a vaccine could save lives and speed economic recovery. The United States is funding multiple efforts to develop vaccines. Developing a vaccine is a complicated process that is costly, typically requires 10 years or more, and has a low success rate, although efforts are underway to accelerate the process.

THE TECHNOLOGY

What Is It?

Vaccines protect people from disease by triggering the immune system to produce antibodies that will fight the pathogen attacking the body. In the

* This is an edited, reformatted and augmented version of the United States Government Accountability Office Report, Publication No. GAO-20-583SP, dated May 2020.

case of COVID-19, the pathogen is the virus SARS-CoV-2. Developing a vaccine is an expensive, lengthy process that involves a rigorous series of steps to first identify a potential vaccine "candidate" and then assess it for safety and effectiveness.

How Does It Work?

A vaccine can use a virus that has been modified to be safe or a molecule that resembles a part of the virus. Once antibodies are produced, if the vaccinated person is exposed later to the virus, their body will produce those antibodies again, increasing their chances of fighting off infection.

Development starts with identifying a "target," such as a protein, that can induce an immune reaction. Researchers create a vaccine candidate similar to that target that will induce production of antibodies effective against the virus. The vaccine candidate is then moved through phases of development, assessment, and approvals (figure 1).

Under normal circumstances, the entire process typically takes 10 to 15 years, with more than 65 percent of candidates failing, according to an MIT study. There is an effort to expedite this process for SARS-CoV-2. As of May 15, 2020, there are more than 110 COVID-19 vaccines in development globally; of those, at least three are being developed in the United States with federal funding. These three use different mechanisms to prompt the body to produce antibodies (figure 2).

The first candidate, developed by National Institute of Allergy and Infectious Diseases scientists and their collaborators, uses a molecule called mRNA specifically coded to generate proteins that will induce an immune response. This is a newer method of vaccine development that has shown promise in animals during the preclinical phase.

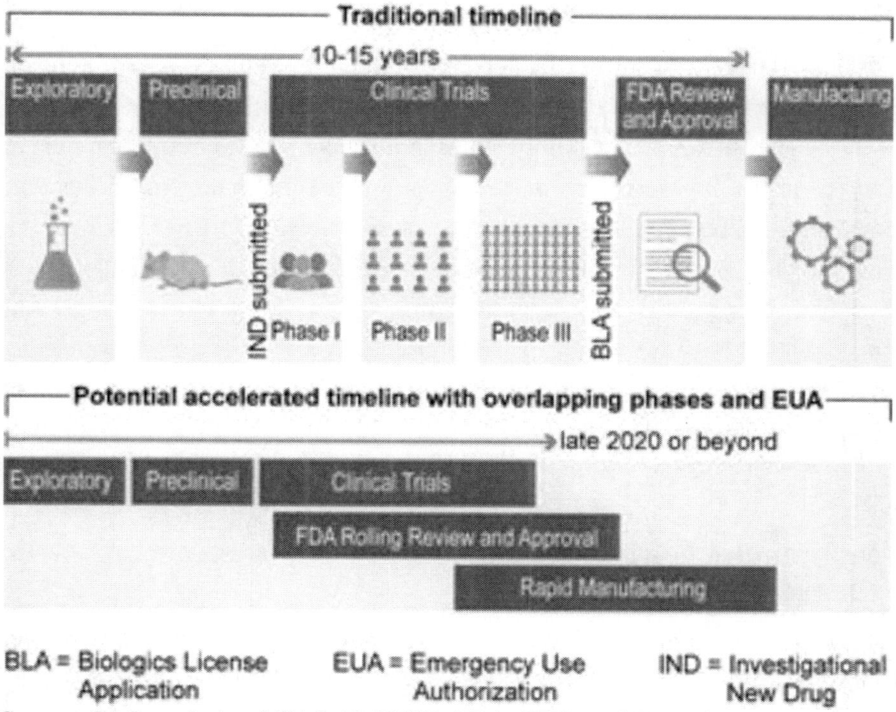

Source: GAO analysis of GAO-20-215SP. FDA, HHS, and Pharmaceutical Research and Manufacturers of America (PhRMA) documentation. | GAO-20-583SP.

Figure 1. The vaccine development process typically takes 10 to 15 years under a traditional timeline. Multiple regulatory pathways, such as Emergency Use Authorization, can be used to facilitate bringing a vaccine for COVID-19 to market sooner.

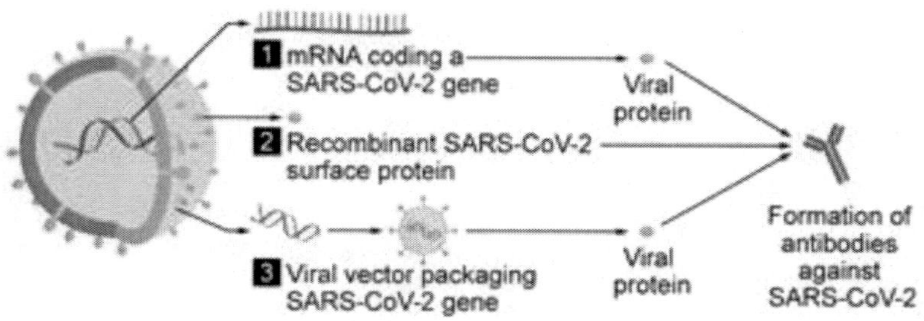

Source: GAO. | GAO-20-583SP.

Figure 2. Vaccine candidates use different mechanisms, such as those shown above, to prompt the body to produce antibodies against SARS-CoV-2.

The second candidate uses a recombinant protein, which is produced by genetically engineering bacteria or other cells to produce a protein that mimics part of the spike protein found on the surface of the SARS-CoV-2 virus. The spike protein alone does not cause an infection but may be sufficient to produce an immune response. Recombinant protein vaccines are already being used successfully against other viruses, such as the human papillomavirus (HPV), which can cause cervical cancer.

The third candidate uses a virus—adenovirus 26, or Ad26—but researchers have removed its infectious aspects, making it safe as a "vector" to deliver a piece of SARS-CoV-2 to trigger a protective immune response. This method is also in clinical trials against HIV and Ebola.

How Mature Is It?

The process for developing a new vaccine as outlined by the Food and Drug Administration (FDA) is well established. In the exploratory phase, the target and candidate vaccine are identified. In the preclinical phase, researchers use cells and animals to assess safety and produce evidence of clinical promise, evaluated by the candidate's ability to elicit a protective immune response.

During clinical trials, more human subjects are added at each successive phase. Safety, efficacy, proposed doses, schedule of immunizations, and method of delivery are evaluated.

The next phase is FDA approval and licensure, which includes oversight of manufacturing and postmarket surveillance, and may include Phase IV trials to monitor safety and efficacy, potency, purity, and other potential uses.

At any phase, the process can be terminated for various reasons including detection of adverse events, such as serious side effects.

FDA has four programs to facilitate and expedite the review and approval of new therapies for the treatment and prevention of serious or life- threatening conditions, such as COVID-19. Fast Track, Breakthrough Therapy, Accelerated Approval, and Priority Review allow for expedited processes, such as overlapping vaccine development phases, to bring vaccines to market more quickly. Vaccine developers could potentially use any or all of these programs for vaccine candidates in the United States.

FDA can also issue Emergency Use Authorizations (EUA) for review of vaccine candidates that have not completed all phases of development if there is sufficient scientific evidence on the product's safety, effectiveness, risks, and benefits.

Opportunities

Several technologies and initiatives offer opportunities to accelerate vaccine development. For example:

- Genomic tools. Tools that provide information about a pathogen's genetic makeup can reduce the length of time for target selection.
- Collaboration and partnerships. The National Institutes of Health's Accelerating COVID-19 Therapeutic Interventions and Vaccines (ACTIV) effort is a public-private partnership intended to provide a collaborative framework for vaccine development.
- Multiple vaccine mechanisms. Simultaneous testing of multiple vaccine mechanisms can improve the chances of developing a successful vaccine faster.

Challenges

- *Virus mutations.* RNA viruses, such as SARS-CoV-2, can mutate and potentially reduce or eliminate a vaccine's effectiveness, potentially creating a need for new vaccines.
- *Risk from accelerated process.* According to FDA, accelerating vaccine development could increase risk of adverse effects, since less time would be allocated to proving safety and effectiveness.

- *Manufacturing and supply issues.* Some production process and materials needs vary by vaccine type, complicating early expansion of manufacturing. Increasing export restrictions, dependence on imported supplies, and competition for materials may constrain access to supplies.

POLICY CONTEXT AND QUESTIONS

- What mechanisms could be used for quickly scaling up vaccine manufacturing, production, and distribution?
- If a vaccine becomes available, who will have priority to be vaccinated? How will the vaccine be purchased and distributed, particularly if distribution requires special handling (e.g., maintaining a specific temperature)?
- How could vaccines developed or manufactured internationally be made more accessible for use within the United States?
- If a vaccine is not developed and widely available soon, what preparations are needed for a possible second wave of the COVID-19 outbreak this fall and winter?

In: Vaccines
Editor: Oliver Huerta

ISBN: 978-1-53619-059-5

Chapter 7

COVID-19: LEGAL CONSIDERATIONS FOR BRINGING A NEW VACCINE TO MARKET*

Erin H. Ward

As the number of confirmed COVID-19 cases increases at an accelerating rate, interest has grown in developing a COVID-19 vaccine as an avenue for addressing the pandemic. Media reports indicate that a number of countries and companies are working on developing a vaccine. The National Institute of Allergy and Infectious Diseases (NIAID) and the biotechnology company Moderna, Inc., recently initiated the first clinical trials of a potential vaccine in the United States at a hospital in Seattle. However, developing a new vaccine and obtaining approval to market it can take a long time. This Sidebar discusses the licensure (i.e., approval) process for vaccines under the Public Health Service Act (PHS Act) and the federal Food, Drug, and Cosmetic Act (FD&C Act), as well as potential legal avenues for expediting that process to bring a new vaccine to market sooner.

---

* This is an edited, reformatted and augmented version of Congressional Research Service Publication No. LSB10427, dated March 24, 2020.

FDA Approval of New Vaccines

Vaccines are intended to prevent diseases and generally work by introducing pathogens to the human body (usually by injection) to trigger an immune response to the disease (i.e., producing antibodies to the pathogen). Vaccines are biological products approved and regulated by the U.S. Food and Drug Administration's (FDA's) Center for Biologics Evaluation and Research (CBER) under Section 351 of the Public Health Service Act. A biologic such as a vaccine generally cannot be introduced into commerce unless FDA approves it. To be approved, FDA must determine that the vaccine is safe, potent, and pure based on data from laboratory studies and clinical trials. In general, this requirement means that the vaccine must achieve the desired effect (i.e., prevents the targeted disease or condition) and that the risk of adverse side effects is outweighed by the expected benefits.

Developing a new vaccine, or any other drug or biological product, begins in a laboratory. When a company (i.e., sponsor) is ready to test its new vaccine on humans in clinical trials, the sponsor submits an investigational new drug application (IND) to FDA. The IND contains information known about the vaccine so far and the sponsor's plan for the clinical studies, including the investigational plan and protocols for the studies. FDA uses the IND to ensure that clinical trials will protect the safety and rights of the participants and yield data with enough scientific integrity to evaluate the safety and effectiveness of the vaccine. The sponsor generally cannot begin clinical trials until FDA approves the IND.

If the clinical trials are successful, the sponsor may seek FDA approval to market its new vaccine. FDA approves new vaccines through biologics license applications (BLAs) reviewed by CBER. BLAs contain data from the laboratory and clinical studies and information about how and where the biologic will be manufactured. As courts have recognized, FDA exercises its scientific judgment when deciding whether to license vaccines based on such studies. Biologics that are approved through a BLA receive 12 years of regulatory exclusivity, during which time FDA cannot approve any biosimilars (i.e., abbreviated applications for the same biologic that depend on the clinical data in the BLA to demonstrate safety, potency, and purity). (These exclusivity rights and separate patent rights raise potential intellectual property questions that are discussed in more detail in this Sidebar.)

OPTIONS FOR BRINGING A NEW VACCINE TO MARKET FASTER

The process of developing and testing a new vaccine to the point where it meets the safety, purity, and potency standard can be a lengthy process. The FD&C Act provides several options that may allow a sponsor to bring a new vaccine to market faster. Generally, these options use one of two approaches. First, FDA can direct more of its resources to the product to accelerate the development and/or review processes (e.g., fast track product designation, breakthrough therapy designation, and priority review). Second, FDA can modify how it evaluates the risks and benefits of the vaccine before allowing its use, either by relying on different types of evidence (e.g., the accelerated approval process) or lowering the evidentiary standard in emergency situations (e.g., emergency use authorization). (For ease of reference, this section uses the general term "biologic" because vaccines are biological products, but the pathways discussed below are also available for traditional small molecule drugs.)

SHORTENING THE DEVELOPMENT AND REVIEW PROCESSES

Several avenues are available for expediting the development and review processes for biologics used to treat or prevent serious or life-threatening conditions and diseases. In its guidance, FDA generally considers a condition or disease *serious* if it substantially affects day-to-day functioning and is irreversible, persistent, or recurrent. A condition or disease may be found to be serious as a matter of clinical judgment based on its effect on survival, day-to-day functioning, or the likelihood that it will progress to a more serious condition if left untreated. As a matter of course, FDA considers any life- threatening condition or disease to be serious. The drug must also be intended to *treat* the serious condition or disease by having an effect on the disease itself or a serious aspect of the disease, such as a symptom or other manifestation. Among the examples FDA provides in its guidance is a product intended to *prevent* the serious condition. Given that COVID-19 is life-threatening, a vaccine intended to prevent COVID-19 seems likely to qualify as a drug used to treat or prevent a serious or life-threatening condition or disease—making it eligible for the following designations to accelerate the approval process.

Fast Track Product Designation

Section 506 of the FD&C Act allows FDA to designate certain biologics as fast track products, which receive FDA assistance in expediting development and review. A biologic may be designated as a fast track product if FDA determines that the biologic will treat or prevent a serious or life-threatening disease or condition and fill an unmet medical need. An unmet medical need exists when available therapies do not adequately address treating or diagnosing a condition or disease. FDA recognizes in its guidance that an unmet medical need necessarily exists if there is no available therapy. Sponsors may provide FDA with nonclinical or clinical data to demonstrate that the drug has the potential to fill that unmet medical need. Given that there are no approved vaccines for COVID-19, any vaccine that showed potential to prevent COVID-19 in laboratory or clinical trials would seem likely to qualify for fast track designation.

At its discretion, the biologic's sponsor requests fast track designation for its product. It may request fast track designation when it submits an IND or any time thereafter. FDA has 60 days to determine if the biologic qualifies for the designation. Once FDA designates a biologic as a fast track product, FDA must facilitate its development and expedite review of the biologic. In practice, this process generally means that the biologic's sponsor has greater access to FDA through written and in-person communications during the development and testing process to improve efficiency and ensure that appropriate data are collected. FDA may also review the BLA for a fast track product on a rolling basis as sections are complete (rather than waiting for a completed application) if initial clinical testing shows the biologic may be effective.

Breakthrough Therapy Designation

Section 506 of the FD&C Act also allows FDA to designate certain biologics as breakthrough therapies, which similarly heightens FDA involvement in the development and review process. Breakthrough therapy designation is based on preliminary clinical evidence showing the biologic may be a substantial improvement over available therapies for one or more clinically significant endpoints. Endpoints measure the outcome of a clinical trial. Under FDA guidance, a clinically significant endpoint generally measures an effect on irreversible morbidity or mortality or on symptoms representing serious consequences of the disease or condition. Unlike fast track product designation, which can be based on laboratory data, breakthrough therapy designation requires evidence from clinical trials. FDA exercises its judgment in determining whether the data show a substantial improvement over existing therapies, taking into consideration both the magnitude of the biologic's effects on the endpoint and the importance of the effect measured by that endpoint to treating the disease or condition. When there are no existing therapies, such as with a COVID-19 vaccine, FDA compares the biologic to a placebo or well-documented historical control. A COVID-19 vaccine may be eligible for breakthrough therapy designation if the sponsor can demonstrate potential effectiveness in early clinical trials.

At its discretion, the sponsor requests breakthrough therapy designation and may do so with submission of an IND or at any time thereafter. FDA must determine whether the biologic qualifies as a breakthrough therapy within 60 days of receipt. As with fast track product designation, the FD&C Act directs FDA to expedite the development and review of applications for breakthrough therapies. Per FDA guidance, expedited development and review of breakthrough therapies entails (1) intensive assistance from FDA on efficient development and clinical trial design; (2) organizational commitment from FDA, including senior management and experienced staff; (3) rolling review of the BLA; and (4) other actions to expedite review, such as priority review discussed below. Extensive FDA assistance during the development process and the involvement of senior managers distinguishes breakthrough therapy designation from fast track product designation.

Accelerated Approval

Section 506 of the FD&C Act also allows FDA to approve certain biologics based on surrogate or intermediate endpoints, referred to as accelerated approval. In general, sponsors select endpoints that directly measure the clinical outcome (i.e., the benefits expected from the biologic), such as whether the patient feels better or lives longer. Surrogate and intermediate endpoints do not measure the clinical benefit directly but instead measure an effect that is expected to predict a clinical benefit. For example, a drug to treat strokes would have an intended clinical outcome of reducing the incidence or severity of strokes. But rather than measuring the incidence of strokes directly, an investigator might measure the drug's effect on blood pressure as a surrogate endpoint due to the strong correlation between strokes and blood pressure.

To qualify for accelerated approval, (1) the biologic must treat a serious or life-threatening condition or disease and (2) FDA must determine that the biologic has an effect on a surrogate or intermediate endpoint that is reasonably likely to predict a clinical benefit. When deciding whether to approve a biologic on this basis, FDA must consider how severe, rare, or prevalent the condition is and the availability of alternative treatments. A vaccine for COVID-19 could qualify for accelerated approval if investigators identified a surrogate or intermediate endpoint that could reasonably predict the vaccine would be effective against the virus.

Priority Review

Once a BLA is submitted, FDA can designate the BLA for standard review or priority review. FDA aims to act on priority review applications within 6 months, compared to 10 months or more for standard review applications. FDA makes this determination for every application, though a sponsor can expressly request priority review. FDA may designate a BLA for priority review if it represents a "significant improvement" over existing treatments in terms of safety or effectiveness in treating, diagnosing, or preventing the disease or condition. In the absence of any approved vaccine for COVID-19, FDA would likely designate for priority review any BLA for such a vaccine.

Emergency Use Authorizations Before Approval

In certain emergency situations, Section 564 of the FD&C Act allows FDA to authorize the use of a drug or biologic (e.g., a vaccine) before it is approved (i.e., an Emergency Use Authorization or EUA). FDA may issue an EUA only if the Secretary of Health and Human Services has declared that circumstances exist justifying emergency authorized use of the medical product. Of relevance to the COVID-19 pandemic, on February 4, 2020, the Secretary determined that there is a public health emergency that has a significant potential to affect national security or the health and security of U.S. citizens living abroad, and that involves a biological, chemical, radiological, or nuclear agent (BCRN agent)—namely, the virus that causes COVID-19. Based on this determination, the Secretary has authorized the emergency use of several diagnostic tests. On March 2,

2020, the Secretary determined that circumstances exist to allow for the emergency use of certain respirators not approved by the agency, and FDA issued an EUA allowing for the emergency use of such respirators.

After the Secretary determines a public health emergency exists (one of four bases for declaring an emergency or threat), FDA may issue an EUA for a specific product if the Secretary concludes that:

- the BCRN agent can cause a serious or life-threatening disease or condition;
- it is reasonable to believe, based on the totality of the scientific evidence available, that:
  - The product may be effective in diagnosing, treating, or preventing the disease or condition caused by the BCRN agent; and
  - The known and potential benefits of the product outweigh the known and potential risks; and
- there is no adequate, approved, and available alternative to the product.

In evaluating a product for an EUA, FDA uses a lower evidentiary standard, determining whether the product "may be effective" in diagnosing, treating, or preventing a disease rather than evaluating its "effectiveness" in doing so. As discussed above, COVID-19 is a serious or life-threatening disease, confirmed by the fact that FDA has already issued EUAs in connection with COVID-19 for diagnostic tests and certain personal protective equipment. There is also no alternative to a COVID-19 vaccine at this time. Any decision by FDA to issue an EUA for a COVID-19 vaccine would accordingly depend on whether the totality of the evidence available to FDA shows that it is reasonable to believe (1) the vaccine may be effective in preventing COVID-19 and (2) that those benefits outweigh any known or potential risks from the vaccine. FDA would have to conduct this evaluation for each vaccine that is developed and submitted for an EUA.

The FD&C Act requires FDA to impose certain conditions on EUAs as necessary and appropriate to protect the public health. The conditions vary depending on whether the product is unapproved or approved but for a different use. In general, the conditions provide for monitoring, reporting, and recordkeeping as well as ensuring that the health care professionals administering the product and the individuals being treated with the product are informed about the benefits and risks of using the product.

FDA may also waive good manufacturing practices (GMP) and certain prescription requirements when issuing an EUA and may impose conditions related to advertising the product.

Considerations for Congress

The current legal regime for approving new pharmaceutical products such as vaccines generally aims to strike a balance between bringing products to market sooner and ensuring that products on the market are safe and effective. For serious or life-threatening diseases and conditions or in emergency situations, the law gives FDA a certain amount of discretion to shift that balance. FDA generally expedites the process one of two ways: shifting its resources or shifting its standard in evaluating the risks and benefits.

In considering avenues to facilitate the development of a COVID-19 vaccine, Congress has similar options. Congress could consider providing additional resources to FDA to exercise its existing authorities. Congress is already employing this approach: The Coronavirus Preparedness and Response Supplemental Appropriations Act, 2020, enacted on March 6, appropriated $61 million to FDA "to prevent, prepare for, and respond to coronavirus, domestically or internationally, including the development of necessary medical countermeasures and vaccines, advanced manufacturing for medical products, the monitoring of medical product supply chains, and related administrative activities." Alternatively, Congress could direct FDA to strike a different balance when evaluating the risks versus the benefits specifically in the context of potential COVID-19 vaccines. In assessing that balance, Congress and FDA would face weighing the benefits from disseminating a vaccine to the public sooner (e.g., limiting the spread of the virus or reducing the economic consequences) against the risk that the vaccine may have been authorized prematurely and prove ineffective or unsafe, potentially leading to worse public health outcomes. Any alteration to this balance that requires FDA to exceed or contradict its existing authority would require an act of Congress to amend the agency's statutory authority.

Should FDA authorize or approve a COVID-19 vaccine, other considerations may come to bear. For example, registered manufacturers may not be able to produce an adequate supply of the vaccine. FDA is currently addressing hand sanitizer shortages by exercising its enforcement discretion with respect to production by over-the-counter drug manufacturers and compounders. Congress may consider other avenues for increasing supply of the vaccine. In addition, existence of a vaccine would raise questions of mandatory vaccination to address the public health crisis, which is addressed in a separate Sidebar.

In: Vaccines
Editor: Oliver Huerta
ISBN: 978-1-53619-059-5

Chapter 8

LEGAL ISSUES IN COVID-19 VACCINE DEVELOPMENT*

Kevin J. Hickey and Erin H. Ward

SUMMARY

Private companies, universities, and governmental entities are working to develop a vaccine for coronavirus disease 2019 (COVID-19). Vaccines are biological products regulated under the Public Health Service Act (PHSA) and the Federal Food, Drug, and Cosmetic Act (FD&C Act). New vaccines must generally be licensed by the U.S. Food & Drug Administration (FDA) before they can be marketed and used in the United States. To obtain licensure, the vaccine must be tested in human subjects through clinical trials. The clinical trials inform the dosing schedule and labeling that will be used for the approved vaccine. Sponsors use the data from clinical trials, along with other information, to prepare a biologics license application (BLA) to submit to FDA. FDA approves the BLA if it determines that the vaccine is safe, potent, and pure.

Because the development and review process can be lengthy, the FD&C Act provides several avenues to accelerate this process for

* This is an edited, reformatted and augmented version of Congressional Research Service, Publication No. R46399, dated June 8, 2020.

pharmaceutical products intended to treat or prevent serious diseases or conditions. FDA may grant fast track product and breakthrough-therapy designation at the sponsor's request for products that are intended to fill an unmet need or improve on existing therapies. Both designations entitle the sponsor to increased communication with FDA regarding the clinical trial design and data collected, as well as rolling review of the BLA. Products may also qualify for accelerated approval based on intermediate or surrogate endpoints likely to predict a clinical benefit. In addition, FDA may designate products for priority review.

In certain emergency situations, FDA may temporarily authorize the use of unapproved products or approved products for unapproved uses through an emergency use authorization (EUA). For FDA to issue an EUA, the Secretary of Health and Human Services (HHS) must determine (1) that a qualifying emergency exists caused by a biological, chemical, radiological, or nuclear (BCRN) agent and (2) that the BCRN agent can cause a serious or life-threatening disease. The Secretary, through FDA, must also determine for each product that (3) it is reasonable to believe, based on the totality of the evidence available, that the product may treat or prevent the disease caused by the BCRN agent and that the known and potential benefits outweigh the known and potential risks, and (4) there are no approved, adequate, and available alternatives. If FDA issues an EUA, the product may be marketed and used for the authorized use while the emergency persists unless FDA revokes the EUA. FDA may also modify or waive good manufacturing practice and prescription requirements when issuing an EUA.

FDA approval of a vaccine allows for its marketing, but does not guarantee that the vaccine will be widely available or affordable. Because patents grant inventors the exclusive rights in a patented invention, patents may influence COVID-19 vaccine affordability and access. Federal agencies and funding support many of the COVID-19 vaccine candidates in development, which may affect the allocation and scope of patent rights. The Bayh-Dole Act allows a federal contractor to obtain the patent on a federally funded invention, but the government retains a free license to use the invention and may "march in" to grant patent licenses to third-party manufacturers in limited circumstances. If federal support is provided through an "other transaction" agreement, however, the allocation of patent rights will depend on the terms of that contract.

The federal government has several authorities that it could exercise should patent rights limit the affordability of or access to a COVID-19 vaccine. For vaccines developed with federal funding or support, the government may secure up-front guarantees on pricing or distribution via funding or purchasing contracts with vaccine developers. For vaccines protected by patents subject to the Bayh-Dole Act, the funding agency could seek to invoke march-in rights to enable other producers to manufacture the vaccine. For any U.S. patent, the federal government could use its "eminent domain" powers under 28 U.S.C. § 1498, which allows the government to make and use patented inventions without license—so long as the use is by or for the United States and compensation is provided to the patent holder. As U.S. patent rights are a creation of Congress, targeted legislation is another option, subject to the constraints of the U.S. Constitution and international treaties.

A COVID-19 vaccine is likely to be subject to specialized rules limiting legal liability under the Public Readiness and Emergency Preparedness (PREP) Act. To encourage the expeditious development and deployment of medical countermeasures, the Secretary of HHS has declared COVID-19 to be a public health emergency and invoked the PREP Act to limit liability for losses relating to the use of covered medical countermeasures during the public health emergency. Under HHS's declaration, covered persons—including COVID-19 vaccine developers, manufacturers, distributors, and health care professionals who administer a vaccine—are generally immune from legal liability for losses relating to administration or use of an FDA-approved COVID-19 vaccine, except for willful misconduct resulting in death or serious physical injury. However, individuals who are injured or die as a result of receiving a COVID-19 vaccine may seek compensation through the Countermeasures Injury Compensation Program, a regulatory process administered by HHS.

INTRODUCTION

Around the world, private companies, universities, and governmental entities are rapidly working to develop a vaccine for coronavirus disease 2019 (COVID-19).[1] In the United States alone, private industry and universities are developing and testing dozens of COVID-19 vaccine candidates,[2] often in collaboration with federal agencies and/or supported by federal funding. For example, the Biomedical Advanced Research and

---

[1] *See Draft Landscape of COVID-19 Candidate Vaccines*, WORLD HEALTH ORGANIZATION (June 2, 2020), https://www.who.int/who-documents-detail/draft-landscape-of-covid-19-candidate-vaccines (listing 133 COVID-19 vaccine candidates in various stages of development worldwide); Jeff Craven, *COVID-19 Vaccine Tracker*, REG. AFF. PROFS. SOC'Y (June 1, 2020), https://www.raps.org/news-and-articles/news-articles/2020/3/covid-19-vaccine-tracker (tracking COVID-19 vaccine candidates currently in clinical trials).

[2] *See* Tung Thanh Le et al., *The COVID-19 Vaccine Development Landscape*, NATURE REV. DRUG DISCOVERY (Apr. 9, 2020), https://www.nature.com/articles/d41573-020-00073-5 (breaking down COVID-19 vaccine candidates by geographical location of lead developer).

Development Authority (BARDA) has partnered with Janssen Pharmaceuticals (a Johnson & Johnson subsidiary) and Sanofi to help develop and scale up manufacturing capacity for each company's COVID-19 vaccine candidate.[3] Together with the National Institute of Allergy and Infectious Diseases (NIAID), BARDA is also collaborating with Moderna to support the development of its COVID- 19 vaccine candidate.[4]

More generally, the Trump Administration recently announced the creation of a program called Operation Warp Speed, which seeks to use coordinated government support to accelerate the development, manufacturing, and distribution of COVID-19 vaccines and other medical countermeasures.[5] With respect to vaccines, the program initially selected fourteen promising vaccine candidates, which was subsequently narrowed to five candidates.[6] Under Operation Warp Speed, the federal government is investing in scaling up manufacturing and distribution for selected COVID-19 vaccine candidates "at risk" (that is, before safety and efficacy is demonstrated).[7] For example, under the program, BARDA has entered into agreements to accelerate the development and manufacturing of a vaccine candidate being developed by the University of Oxford and AstraZeneca.[8]

---

[3] *See* Press Release, U.S. Department of Health and Human Services, HHS, Janssen Join Forces On Coronavirus Vaccine (Feb. 11, 2020), https://www.hhs.gov/about/news/2020/02/11/hhs-janssen-join-forces-on-coronavirus- vaccine.html; Press Release, U.S. Department of Health and Human Services, HHS Engages Sanofi's Recombinant Technology for 2019 Novel Coronavirus Vaccine (Feb. 18, 2020), https://www.hhs.gov/about/news/2020/02/18/hhs-engages-sanofis-recombinant-technology-for-2019-novel-coronavirus-vaccine.html.

[4] *See* Press Release, U.S. Department of Health and Human Services, HHS Accelerates Clinical Trials, Prepares for Manufacturing of COVID-19 Vaccines (Mar. 30, 2020).

[5] *See* Press Release, U.S. Department of Health and Human Services, Trump Administration Announces Framework and Leadership for "Operation Warp Speed" (May 15, 2020), https://www.hhs.gov/about/news/2020/05/15/trump- administration-announces-framework-and-leadership-for-operation-warp-speed.html.

[6] *See* Noah Weiland & David E. Sanger, *Trump Administration Selects Five Coronavirus Vaccine Candidates as Finalists*, N.Y. TIMES (June 3, 2020), https://www.nytimes.com/2020/06/03/us/politics/coronavirus-vaccine-trump- moderna.html. The five candidates are vaccines being developed by (1) Moderna/NIAID; (2) University of Oxford/AstraZeneca; (3) Johnson & Johnson; (4) Merck; and (5) Pfizer/BioNTech. *See id.*

[7] *See* Jennifer Jacobs and Drew Armstrong, *Trump's 'Operation Warp Speed' Aims to Rush Coronavirus Vaccine*, BLOOMBERG (Apr. 29, 2020), https://www.bloomberg.com/news/articles/2020-04-29/trump-s-operation-warp-speed- aims-to-rush-coronavirus-vaccine.

[8] Press Release, U.S. Department of Health and Human Services, Trump Administration's Operation Warp Speed Accelerates AstraZeneca COVID-19 Vaccine to be Available

This chapter overviews certain legal issues in COVID-19 vaccine development, testing, licensing, production, and administration, focusing on three areas: (1) vaccine testing, authorization, and licensure by the U.S. Food and Drug Administration (FDA); (2) patent and other intellectual property (IP) rights that may protect a COVID-19 vaccine; and (3) liability and compensation issues for individuals harmed by the testing or administration of a vaccine.

First, this chapter explains the existing legal requirements for clinical trials and FDA authorization or licensure of new vaccines, including different options to accelerate those processes. Second, it analyzes who might own the patent rights in a potential COVID-19 vaccine, and the federal government's legal options should patent rights restrict the affordability or availability of a vaccine. Third, it reviews the protections from legal liability available to vaccine developers, manufacturers, administrators, and health care professionals under the Public Readiness and Emergency Preparedness (PREP) Act.

FDA LAW CONSIDERATIONS: BRINGING A NEW VACCINE TO MARKET

Vaccines are intended to prevent diseases and generally work by introducing pathogens to the human body (usually by injection) to trigger an immune response to the disease (i.e., producing antibodies to the pathogen).[9] Vaccines are biological products approved and regulated by FDA's Center for Biologics Evaluation and Research (CBER) under

---

Beginning in October (May 21, 2020), https://www.hhs.gov/about/news/2020/05/21/trump-administration-accelerates-astrazeneca-covid-19-vaccine-to-be-available-beginning-in-october.html.

9 *Vaccines: The Basics*, CTRS. FOR DISEASE CONTROL & PREVENTION, https://www.cdc.gov/vaccines/vpd/vpd-vac- basics.html (last updated Mar. 14, 2012); *Understanding How Vaccines Work*, CTRS. FOR DISEASE CONTROL & PREVENTION, https://www.cdc.gov/vaccines/hcp/conversations/understanding-vacc-work.html (last updated Aug. 17, 2018).

Section 351 of the Public Health Service Act (PHSA).[10] A biologic such as a vaccine generally cannot be introduced into commerce unless FDA approves it.[11] To be approved, FDA must determine that the vaccine is safe, potent, and pure based on data from laboratory studies and clinical trials.[12] This section discusses the legal framework for developing, testing, and licensing (i.e., approving) new vaccines under the PHSA and the Federal Food, Drug, and Cosmetic Act (FD&C Act), as well as existing legal avenues that would allow that process to be expedited to bring a new vaccine to market sooner.

Clinical Trials of Investigational New Drugs

Sponsors use clinical trials to generate the data needed to obtain FDA approval to market their products. Because clinical trials expose human subjects to unapproved pharmaceutical products, they risk causing unanticipated serious adverse side effects in the participants. To manage these risks, the FD&C Act and FDA regulations have imposed procedural requirements, such as advance and ongoing scientific and ethical review, on clinical trials to help protect the participants by minimizing risks, requiring informed consent, and ensuring that the studies collect the data needed to determine whether to approve the product.

Using Clinical Trials to Collect Substantial Evidence

Sponsors must submit "substantial evidence" to FDA that their products are safe and effective (or safe, potent, and pure) to obtain FDA approval.[13] Section 505(d) of the FD&C Act defines substantial evidence to mean adequately and well-controlled investigations on the basis of

---

[10] 42 U.S.C. § 262; *Vaccine Product Approval Process,* U.S. FOOD & DRUG ADMIN., https://www.fda.gov/vaccines-blood-biologics/development-approval-process-cber/vaccine-product-approval-process (last updated Jan. 30, 2018) [hereinafter *FDA Vaccine Approval Process*].

[11] 42 U.S.C. § 262(a)(1).

[12] *Id.* § 262(a)(2); 21 C.F.R. § 601.2.

[13] 21 U.S.C. § 355(d).

which qualified scientific experts could fairly and responsibly conclude that the product has the purported effect.[14] FDA assesses both the quality and quantity of the data provided when determining whether a product meets this standard.[15]

Quality refers to the strength of the evidence and the amount of certainty it provides as to the product's safety and effectiveness—that is, whether the investigation is "adequate" and "well- controlled."[16] The quality of the evidence depends on how the clinical trial is designed and how the study is conducted.[17] Under FDA regulations, the design must allow for a valid comparison of the product to a control, such as a placebo, an existing therapy, or no treatment.[18] FDA also evaluates whether the study's method for selecting participants and assigning them to groups is adequate to ensure that meaningful data are collected.[19] The methodology must also include a well-defined and reliable means of assessing the participants' responses and explain the analytical and statistical methods used to assess the results.[20] Finally, sponsors must provide a clear statement of the investigation's objectives and take adequate measures to minimize bias in the study.[21] FDA may, however, waive any of these criteria for a specific investigation if the sponsor can show that the criteria are not reasonably applicable to the study and an alternative approach yields substantial evidence of effectiveness.[22] FDA guidance further clarifies how sponsors should select their clinical trial design, endpoints, and statistical methods.[23]

As for quantity, FDA generally requires that sponsors complete two "adequate and well- controlled clinical investigations" to meet the

---

[14] *Id.*

[15] U.S. FOOD & DRUG ADMIN., DEMONSTRATING SUBSTANTIAL EVIDENCE OF EFFECTIVENESS FOR HUMAN DRUG AND BIOLOGICAL PRODUCTS: DRAFT GUIDANCE FOR INDUSTRY 3 (Dec. 2019), https://www.fda.gov/media/133660/download [hereinafter DEMONSTRATING SUBSTANTIAL EVIDENCE].

[16] *Id.* at 5.

[17] 21 C.F.R. § 314.126.

[18] *Id.* § 314.126(b)(2).

[19] *Id.* § 314.126(b)(3) & (4).

[20] *Id.* § 314.126(b)(6) & (7).

[21] *Id.* § 314.126(b)(1) & (5).

[22] *Id.* § 314.126(c).

[23] DEMONSTRATING SUBSTANTIAL EVIDENCE, *supra* note 15, at 5.

substantial evidence standard.[24] FDA notes in its guidance that completing two studies, particularly if they are designed and conducted differently, reduces the likelihood of a design flaw, bias, or other issue or anomaly that could result in erroneous conclusions.[25] However, under the Food and Drug Modernization Act of 1997,[26] FDA may allow sponsors to rely on one large multicenter adequate and well-controlled clinical investigation supported by another form of additional data,[27] such as data regarding the effectiveness of other drugs in the same pharmacological class.[28] In deciding whether to allow a sponsor to rely on a single study, FDA states that it considers, among other factors, the seriousness of the disease, whether there is an unmet medical need, and whether additional trials would be ethical and practicable.[29]

Given the flexibility afforded sponsors in designing and conducting their clinical trials, FDA uses written guidance and individual meetings to help sponsors ensure that their investigations will generate the substantial evidence needed for approval.[30] Sponsors that obtain fast track product or breakthrough therapy designation for their products are entitled to additional assistance from and communication with FDA staff to craft efficient and effective clinical trial designs.[31]

Submitting an Investigational New Drug Application to FDA

New drugs and biological products that are being tested in clinical trials are referred to as investigational new drugs.[32] Section 505(i) of the FD&C Act, Section 351(a)(3) of the PHSA, and their implementing regulations allow investigational new drugs to be used for research before they are approved.[33] To conduct clinical trials of investigational new drugs,

[24] *Id.* at 8.
[25] *Id.* at 9-10.
[26] Pub. L. No. 105-115 § 115, 111 Stat. 2313 (1997).
[27] 21 U.S.C. § 355(d).
[28] DEMONSTRATING SUBSTANTIAL EVIDENCE, *supra* note 15, at 12.
[29] *Id.* at 10.
[30] *See, e.g.*, 21 C.F.R. § 312.47; DEMONSTRATING SUBSTANTIAL EVIDENCE, *supra* note 15.
[31] *See* "Shortening the Development and Review Processes."
[32] 21 C.F.R. § 312.3.
[33] 21 U.S.C. § 355(i); 42 U.S.C. § 262(a)(3); 21 C.F.R. § 312.2(a).

the company developing the product (i.e., sponsor) must generally receive FDA approval for the investigation and comply with regulatory requirements for human subjects research.[34]

Sponsors obtain FDA approval to test an investigational new drug on human subjects through an investigational new drug application (IND).[35] The IND gives FDA an opportunity to ensure that the study will protect the safety and rights of its human subjects and gather scientific data that adequately show the product's safety and effectiveness.[36] The sponsor may begin its clinical trials 30 days after submitting an IND unless FDA notifies the sponsor that it is either (1) authorizing the IND and the study can begin immediately or (2) imposing a clinical hold due to concerns about the study.[37] If FDA imposes a clinical hold, the study cannot begin (or resume, for ongoing investigations) pending further notification.[38]

FDA regulations prescribe the information that sponsors must include in an IND.[39] The IND must contain information about the product, such as the substance and formulation; existing data on use in animals or humans if available; and anticipated risks and side effects.[40] The IND must also contain a general investigational plan, which explains why the sponsor is undertaking the study and includes, among other things, the indications being studied, the sponsor's approach to evaluating the product, the kinds of clinical trials being conducted, the anticipated number of participants, and any anticipated risks.[41] Along with the general investigational plan, the IND must include specific protocols for each clinical trial phase.[42] The sponsor must also generally certify that an institutional review board (IRB) will provide initial and continuing review of each study, including the

---

[34] *See generally* 21 C.F.R. Parts 50, 56, & 312.

[35] 21 C.F.R. § 312.20; *Investigational New Drug (IND) Application*, U.S. FOOD & DRUG ADMIN., https://www.fda.gov/drugs/types-applications/investigational-new-drug-ind-application (last updated May 12, 2020).

[36] 21 C.F.R. § 312.22.

[37] *Id.* §§ 312.40 & 312.42.

[38] *Id.* § 312.42(a) & (e).

[39] *Id.* § 312.23.

[40] *Id.*

[41] *Id.*

[42] *Id.*

proposed protocols and any subsequent changes to the study.[43] FDA may, however, waive any IRB requirements, including the requirement of IRB review itself.[44]

Institutional Review Board Review and Approval

An IRB is a group convened by an institution to review and approve biomedical research involving humans.[45] IRBs evaluate the initial clinical study design and protocols, along with any changes implemented during the investigation, in an effort to ensure that the rights and well-being of the human subjects are protected.[46] To that end, IRBs assess whether risks to the participants are minimized and reasonable in relation to the anticipated benefits, both to the participants directly and from the knowledge expected to be gained through the study.[47] IRBs also aim to ensure that the researchers will obtain adequate informed consent from all participants (unless an exemption applies) and that selection of the participants will be equitable.[48] IRBs may also require (as appropriate) that the research plan provide for monitoring of the collected data to protect the participants' safety and privacy.[49] To the extent the study may include participants from populations that may be vulnerable to coercion or undue influence (e.g., children, prisoners), IRBs must ensure that sufficient safeguards are in place to protect these populations in participant selection and during the clinical trials.[50]

IRBs review clinical trial plans and protocols from various standpoints, including ensuring that the study complies with legal, ethical, and professional standards; is scientifically sound; and is free from illicit discrimination. Accordingly, to ensure adequate and independent review, IRBs must have at least five members from multiple backgrounds, including at least one member with a scientific background and at least one

---

[43] *Id.*
[44] 21 C.F.R. § 56.105(c).
[45] *Id.* § 56.102(g).
[46] *Id.*
[47] *Id.* § 56.111(a)(1)-(2).
[48] *Id.* § 56.111(a)(3)-(5).
[49] *Id.* § 56.111(a)(6)-(7).
[50] *Id.* § 56.111(b) & (c).

with a nonscientific background.[51] At least one member must be independent from the institution running the clinical trials, and the IRB members cannot have any financial or other conflicting interests in the project.[52] IRB review must comply with any other requirements relating to IRBs and human subject research found in Parts 50 and 56 of Chapter 21 of the Code of Federal Regulation.

Clinical Trial Phases

Clinical trials for a new pharmaceutical product generally proceed in three phases, transitioning from smaller trials focused on initial safety early on to larger trials assessing safety and effectiveness to inform approval and labeling.[53] The size, duration, and specific purpose of each clinical trial phase varies from product to product depending on such factors as the type of product (e.g., a vaccine, treatment, or preventative medication), how the product works, and the relevant underlying patient population. However, as defined by FDA regulations, a clinical investigation generally proceeds as follows:

- *Phase 1 Trials.* Phase 1 trials are the first time the product is introduced in human subjects.[54] These carefully controlled trials typically involve 20 to 80 patients or volunteer subjects, though the exact numbers may vary depending on the product.[55] Phase 1 trials generally assess how the product acts in the body and evaluate initial safety (i.e., side effects).[56] They may also be used to determine the dosing levels to use in phase 2 (e.g., the maximum safe dose or what dose is required to have an effect).[57] Depending on the product, phase 1 trials may also provide some initial indication as to whether the product may be effective.[58] In

[51] *Id.* § 56.107(a)-(c).
[52] *Id.* § 56.107(d)-(e).
[53] *Id.* § 312.21.
[54] *Id.* § 312.21(a).
[55] *Id.*
[56] *Id.*
[57] *Id.*
[58] *Id.*

the case of vaccines specifically, phase 1 trials also assess their ability to provoke an immune response in the body (i.e., immunogenicity).[59]

- *Phase 2 Trials.* Phase 2 trials continue to assess safety but also evaluate the product's effectiveness and common short-term side effects or other risks associated with the product.[60] Phase 2 trials are also used to determine the optimal dose of the product.[61] For vaccines, phase 2 assesses how much of the vaccine to administer and on what dosing schedule (e.g., whether a boost is needed to maximize its effectiveness or whether the vaccine must be administered on a regular schedule to maintain immunity).[62] As with phase 1 studies, phase 2 studies are carefully controlled.[63] However, phase 2 involves a larger (though still relatively limited) number of volunteer subjects—generally no more than a few hundred participants.[64]
- *Phase 3 Trials.* Phase 3 trials involve an expanded number of participants—from several hundred to thousands—and are used to assess the product's safety and effectiveness across a wide range of patient categories through controlled and uncontrolled studies.[65] These trials are intended to present a clearer picture of expected risks and benefits under real-world conditions.[66] The information obtained from phase 3 trials also forms the basis for the product's labeling.[67]

---

[59] *FDA Vaccine Approval Process*, *supra* note 10.
[60] 21 C.F.R. § 312.21(b).
[61] *See, e.g.*, Kert Viele & Jason T. Connor, *Dose Finding Trials: Optimizing Phase 2 Data in the Drug Development Process*, 314 J. AM. MED. ASS'N 2294, 2294 (2015), https://jamanetwork.com/journals/jama/fullarticle/2473474.
[62] *FDA Vaccine Approval Process*, *supra* note 10.
[63] 21 C.F.R. § 312.21(b).
[64] *Id.*
[65] *Id.* § 312.21(c).
[66] *Id.*
[67] *Id.*

Sponsors must generally complete all three phases to obtain FDA approval unless they obtain accelerated approval,[68] in which case FDA requires postapproval trials to confirm the expected clinical benefit.[69] FDA may also require, at its discretion, additional clinical trials after approval (i.e., phase 4 trials) for any approved product to continue assessing the product's safety and effectiveness once on the market.[70]

Considerations for Congress

The current legal framework seeks to balance various competing interests, which may be amplified in the current crisis. The FD&C Act and implementing regulations provide standards and factors to consider but otherwise give FDA and IRBs discretion to evaluate investigational plans and clinical trial protocols for investigational new drugs. FDA may also waive requirements relating to IRB review and clinical trial design. To the extent Congress may seek to direct how FDA and IRBs exercise that discretion with respect to any potential COVID-19 vaccine, Congress could consider implementing legislation that provides more specific direction on how to approach clinical trials either specifically for the current COVID-19 pandemic or in epidemic, pandemic, or other emergency situations more generally. For example, courts have determined that Congress can cabin FDA's discretion by imposing mandatory (e.g., "shall") rather than permissive (e.g., "may") language in a statute.[71]

In light of the multiple companies involved in developing potential COVID-19 vaccines, Congress could also consider facilitating the coordination of any clinical trials or appointing a neutral scientific body to consider the ethical and scientific considerations and generate guidelines or a master protocol. The World Health Organization (WHO) employed this approach to facilitate development of an Ebola vaccine following the 2014

---

[68] *Accelerated Approval*, U.S. FOOD & DRUG ADMIN., https://www.fda.gov/patients/fast-track-breakthrough-therapy-accelerated-approval-priority-review/accelerated-approval (last updated Jan. 4, 2018).

[69] DEMONSTRATING SUBSTANTIAL EVIDENCE, *supra* note 15, at 2.

[70] 21 C.F.R. § 312.85.

[71] *See, e.g.*, Cook v. FDA, 733 F.3d 1, 8 (D.C. Cir. 2013).

to 2016 Ebola epidemic.[72] Congress could also direct or fund increased global collaboration between regulators to promote information sharing, which could potentially result in more streamlined clinical investigations with fewer participants being exposed to investigational vaccines.[73] Congress could also consider providing additional funding or other resources to facilitate the clinical trials themselves or any research directed toward understanding the SARS-CoV-2 virus or COVID-19 disease to allow for improved risk minimization in future clinical trials.

FDA Approval and Options for Bringing a New Vaccine to Market Faster

If the clinical trials are successful, the sponsor may seek FDA approval to market its new vaccine. FDA approves new vaccines through biologics license applications (BLAs) reviewed by CBER.[74] BLAs contain data from the laboratory and clinical studies and information about how and where the biologic will be manufactured.[75] As courts have recognized, FDA exercises its scientific judgment when deciding whether to license vaccines based on such studies.[76] Biologics that are approved through a BLA receive 12 years of regulatory exclusivity, during which time FDA cannot approve any biosimilars (i.e., abbreviated applications for the same

[72] WORLD HEALTH ORG., WHO R&D BLUEPRINT – AD-HOC WORKSHOP ON EBOLA VACCINES: DELIBERATIONS ON DESIGN OPTIONS FOR CLINICAL TRIALS TO ASSESS THE SAFETY AND EFFICACY OF INVESTIGATIONAL EBOLA VACCINES (Jan. 23, 2019), https://www.who.int/docs/default-source/blue-print/ebola-vaccine-meeting-report.pdf?sfvrsn=9dd492f4_2.

[73] *See, e.g.*, *Summary of FDA & EMA Global Regulators Meeting on Data Requirements Supporting First-in-Human Clinical Trials with SARS-CoV-2 Vaccines*, U.S. FOOD & DRUG ADMIN., https://www.fda.gov/news-events/fda-meetings-conferences-and-workshops/summary-fda-ema-global-regulators-meeting-data-requirements-supporting-first-human-clinical-trials (last updated Mar. 18, 2020).

[74] 21 U.S.C. § 262(a); *FDA Vaccine Approval Process*, *supra* note 10. For additional information about the biologics licensing process, see CRS Report R45666, *Drug Pricing and Intellectual Property Law: A Legal Overview for the 116th Congress*, coordinated by Kevin J. Hickey, at 17-27.

[75] 21 C.F.R. § 601.2.

[76] Rempfer v. Sharfstein, 583 F.3d 860, 868 (D.C. Cir. 2009).

biologic that depend on the clinical data in the BLA to demonstrate safety, potency, and purity).[77]

The process of developing and testing a new vaccine to the point where it meets the safety, purity, and potency standard can be a lengthy process. The FD&C Act provides several options that may allow a sponsor to bring a new vaccine to market faster.[78] Generally, these options use one of two approaches. First, FDA can direct more of its resources to the product to accelerate the development and/or review processes (e.g., fast track product designation, breakthrough therapy designation, and priority review). Second, FDA can modify how it evaluates the risks and benefits of the vaccine before allowing its use, either by relying on different types of evidence (e.g., the accelerated approval process) or lowering the evidentiary standard in emergency situations (e.g., emergency use authorization). (For ease of reference, this section uses the general term "biologic" because vaccines are biological products, but the pathways discussed below are also available for traditional small molecule drugs.)

Shortening the Development and Review Processes

Several avenues are available for expediting the development and review processes for biologics used to treat or prevent serious or life-threatening conditions and diseases. In its guidance, FDA generally considers a condition or disease *serious* if it substantially affects day-to-day functioning and is irreversible, persistent, or recurrent.[79] A condition or disease may be found to be serious as a matter of clinical judgment based on its effect on survival, day-to-day functioning, or the likelihood that it will progress to a more serious condition if left untreated.[80] As a matter of course, FDA considers any life-threatening condition or disease to be

---

[77] 21 U.S.C. § 262(k)(7)(A).

[78] *See generally* 21 U.S.C. § 356.

[79] U.S. FOOD & DRUG ADMIN., GUIDANCE FOR INDUSTRY: EXPEDITED PROGRAMS FOR SERIOUS CONDITIONS – DRUGS AND BIOLOGICS 2-3 (2014), https://www.fda.gov/media/86377/download [hereinafter EXPEDITED PROGRAMS FOR SERIOUS CONDITIONS: FDA GUIDANCE].

[80] 21 C.F.R. § 312.300(b)(1).

serious.[81] The drug must also be intended to *treat* the serious condition or disease by having an effect on the disease itself or a serious aspect of the disease, such as a symptom or other manifestation.[82] Among the examples FDA provides in its guidance is a product intended to *prevent* the serious condition.[83] Given that COVID-19 is life threatening, a vaccine intended to prevent COVID-19 seems likely to qualify as a drug used to treat or prevent a serious or life-threatening condition or disease— making it eligible for the following designations to accelerate the approval process.

Fast Track Product Designation

Section 506 of the FD&C Act allows FDA to designate certain biologics as fast track products, which receive FDA assistance in expediting development and review.[84] A biologic may be designated as a fast track product if FDA determines that the biologic will treat or prevent a serious or life-threatening disease or condition and fill an unmet medical need.[85] An unmet medical need exists when available therapies do not adequately address treating or diagnosing a condition or disease.[86] FDA recognizes in its guidance that an unmet medical need necessarily exists if there is no available therapy.[87] Sponsors may provide FDA with nonclinical or clinical data to demonstrate that the drug has the potential to fill that unmet medical need.[88] Given that there are no approved vaccines for COVID-19, any vaccine that showed potential to prevent COVID-19 in laboratory or clinical trials would seem likely to qualify for fast track designation. On May 12, 2020, FDA designated Moderna's COVID-19 vaccine as a fast track product after it completed its Phase 1 trials.[89]

---

[81] EXPEDITED PROGRAMS FOR SERIOUS CONDITIONS: FDA GUIDANCE, *supra* note 79, at 3.

[82] *Id.*

[83] *Id.*

[84] 21 U.S.C. § 356(b).

[85] *Id.*

[86] EXPEDITED PROGRAMS FOR SERIOUS CONDITIONS: FDA GUIDANCE, *supra* note 79, at 4.

[87] *Id.* at 5.

[88] *Id.* at 9.

[89] Press Release, Moderna, Moderna Receives FDA Fast Track Designation for mRNA Vaccine (mRNA-1273) Against Novel Coronavirus (May 12, 2020), https://investors.modernatx.

At its discretion, the biologic's sponsor requests fast track designation for its product.[90] It may request fast track designation when it submits an IND or any time thereafter.[91] FDA has 60 days to determine if the biologic qualifies for the designation.[92] Once FDA designates a biologic as a fast track product, FDA must facilitate its development and expedite review of the biologic.[93] In practice, this process generally means that the biologic's sponsor has greater access to FDA through written and in-person communications during the development and testing process to improve efficiency and ensure that appropriate data are collected.[94] FDA may also review the BLA for a fast track product on a rolling basis as sections are complete (rather than waiting for a completed application) if initial clinical testing shows the biologic may be effective.[95]

Breakthrough Therapy Designation

Section 506 of the FD&C Act also allows FDA to designate certain biologics as breakthrough therapies, which similarly heightens FDA involvement in the development and review process.[96] Breakthrough therapy designation is based on preliminary clinical evidence showing the biologic may be a substantial improvement over available therapies for one or more clinically significant endpoints.[97] Endpoints measure the outcome of a clinical trial.[98] Under FDA guidance, a clinically significant endpoint

---

com/news-releases/news-release-details/moderna- receives-fda-fast-track-designation-mrna-vaccine-mrna.

[90] 21 U.S.C. § 356(b)(2).

[91] *Id.*

[92] *Id.* § 356(b)(3).

[93] *Id.*

[94] EXPEDITED PROGRAMS FOR SERIOUS CONDITIONS: FDA GUIDANCE, *supra* note 79, at 9; *Fast Track*, U.S. FOOD & DRUG ADMIN., https://www.fda.gov/patients/fast-track-breakthrough-therapy-accelerated-approval-priority-review/fast- track (last updated Jan. 4, 2018).

[95] EXPEDITED PROGRAMS FOR SERIOUS CONDITIONS: FDA GUIDANCE, *supra* note 79, at 10; U.S. Food & Drug Admin., Fast Track (Jan. 4, 2018), https://www.fda.gov/patients/fast-track-breakthrough-therapy-accelerated-approval-priority-review/fast-track.

[96] 21 U.S.C. § 356(a).

[97] *Id.* § 356(a)(1).

[98] *Surrogate Endpoint Resources for Drug and Biologic Development*, U.S. FOOD & DRUG ADMIN., https://www.fda.gov/drugs/development-resources/surrogate-endpoint-resources-drug-and-biologic-development (la updated July 24, 2018).

generally measures an effect on irreversible morbidity or mortality or on symptoms representing serious consequences of the disease or condition.[99] Unlike fast track product designation, which can be based on laboratory data, breakthrough therapy designation requires evidence from clinical trials.[100] FDA exercises its judgment in determining whether the data show a substantial improvement over existing therapies, taking into consideration both the magnitude of the biologic's effects on the endpoint and the importance of the effect measured by that endpoint to treating the disease or condition.[101] When there are no existing therapies, such as with a COVID-19 vaccine, FDA compares the biologic to a placebo or well-documented historical control.[102] A COVID-19 vaccine may be eligible for breakthrough therapy designation if the sponsor can demonstrate potential effectiveness in early clinical trials.

At its discretion, the sponsor requests breakthrough therapy designation and may do so with submission of an IND or at any time thereafter.[103] FDA must determine whether the biologic qualifies as a breakthrough therapy within 60 days of receipt.[104] As with fast track product designation, the FD&C Act directs FDA to expedite the development and review of applications for breakthrough therapies.[105] Per FDA guidance, expedited development and review of breakthrough therapies entails (1) intensive assistance from FDA on efficient development and clinical trial design; (2) organizational commitment from FDA, including senior management and experienced staff; (3) rolling review of the BLA; and (4) other actions to expedite review, such as priority review discussed below.[106] Extensive FDA assistance during the development process and the involvement of senior managers distinguishes breakthrough therapy designation from fast track product designation.

---

[99] EXPEDITED PROGRAMS FOR SERIOUS CONDITIONS: FDA GUIDANCE, *supra* note 79, at 12.

[100] *Id.* at 11-12; *compare* 21 U.S.C. § 356(a)(1), *with id.* § 356(b)(1).

[101] EXPEDITED PROGRAMS FOR SERIOUS CONDITIONS, *supra* note 79, at 12.

[102] *Id.*

[103] 21 U.S.C. § 356(a)(2).

[104] *Id.* § 356(a)(3)(A).

[105] *Id.* § 356(a)(3)(B).

[106] EXPEDITED PROGRAMS FOR SERIOUS CONDITIONS: FDA GUIDANCE, *supra* note 79, at 13-15.

Accelerated Approval

Section 506 of the FD&C Act also allows FDA to approve certain biologics based on surrogate or intermediate endpoints, referred to as accelerated approval.[107] In general, sponsors select endpoints that directly measure the clinical outcome (i.e., the benefits expected from the biologic), such as whether the patient feels better or lives longer.[108] Surrogate and intermediate endpoints do not measure the clinical benefit directly but instead measure an effect that is expected to predict a clinical benefit.[109] For example, a drug to treat strokes would have an intended clinical outcome of reducing the incidence or severity of strokes.[110] But rather than measuring the incidence of strokes directly, an investigator might measure the drug's effect on blood pressure as a surrogate endpoint due to the strong correlation between strokes and blood pressure.[111]

To qualify for accelerated approval, (1) the biologic must treat a serious or life-threatening condition or disease and (2) FDA must determine that the biologic has an effect on a surrogate or intermediate endpoint that is reasonably likely to predict a clinical benefit. When deciding whether to approve a biologic on this basis, FDA must consider how severe, rare, or prevalent the condition is and the availability of alternative treatments. A vaccine for COVID-19 could qualify for accelerated approval if investigators identified a surrogate or intermediate endpoint that could reasonably predict the vaccine would be effective against the virus.

---

[107] 21 U.S.C. § 356(c); *see also Accelerated Approval*, U.S. FOOD & DRUG ADMIN., https://www.fda.gov/patients/fast-track-breakthrough-therapy-accelerated-approval-priority-review/accelerated-approval (updated Jan. 4, 2018).

[108] *See Surrogate Endpoint Resources for Drug and Biologic Development*, U.S. FOOD & DRUG ADMIN., https://www.fda.gov/drugs/development-resources/surrogate-endpoint-resources-drug-and-biologic-development (last updated July 24, 2018).

[109] *Id.*

[110] *Id.*

[111] *Id.*

Priority Review

Once a BLA is submitted, FDA can designate the BLA for standard review or priority review.[112] FDA aims to act on priority review applications within 6 months, compared to 10 months or more for standard review applications.[113] FDA makes this determination for every application, though a sponsor can expressly request priority review.[114] FDA may designate a BLA for priority review if it represents a "significant improvement" over existing treatments in terms of safety or effectiveness in treating, diagnosing, or preventing the disease or condition.[115] In the absence of any approved vaccine for COVID-19, FDA would likely designate for priority review any BLA for such a vaccine.

Emergency Use Authorizations before Approval

In certain emergency situations, Section 564 of the FD&C Act allows FDA to authorize the use of a drug or biologic (e.g., a vaccine) before it is approved (i.e., an Emergency Use Authorization or EUA).[116] FDA may issue an EUA only if the Secretary of Health and Human Services (HHS) has declared that circumstances exist justifying emergency authorized use of the medical product.[117] Of relevance to the COVID-19 pandemic, on February 4, 2020, the Secretary determined that there is a public health emergency that has a significant potential to affect national security or the health and security of U.S. citizens living abroad, and that involves a biological, chemical, radiological, or nuclear agent (BCRN agent)—

---

[112] Prescription Drug User Fee Act of 1992, Pub. L. No. 102-571, 106 Stat. 4491 (1992); *Priority Review*, U.S. FOOD & DRUG ADMIN., https://www.fda.gov/patients/fast-track-breakthrough-therapy-accelerated-approval-priority- review/priority-review. (last updated Jan. 4, 2018) [hereinafter *Priority Review*].

[113] *Priority Review*, *supra* note 112; EXPEDITED PROGRAMS FOR SERIOUS CONDITIONS: FDA GUIDANCE, *supra* note 79, at 24-25.

[114] *Priority Review*, *supra* note 112.

[115] *Priority Review*, *supra* note 112; EXPEDITED PROGRAMS FOR SERIOUS CONDITIONS: FDA GUIDANCE, *supra* note 79, at 24-25.

[116] 21 U.S.C. § 360bbb-3; *see also Emergency Use Authorization*, U.S. FOOD & DRUG ADMIN., https://www.fda.gov/emergency-preparedness-and-response/mcm-legal-regulatory-and-policy-framework/emergency- use-authorization#2019-ncov (last updated May 22, 2020).

[117] *See* 21 U.S.C. § 360bbb-3(b).

namely, the virus that causes COVID-19.[118] Based on this determination, the Secretary has authorized the emergency use of several diagnostic tests.[119] On March 2, 2020, the Secretary determined that circumstances exist to allow for the emergency use of certain respirators not approved by the agency,[120] and FDA issued an EUA allowing for the emergency use of such respirators.[121]

After the Secretary determines a public health emergency exists (one of four bases for declaring an emergency or threat), FDA may issue an EUA for a specific product if the Secretary concludes that

1) the BCRN agent can cause a serious or life-threatening disease or condition;
2) it is reasonable to believe, based on the totality of the scientific evidence available, that
   a) the product may be effective in diagnosing, treating, or preventing the disease or condition caused by the BCRN agent; and
   b) the known and potential benefits of the product outweigh the known and potential risks; and
3) there is no adequate, approved, and available alternative to the product.[122]

---

[118] Alex M. Azar II, Sec'y of the Dep't of Health & Human Servs., Determination of a Public Health Emergency and Declaration that Circumstances Exist Justifying Authorizations Pursuant to Section 564(b) of the Federal Food, Drug, and Cosmetic Act, 21 U.S.C. § 360bbb-3 (Feb. 4, 2020), https://www.fda.gov/media/135010/download.

[119] *See Emergency Use Authorization*, U.S. FOOD & DRUG ADMIN., https://www.fda.gov/emergency-preparedness-and-response/mcm-legal-regulatory-and-policy-framework/emergency-use-authorization#2019-ncov (last updated May 22, 2020).

[120] Alex M. Azar II, Sec'y of the Dep't of Health & Human Servs., Declaration that Circumstances Exist Justifying Authorizations Pursuant to Section 564(b) of the Federal Food, Drug, and Cosmetic Act, 21 U.S.C. § 360bbb-3 (Mar. 2, 2020), https://www.fda.gov/media/135787/download.

[121] Letter from Denise M. Hinton, Chief Scientist, U.S. Food & Drug Admin., to Dr. Redfield, Director, Ctrs. for Disease Control & Prevention (Mar. 28, 2020), https://www.fda.gov/media/135763/download.

[122] 21 U.S.C. § 360bbb-3(c).

In evaluating a product for an EUA, FDA uses a lower evidentiary standard, determining whether the product "may be effective" in diagnosing, treating, or preventing a disease rather than evaluating its "effectiveness" in doing so.[123] As discussed above, COVID-19 is a serious or life- threatening disease, confirmed by the fact that FDA has already issued EUAs in connection with COVID-19 for diagnostic tests and certain personal protective equipment.[124] There is also no alternative to a COVID-19 vaccine at this time.[125] Any decision by FDA to issue an EUA for a COVID-19 vaccine would accordingly depend on whether the totality of the evidence available to FDA shows that it is reasonable to believe that (1) the vaccine may be effective in preventing COVID-19 and (2) those benefits outweigh any known or potential risks from the vaccine. FDA would have to conduct this evaluation for each vaccine that is developed and submitted for an EUA.

The FD&C Act requires FDA to impose certain conditions on EUAs as necessary and appropriate to protect the public health.[126] The conditions vary depending on whether the product is unapproved or approved but for a different use.[127] In general, the conditions provide for monitoring, reporting, and recordkeeping as well as ensuring that the health care professionals administering the product and the individuals being treated with the product are informed about the benefits and risks of using the product.[128] FDA may also waive good manufacturing practices (GMP) and certain prescription requirements when issuing an EUA and may impose conditions related to advertising the product.[129]

---

[123] U.S. FOOD & DRUG ADMIN., EMERGENCY USE AUTHORIZATION OF MEDICAL PRODUCTS AND RELATED AUTHORITIES: GUIDANCE FOR INDUSTRY AND OTHER STAKEHOLDERS 12 (Jan. 2017), https://www.fda.gov/media/97321/download.

[124] *Emergency Use Authorization*, U.S. FOOD & DRUG ADMIN., https://www.fda.gov/emergency-preparedness-and-response/mcm-legal-regulatory-and-policy-framework/emergency-use-authorization#2019-ncov (last updated May 22, 2020).

[125] Press Release, Nat'l Insts. of Health, NIH Clinical Trial of Investigational Vaccine for COVID-19 Begins (Mar. 16, 2020), https://www.nih.gov/news-events/news-releases/nih-clinical-trial-investigational-vaccine-covid-19-begins; *WHO Draft Landscape of COVID-19 Candidate Vaccines*, *supra* note 1.

[126] 21 U.S.C. § 360bbb-3(e).

[127] *Id.* § 360bbb-3(e)(1) & (2).

[128] *Id.*

[129] Id. § 360bbb-3(e)(3) & (4).

Considerations for Congress

The current legal regime for approving new pharmaceutical products such as vaccines generally aims to strike a balance between bringing products to market sooner and ensuring that products on the market are safe and effective. For serious or life-threatening diseases and conditions or in emergency situations, the law gives FDA a certain amount of discretion to shift that balance. FDA generally expedites the process one of two ways: shifting its resources or shifting its standard in evaluating the risks and benefits.

In considering avenues to facilitate the development of a COVID-19 vaccine, Congress has similar options. Congress could consider providing additional resources to FDA to exercise its existing authorities. Congress is already employing this approach: The Coronavirus Preparedness and Response Supplemental Appropriations Act, 2020, enacted on March 6, appropriated $61 million to FDA "to prevent, prepare for, and respond to coronavirus, domestically or internationally, *including the development of necessary medical countermeasures and vaccines*, advanced manufacturing for medical products, the monitoring of medical product supply chains, and related administrative activities."[130] Alternatively, Congress could direct FDA to strike a different balance when evaluating the risks versus the benefits specifically in the context of potential COVID-19 vaccines. In assessing that balance, Congress and FDA would face weighing the benefits from disseminating a vaccine to the public sooner (e.g., limiting the spread of the virus or reducing the economic consequences) against the risk that the vaccine may have been authorized prematurely and prove ineffective or unsafe, potentially leading to worse public health outcomes. Any alteration to this balance that requires FDA to exceed or contradict its existing authority would require an act of Congress to amend the agency's statutory authority.

Should FDA authorize or approve a COVID-19 vaccine, other considerations may come to bear. For example, registered manufacturers may not be able to produce an adequate supply of the vaccine. FDA is

---

[130] Pub. L. No. 116-123, 134 Stat. 146 (2020) (emphasis added).

currently addressing hand sanitizer shortages by exercising its enforcement discretion with respect to production by over-the-counter drug manufacturers and compounders.[131] Congress may consider other avenues for increasing supply of the vaccine. In addition, existence of a vaccine would raise questions of mandatory vaccination to address the public health crisis, which is addressed in a CRS Legal Sidebar.[132]

PATENT RIGHTS IN COVID-19 VACCINES: INCENTIVES, ACCESS, AND AFFORDABILITY

FDA authorization or licensure of a COVID-19 vaccine would permit the manufacturer to market the vaccine, but does not guarantee that the vaccine will be widely available or affordable. A significant factor that may influence COVID-19 vaccine affordability and access is the existence and allocation of IP rights in a vaccine, such as patent rights.[133] If some

---

[131] Press Release, U.S. Food & Drug Admin., Coronavirus (COVID-19) Update: FDA Provides Guidance on Production of Alcohol-Based Hand Sanitizer to Help Boost Supply, Protect Public Health (Mar. 20, 2020), https://www.fda.gov/news-events/press-announcements/coronavirus-covid-19-update-fda-provides-guidance-production-alcohol-based-hand-sanitizer-help-boost; U.S. FOOD & DRUG ADMIN., TEMPORARY POLICY FOR PREPARATION OF CERTAIN ALCOHOL-BASED HAND SANITIZER PRODUCTS DURING THE PUBLIC HEALTH EMERGENCY (COVID-19): GUIDANCE FOR INDUSTRY, https://www.fda.gov/media/136289/download (updated June 1, 2020); U.S. FOOD & DRUG ADMIN., POLICY FOR TEMPORARY COMPOUNDING OF CERTAIN ALCOHOL-BASED HAND SANITIZER PRODUCTS DURING THE PUBLIC HEALTH EMERGENCY: IMMEDIATELY IN EFFECT GUIDANCE FOR INDUSTRY https://www.fda.gov/media/136118/download (updated June 1, 2020).

[132] CRS Legal Sidebar LSB10300, *An Overview of State and Federal Authority to Impose Vaccination Requirements*, by Wen S. Shen.

[133] *See, e.g.*, Médecins Sans Frontières/Doctors Without Borders, *MSF Calls for No Patents or Profiteering on COVID- 19 Drugs, Tests, and Vaccines in Pandemic*, MSF ACCESS CAMPAIGN (Mar. 27, 2020), https://msfaccess.org/msf-calls- no-patents-or-profiteering-covid-19-drugs-tests-and-vaccines-pandemic (urging suspension of patent rights in COVID-19 countermeasures to ensure affordability and access); Jennifer Hillman, *Drugs and Vaccines Are Coming—But to Whom?*, FOREIGN AFF. (May 19, 2020), https://www.foreignaffairs.com/articles/world/2020-05-19/drugs-and-vaccines- are-coming-whom (expressing concern that "intellectual property rights could prevent vaccines or drugs from reaching the poor and vulnerable"); *but see* Daniel Hemel & Lisa Larrimore Ouellette, *Pharmaceutical Profits and Public Health Are Not Incompatible*, N.Y. TIMES (Apr. 8, 2020) (arguing that encouraging COVID-19 countermeasure development need not come at the cost of reducing patient access).

element of a successful COVID-19 vaccine was patented, for example, the patent holder would have the exclusive right to make and use that COVID-19 vaccine within the United States.[134]

Some Members of Congress have raised concerns about whether a COVID-19 vaccine and other medical countermeasures, if shown to be safe and effective, will be affordable and accessible to the public—especially if federal funds contribute to their development.[135] Several of the congressional responses to the COVID-19 pandemic contain provisions that relate to this issue. First, under the Coronavirus Aid, Relief, and Economic Security (CARES) Act, most private health insurance plans must cover a COVID-19 vaccine and other COVID-19 preventative services without cost sharing (e.g., deductibles or co-pays).[136] Although this provision aims to ensure that consumers with private health insurance will not pay co-payments for accessing a COVID-19 vaccine, it does not directly address other pricing issues, such as the potential cost to health care providers, health insurance companies, persons without health insurance, or the federal government.[137]

---

[134] *See* 35 U.S.C. § 271(a).

[135] *See* Ariel Cohen, *Senators Worry About COVID-19 Vaccine Affordability, Distribution*, INSIDE HEALTH POLICY (May 14, 2020), https://insidehealthpolicy.com/daily-news/senators-worry-about-covid-19-vaccine-affordability- distribution; Letter from Reps. James E. Clyburn & Carolyn Maloney to Sec. Alex M. Azar II (June 2, 2020), https://oversight.house.gov/sites/democrats.oversight.house.gov/files/2020-06-02.Clyburn%20CBM%20to%20HHS%20re%20Vaccine%20and%20Treatment%20Contracts.pdf; Letter from Rep. Jan Schakowsky et al. to President Donald J. Trump (Feb. 20, 2020), https://freepdfhosting.com/20bf1d75af.pdf.

[136] Pub. L. No. 116-136, § 3203 (2020). Most specifically, this requirement applies to COVID-19 vaccines recommended by the Advisory Committee on Immunization Practices of the Centers for Disease Control and Prevention and to group health plans and health insurance issuers offering group or individual health insurance as defined by PHSA Section 2791. *See id.* § 3203(b)(1), (3). For an analysis of the current federal insurance coverage requirements for COVID-19 testing, treatments, and vaccinations, *see* CRS Report R46359, *COVID-19 and Private Health Insurance Coverage: Frequently Asked Questions*, by Vanessa C. Forsberg.

[137] It is likely that the federal government will be a primary purchaser and distributor of a COVID-19 vaccine. The federal government currently purchases over half of the pediatric vaccines administered in the United States (primarily for children who are uninsured or eligible for Medicaid). *See* Christoph Diasio, *Pediatric Vaccination: Who Bears The Burden?*, HEALTH AFF. (Feb. 6, 2016), https://www.healthaffairs.org/do/10.1377/hblog20160209.053058/full/; *see generally Vaccines for Children Program (VFC)*, CTRS. FOR DISEASE CONTROL & PREVENTION (Feb. 18, 2016), https://www.cdc.gov/vaccines/programs/vfc/index.html; COMMITTEE ON THE

The Coronavirus Preparedness and Response Supplemental Appropriations Act (CPRSA) contains two general provisions related to the affordability of COVID-19 countermeasures. First, products purchased by the federal government using funds appropriated by CPRSA, including vaccines, therapeutics, and diagnostics for COVID-19, "shall be purchased in accordance with Federal Acquisition Regulation guidance on fair and reasonable pricing."[138] Second, CPRSA states that the Secretary of HHS "may take such measures authorized under current law to ensure that vaccines, therapeutics, and diagnostics developed from funds provided in [CPRSA] will be affordable in the commercial market."[139] These general statements were repeated in the appropriations for COVID-19 vaccines and other medical countermeasures in the CARES Act.[140]

This section reviews IP rights provisions under current law that the federal government could use to try to ensure that COVID-19 countermeasures such as a vaccine are accessible and affordable. Other actions that the federal government might hypothetically take—such as additional spending, direct production by federal agencies, contractual guarantees from vaccine manufacturers, governmental negotiation, or price controls—are not discussed, in that such measures do not implicate IP rights and may require additional legislative action beyond the "current law" referenced in CPRSA and the CARES Act.

EVALUATION OF VACCINE PURCHASE FINANCING IN THE UNITED STATES, FINANCING VACCINES IN THE 21ST CENTURY: ASSURING ACCESS AND AVAILABILITY 4 (2003), https://www.ncbi.nlm.nih.gov/books/NBK221813/pdf/Bookshelf_NBK221813.pdf.

During the 2009 to 2010 H1N1 influenza pandemic, the H1N1 vaccine and ancillary supplies (needles, syringes, etc.) were purchased by the federal government and distributed to health care providers, who could charge only for the administration of the vaccine. *See Questions and Answers on 2009 H1N1 Vaccine Financing*, CTRS. FOR DISEASE CONTROL & PREVENTION (Nov. 30, 2009), https://www.cdc.gov/H1N1flu/vaccination/statelocal/vaccine_financing.htm.

[138] Pub. L. No. 116-123, tit. III, 134 Stat. 146, 149 (2020).

[139] *Id.*

[140] *See* Pub. L. No. 116-136, tit. VIII (2020).

Patent Rights in Inventions Made with Federal Assistance

Patent Basics

Under the Patent Act,[141] any person who "invents or discovers any new and useful process, machine, manufacture, or composition of matter" may apply for a patent on the invention with the U.S. Patent and Trademark Office (PTO).[142] PTO patent examiners evaluate the application to ensure it meets all the applicable legal requirements to merit the grant of a patent.[143] If the patent examiner concludes that the claimed invention is new, nonobvious, useful, directed at patentable subject matter, and adequately disclosed and claimed,[144] PTO will issue the patent.[145] If granted, patents typically expire 20 years after the initial patent application is filed.[146]

Patents are available for almost every field of technology, including biotechnology, chemistry, computer hardware, electrical engineering, mechanical engineering, and manufacturing processes.[147] In the pharmaceutical context, if an inventor is the first to synthesize a particular chemical that is useful in treating disease, she may seek a patent claiming the chemical itself.[148] That said, patents on a pharmaceutical's active ingredient are only a subset of patents relating to pharmaceuticals and other medical treatments.[149] Particular drug formulations, methods of using the pharmaceutical to treat a particular disease, methods and technologies

---

[141] *See* Patent Act of 1952, Pub. L. No. 82-593, 66 Stat. 792 (1952) (codified as amended at 35 U.S.C. §§ 1-390).

[142] 35 U.S.C. §§ 101, 111.

[143] *Id.* § 131.

[144] *Id.* §§ 101, 102-103, 112. For a summary of the requirements for patentability, see generally CRS Report R44962, *Patent Law: A Primer and Overview of Emerging Issues*, by Kevin J. Hickey, at 2-4.

[145] 35 U.S.C. § 151, 153.

[146] *Id.* § 154(a)(2).

[147] *See id.* § 101; *Patent Technology Centers Management*, U.S. PATENT & TRADEMARK OFFICE, https://www.uspto.gov/patent/contact-patents/patent-technology-centers-management (last visited May 29, 2020) (listing technological divisions for PTO examiners). For a full discussion of the scope of patentable subject matter, *see generally* CRS Report R45918, *Patent-Eligible Subject Matter Reform in the 116th Congress*, by Kevin J. Hickey.

[148] *See* 35 U.S.C. § 101 (allowing patents on "any new and useful . . . composition of matter").

[149] *See* Amy Kapczynski et al., *Polymorphs and Prodrugs and Salts (Oh My!): An Empirical Analysis of "Secondary" Pharmaceutical Patents*, 7 PLOS ONE 1, 4-6 (2012).

to administer a pharmaceutical, methods and technologies to manufacture a pharmaceutical, as well as methods and technologies for testing for and diagnosing disease, are all patentable if they meet the Patent Act's requirements.[150]

To encourage innovation, a valid patent holder has the exclusive right to make, use, sell, and import (collectively, "practice") the patented invention in the United States.[151] Patents are thus said to confer a "temporary monopoly" on the patent holder: anyone else who wishes to practice the invention needs to obtain permission from the patent holder to do so (and, typically, pays for that permission).[152] In some situations, patent rights can confer substantial market power on patent holders, enabling them to charge higher-than-competitive prices for the patented product, as a monopolist would.[153] Some empirical studies have found patent rights are among the most important factors driving high prices for pharmaceutical products.[154] At least to some extent, higher prices are part of the patent system's design, in that they enable inventors to recoup the costs of research and development necessary to produce the invention in

---

[150] *See* Hickey et al., *supra* note 74, at 12-13.

[151] 35 U.S.C. § 271(a). These actions are the core of *direct* patent infringement. There are also a variety of ways to *indirectly* infringe a patent, such as actively inducing another person to infringe a patent or selling a component especially made or especially adapted for an infringing use. *See id.* § 271(b)-(c), (f)-(g).

[152] *See, e.g.*, Festo Corp. v. Shoketsu Kinzoku Kogyo Kabushiki Co., 535 U.S. 722, 730 (2002) (characterizing patents as a "temporary monopoly"). It should be noted that this usage of "monopoly" is somewhat imprecise, because the exclusive rights provided by IP law do not necessarily confer monopolistic market power in the economic sense—for example, there may be noninfringing substitutes for a patented good in the relevant market. *See* WILLIAM M. LANDES & RICHARD A. POSNER, THE ECONOMIC STRUCTURE OF INTELLECTUAL PROPERTY LAW 22 (2003) ("[IP] protection creates a monopoly, in the literal sense in which a person has a monopoly in the house he owns but [only] occasionally in a meaningful economic sense as well because there may be no good substitutes for a particular intellectual work.").

[153] *See* FTC v. Actavis, Inc., 570 U.S. 136, 147 (2013) ("[Patent rights] may permit the patent owner to charge a higher- than-competitive price for the patented product.").

[154] *See, e.g.*, Aaron S. Kesselheim et al., *The High Cost of Prescription Drugs in the United States: Origins and Prospects for Reform*, 316 JAMA: J. AM. MED. ASS'N 858, 861 (2016) ("The most important factor that allows manufacturers to set high drug prices for brand-name drugs is market exclusivity, which arises from 2 forms of legal protection against competition [i.e., patent rights and FDA regulatory exclusivities.]"); *Generic Competition and Drug Prices*, FOOD & DRUG ADMIN. (Nov. 28, 2017), https://www.fda.gov/aboutfda/centersoffices/officeofmedicalproductsandtobacco/cder/ucm129385.htm (finding association between generic competition and lower drug prices).

the first place.[155] IP law thus seeks to balance the importance of providing incentives to innovate against the costs that IP rights impose on the public in the form of higher prices and reduced competition.[156]

Inventions Made with Federal Assistance

Patent rights initially vest in the individual inventor or inventors, as a general rule.[157] Commonly, however, employees agree by contract to assign their patent rights to inventions made in the course of their employment to their employer, who may seek a patent on an employee's behalf.[158]

When private parties rely on federal assistance to develop an invention, any resulting patent rights will typically be owned by either the U.S. government or the federal contractor, depending on the nature of federal involvement. For inventions made by federal employees during their official duties, the federal government will typically obtain title to the patent.[159] The federal government's general policy for federally owned inventions, under the Stevenson-Wydler Technology Innovation Act[160] and

---

[155] *See, e.g.*, Kewanee Oil Co. v. Bicron Corp., 416 U.S. 470, 480 (1974) ("The patent laws promote [the progress of the useful arts] by offering a right of exclusion for a limited period as an incentive to inventors to risk the often enormous costs in terms of time, research, and development."); Emily Michiko Morris, The *Myth of Generic Pharmaceutical Competition under the Hatch-Waxman Act*, 22 FORDHAM INTELL. PROP. MEDIA & ENT. L.J. 245, 252 (2012) ("[P]harmaceuticals are also widely recognized as one of the industries most dependent on patent protection to recoup its enormous research, development, regulatory, and post-marketing costs …").

[156] *See* Sony Corp. of Am. v. Universal City Studios, Inc., 464 U.S. 417, 429 (1984) ("[D]efining the scope of [patents and copyrights] involves a difficult balance between the interests of authors and inventors in the control and exploitation of their writings and discoveries on the one hand, and society's competing interest in the free flow of ideas, information, and commerce on the other hand …"); Mark A. Lemley, *Property, Intellectual Property, and Free Riding*, 83 TEX. L. REV. 1031, 1031 (2005) ("[Traditionally,] the proper goal of intellectual property law is to give as little protection as possible consistent with encouraging innovation").

[157] Bd. of Trustees of Leland Stanford Junior Univ. v. Roche Molecular Sys., Inc., 563 U.S. 776, 785 (2011) ("Our precedents confirm the general rule that rights in an invention belong to the inventor."); *see* 35 U.S.C. §§ 100(f), 101.

[158] *See Roche*, 563 U.S. at 793 (noting "common practice" of assignment of patent rights in inventions from employees to their employer); 35 U.S.C. §§ 118, 152, 261.

[159] *See* 37 C.F.R. § 501.6(a).

[160] Pub. L. No. 96-480, 94 Stat. 2311 (1980).

the Federal Technology Transfer Act of 1986,[161] is to encourage their commercialization by licensing the federally owned patent rights to private parties—a process called "technology transfer."[162] Under technology transfer agreements, federal agencies grant private parties the exclusive or nonexclusive right to practice the invention,[163] while the U.S. government retains (1) a "nontransferable, irrevocable, paid-up license . . . to practice the invention . . . by or on behalf of" the United States (the "government-use license");[164] and (2) the power "to terminate the license in whole or in part" based on grounds similar to the conditions for "march-in rights" (discussed below).[165]

The Bayh-Dole Act of 1980 (Bayh-Dole),[166] as amended, applies to inventions that a federal contractor conceives or first reduces to practice during the performance of a funding agreement with a federal agency.[167] Under Bayh-Dole, the federal contractor may elect to retain the patent rights for a federally funded invention.[168] In exchange, however, the contractor provides the federal agency with a government-use license,[169] and the United States retains the authority to grant compulsory licenses to third parties in certain circumstances ("march-in rights").[170] Although Bayh-Dole, by its terms, only applies to federal contractors that are nonprofit organizations or small businesses, long-standing executive practice (codified by regulation) has applied Bayh-Dole to all federal contractors, regardless of size.[171]

---

[161] Pub. L. No. 99-502, 100 Stat. 1785 (1986).

[162] *See* 15 U.S.C. § 3710(a) ("The Federal Government shall strive where appropriate to transfer federally owned or originated technology to State and local governments and to the private sector."); 35 U.S.C. § 209 (conditions for licensing of federally owned inventions).

[163] 35 U.S.C. § 209(a).

[164] *Id.* § 209(d)(1).

[165] *Compare id.* § 209(d)(3)(A)-(D) *with* 35 U.S.C. § 203(a)(1)-(4); *see infra* "March-In Rights Under the Bayh-Dole Act (35 U.S.C. § 203)."

[166] Act of Dec. 12, 1980 to Amend the Patent and Trademark Laws (Bayh-Dole Act), Pub. L. No, 96-517, § 6, 94 Stat. 3015, 3018-27 (1980) (codified as amended at 35 U.S.C. ch. 18).

[167] *See* 35 U.S.C. §§ 201(b), (e).

[168] *Id.* § 202(a).

[169] *Id.* § 202(c)(4).

[170] *Id.* § 203; *see generally* Hickey et al., *supra* note 74, at 17.

[171] 37 C.F.R. § 401.1(b) (Bayh-Dole regulations apply "to all funding agreements with business firms regardless of size"); Exec. Order No. 12591, Facilitating Access to Science & Technology, 52 Fed. Reg. 13,414, 13,414 (Apr. 10, 1987) (granting "to all contractors,

Finally, federal laboratories and private parties may enter into cooperative research and development agreements (CRADAs) in which both parties agree to provide services, facilities, equipment, IP, or other resources, but the federal government does not provide federal funding to the nonfederal party.[172] In this situation, ownership of IP rights may depend on the terms of the agreement. That said, the federal laboratory generally has the authority to license existing federally owned IP to a private party as part of a CRADA, as well as to license or assign inventions made in whole or part by a federal employee working under a CRADA.[173] In return, the federal government retains a government-use license[174] and compulsory-licensing authority similar to Bayh-Dole march-in rights.[175]

These general rules for patent ownership are subject to various exceptions and waivers, depending on the agency and circumstances. For example, some agencies (including BARDA and National Institutes of Health [NIH]) have the authority to enter into transactions that are *not* contracts, grants, or cooperative agreements, known as "other transaction" authority.[176] Other transactions are exempt from many statutory provisions and procurement regulations, including Bayh-Dole's requirements.[177]

---

regardless of size, the title to patents made in whole or in part with Federal funds, in exchange for royalty-free use by or on behalf of the government").

[172] 15 U.S.C. § 3710a(a)(1) (CRADA authority); *id.* § 3710a(d)(1) (CRADA definition).

[173] *See id.* § 3710a(a)(2), (b)(1)-(2); 35 U.S.C. §§ 207, 209.

[174] 15 U.S.C. § 3710a(b)(1)(A), (2).

[175] *See id.* § 3710a(b)(1)(C)(i)-(iii) (grounds for compulsory licensing of inventions "made in whole or in part by a [federal] laboratory employee" under a CRADA). In the case of inventions "made solely by [the private collaborating party's] employee" in the course of a CRADA, the federal agency retains a government-use license, but need not impose march-in rights. *Compare id.* § 3710a(b)(1) *with* 3710a(b)(2).

[176] 42 U.S.C. § 247d-7e(c)(5) (granting Secretary of HHS authority to enter into other transactions for BARDA projects); *id.* § 282(n) (granting director of NIH other transaction authority in certain contexts). Because NIAID is one of NIH's research institutes, *see id.* § 281(b)(6), this authority could apply to NIAID projects approved by the Director of NIH. In the case of COVID-19 projects, NIH authority for use of other transactions when "urgently required to respond to a public health threat" appears applicable. *See id.* § 282(n)(1)(C). For a general overview of other transactions, see U.S. GOVERNMENT ACCOUNTABILITY OFFICE, USE OF 'OTHER TRANSACTION' AGREEMENTS LIMITED AND MOSTLY FOR RESEARCH AND DEVELOPMENT ACTIVITIES 3-12 (2016), https://www.gao.gov/assets/680/674534.pdf [hereinafter GAO OTA REPORT].

[177] *See* GAO OTA REPORT, *supra* note 176, at 4-5; 35 U.S.C. § 201(b) (defining "funding agreements" subject to Bayh- Dole to include "any contract, grant, or cooperative agreement").

Thus, for other transactions, the allocation of IP rights between the government and private contracting entities will depend on the agreement. For example, BARDA's template for other transactions includes contractual patent provisions much like those of Bayh-Dole, including march-in rights provisions.[178] These patent provisions are "fluid and negotiable," however, and may be different for particular transactions.[179] In addition, both Stevenson-Wydler's and Bayh- Dole's requirements contain specific exceptions. For example, Bayh-Dole's patent provisions do not apply to contractors located outside the United States, nor in "exceptional circumstances," including if necessary "to meet the needs of the Government and protect the public against nonuse or unreasonable use of inventions."[180]

Governmental Compulsory Patent Licenses

As explained above, a patent holder generally has the exclusive right to make, use, sell, and import an invention.[181] Thus, any other person who wishes to practice that invention will ordinarily need a license (i.e., permission) from the patent holder, or else be exposed to legal liability. In certain cases, however, patents may be subject to a "compulsory license," which allows another person to practice the invention without the consent of the patent holder.[182] Compulsory licenses require the sanction of a governmental entity and the payment of compensation to the patent holder.[183] Compulsory licenses differ from ordinary licenses in two important respects. First, the person seeking to use the invention need not

---

[178] *See* Other Transaction for Advanced Research (OTAR) Template, BIOMEDICAL ADVANCED RESEARCH AND DEVELOPMENT AUTHORITY, https://www.phe.gov/about/amcg/otar/Documents/otar-consortium.pdf (last visited May 31, 2020), at pp. 16-21 [hereinafter BARDA OTA Template]; *see generally* Other Transaction Agreements, BIOMEDICAL ADVANCED RESEARCH AND DEVELOPMENT AUTHORITY, https://www.phe.gov/about/amcg/otar/Pages/default.aspx (last visited May 31, 2020).

[179] BARDA OTAR Template, *supra* note 178, at 16.

[180] *See* 35 U.S.C. §§ 200, 202(a)(ii).

[181] *Id.* § 271(a).

[182] *See generally* Hickey et al., *supra* note 74, at 16-17.

[183] *Id.* at 1.

obtain permission from the patent holder.[184] Second, the compensation paid to the patent holder is determined by operation of law, not by private contractual negotiations between the licensee and the patent holder.[185]

March-in Rights under the Bayh-Dole Act (35 U.S.C. § 203)

Although Bayh-Dole generally allows federal contractors to take title to patents on inventions created with federal funding,[186] the federal government retains the authority to "march in" and grant compulsory licenses to third parties in some circumstances.[187] Specifically, the federal agency that provided the funding may require the federal contractor to grant a patent license to a third party if the agency determines that either

> 1) action is necessary because the contractor or assignee has not taken, or is not expected to take within a reasonable time, effective steps to achieve practical application of the subject invention in such field of use;
> 2) action is necessary to alleviate health or safety needs which are not reasonably satisfied by the contractor, assignee, or their licensees;
> 3) action is necessary to meet requirements for public use specified by federal regulations and such requirements are not reasonably satisfied by the contractor, assignee, or licensees; or
> 4) action is necessary because the agreement [to prefer U.S. manufacturing of the invention by the contractor's exclusive licensees] has not been obtained or waived or because a licensee of the exclusive right to use or sell any subject invention in the United States is in breach of its agreement [to prefer U.S. manufacturing].[188]

---

[184] *See* Hickey et al., *supra* note 74, at 16.
[185] *Id.*
[186] 35 U.S.C. § 202(a)-(b).
[187] *Id.* § 203.
[188] *Id.* § 203(a)(1)-(4).

A license granted under Bayh-Dole's march-in provisions must be "upon terms that are reasonable under the circumstances,"[189] which may require that the licensee pay compensation to the patent holder (i.e., the federal contractor or its assignee).[190]

The federal government has never exercised march-in rights under Bayh-Dole.[191] Advocacy groups have petitioned NIH several times to exercise march-in rights based on the high prices of certain drugs developed with federal funding, such as treatments for HIV/AIDS.[192] NIH has rejected these petitions, contending that pricing concerns alone are insufficient to exercise march- in rights—so long as the invention is on the market and available to patients.[193] In the context of a pandemic like COVID-19, the "health or safety needs" language would appear to provide a possible basis for the exercise of march-in rights, should the funding agency determine that compulsory licensing is necessary to address public health needs unmet by a federal contractor.[194]

Governmental Use Rights (28 U.S.C. § 1498)

A broader statutory authority than march-in rights, 28 U.S.C. § 1498 (Section 1498), applies to any patented invention—not just inventions made with federal funding.[195] Under Section 1498, sometimes described as an "eminent domain" provision for patents,[196] the U.S. government has the authority to use or manufacture any patented invention "without

---

[189] *Id.* § 202(a).

[190] *See id* § 203(a); Jennifer Penman & Fran Quigley, *Better Late than Never: How the U.S. Government Can and Should Use Bayh-Dole March-in Rights to Respond to the Medicines Access Crisis*, 54 WILLAMETTE L. REV. 171, 178 (2017).

[191] *Id.*

[192] *See id.* at 8-10 (reviewing petitions to exercise march-in rights).

[193] *See, e.g.*, National Institutes of Health, Office of the Director, *In the Case of Norvir Manufactured by Abbott Laboratories, Inc.* (July 29, 2004), https://www.ott.nih.gov/sites/default/files/documents/policy/March-In-Norvir.pdf, at pp. 5-6.

[194] 35 U.S.C. § 203(a)(2). A federal contractor adversely affected by the exercise of march-in rights may challenge an agency's determination through an administrative process, *see* 37 C.F.R. § 401.6, and may appeal an adverse determination through a petition in the U.S. Court of Federal Claims, *see* 35 U.S.C. § 203(b).

[195] 28 U.S.C. § 1498(a) (reaching "any invention described in and covered by a patent of the United States"). Section 1498 does not apply to patent rights granted by other nations.

[196] *See, e.g.*, Motorola, Inc. v. United States, 729 F.2d 765, 768 (Fed. Cir. 1984) ("The theoretical basis for [Section 1498] recovery is the doctrine of eminent domain").

license."[197] In practice, this means that if the U.S. government determines that it needs to practice an invention, it need not ask permission from the patent holder to do so, and—despite the existence of the patent—courts will not order the government to cease infringing activity.[198] The patent holder, however, has the right to sue in the U.S. Court of Federal Claims for "reasonable and entire compensation" for the government's use of the patented invention.[199] In effect, then, Section 1498 allows the United States to issue itself a compulsory license to make and use any patented invention without obtaining the permission of the patent holder, in exchange for consenting to liability in a suit seeking reasonable compensation for the government's use.[200]

In the context of COVID-19 medical countermeasures, the U.S. government could rely on Section 1498 to make and use any patented invention without the consent of the patent holder. Because Section 1498 extends to infringement "by a contractor, a subcontractor, or any person, firm, or corporation for the [U.S.] Government and with the authorization or consent of the [U.S.] Government,"[201] the federal government could also extend its Section 1498 authority to the actions of private entities by authorizing them to practice a patented invention on behalf of the government.

Targeted Legislation and the Takings Clause

U.S. patent rights were created by an act of Congress. Thus, should patent rights inhibit access to or affordability of COVID-19 countermeasures such as a vaccine, and should Congress conclude that

---

[197] 28 U.S.C. § 1498(a).

[198] Advanced Software Design Corp. v. Fed. Reserve Bank of St. Louis, 583 F.3d 1371, 1375 (Fed. Cir. 2009); *Motorola*, 729 F.2d at 768 n.3.

[199] 28 U.S.C. § 1498(a); *see generally* Leesona Corp. v. United States, 599 F.2d 958, 966-69 (Ct. Cl. 1979).

[200] *See* Amanda Mitchell, *Tamiflu, the Takings Clause, and Compulsory Licenses: An Exploration of the Government's Options for Accessing Medical Patents*, 95 CAL. L. REV. 535, 541-42 (2007) (analogizing Section 1498 to a compulsory license).

[201] 28 U.S.C. § 1498(a).

existing legal authorities are insufficient, targeted legislation is a possible option. Although the U.S. Constitution grants Congress the authority to create a patent system,[202] it does not require Congress to do so. Congress therefore has wide discretion in designing the patent system's scope and operation.[203] So long as it operates prospectively (and consistent with its international treaty obligations),[204] Congress may exclude certain technologies from patent protection. For example, a provision in the 2011 Leahy-Smith America Invents Act prohibits the PTO from issuing a patent on inventions "directed to or encompassing a human organism."[205]

When legislation operates retroactively to invalidate a patent or diminish patent rights, however, it raises issues under the Takings Clause of the Fifth Amendment to the U.S. Constitution. The Takings Clause states that if "private property [is] taken for public use" by the U.S. government, it must provide "just compensation."[206] The Supreme Court has suggested several times that patents are private property under the Takings Clause,[207] but it has never held so explicitly.

Presuming that patents are private property under the Fifth Amendment,[208] legislation that retroactively impairs patent rights could

---

[202] U.S. CONST. art. I, § 8, cl. 8.

[203] *See, e.g.*, McClurg v. Kingsland, 42 U.S. 202, 206 (1843) ("[T]he powers of Congress to legislate upon the subject of patents is plenary by the terms of the Constitution, and as there are no restraints on its exercise, there can be no limitation of their right to modify them at their pleasure, so that they do not take away the rights of property in existing patents."). There are, of course, some limits on the power granted Congress in the IP Clause. *See generally, e.g.*, Eldred v. Ashcroft, 537 U.S. 186, 199-208 (2003); Graham v. John Deere Co. of Kan. City, 383 U.S. 1, 5-10 (1966).

[204] *See infra* note 211 and accompanying text.

[205] Pub. L. No, 112-29, § 33, 125 Stat. 284, 340 (2011).

[206] U.S. CONST. amend. V.

[207] *Compare* James v. Campbell, 104 U.S. 356, 357-58 (1881) ("[By issuing a patent, the United States] confers on the patentee an exclusive property in the patented invention which cannot be appropriated or used by the government itself, without just compensation ..."), *with* Oil States Energy Servs. v. Greene's Energy Grp., 138 S. Ct. 1365, 1379 (2018) (holding that the grant of a patent is matter of public rights but stating that "our decision should not be misconstrued as suggesting that patents are not property for purposes of the Due Process Clause or the Takings Clause").

[208] Legal academics have debated this point. *Compare* Adam Mossoff, *Patents as Constitutional Private Property: The Historical Protection of Patents Under the Takings Clause*, 87 B.U. L. REV. 689 (2007), *with* Davida H. Isaacs, *Not All Property Is Created Equal: Why Modern Courts Resist Applying the Takings Clause to Patents, and Why They Are Right to Do So*, 15 GEO. MASON L. REV. 1 (2007). Notably, in a recent Federal Circuit case, the

give rise to a constitutional claim for just compensation.[209] Recognizing this, Congress has often provided for compensation in past legislation that has retroactively invalidated patents. For example, the Atomic Energy Act of 1954 "revoked" existing patents on "any invention or discovery which is useful solely in the utilization of special nuclear material or atomic energy in an atomic weapon," while providing a process to provide just compensation to any such patent holder.[210]

If Congress seeks to preclude the exercise of exclusive patent rights over COVID-19 medical countermeasures, it could pass legislation preventing the PTO from issuing such patents, or invalidating already issued patents relating to countermeasures. In the latter case, some mechanism for compensation to the patent holder might be required under the Takings Clause. In either case, such legislation could raise issues under the United States' treaty obligations, including the treaty on Trade-Related Aspects of Intellectual Property Rights of the Marrakesh Agreement establishing the World Trade Organization (WTO), in which WTO members agree to make patents available in "all fields of technology," with some exceptions.[211] In addition, limitations on patent rights could reduce

---

PTO conceded that patents were "private property" under the Takings Clause. *See* Celgene Corp. v. Peter, 931 F.3d 1342, 1358 (Fed. Cir. 2019), *petition for cert. filed,* No. 19-1074 (U.S. Feb. 26, 2020).

[209] *See, e.g., Celgene*, 931 F.3d at 1358 (rejecting claim that retroactive application of inter partes review procedures is an unconstitutional taking of patent rights). For analyses of potential Takings Clause claims as applied to patents, see generally, e.g., Gregory Dolin & Irina D. Manta, *Taking Patents*, 73 WASH. & LEE L. REV. 719 (2016); Joshua I. Miller, *28 U.S.C. § 1498(a) and the Unconstitutional Taking of Patents*, 13 YALE J.L. & TECH. 1 (2010); Christopher S. Storm, *Federal Patent Takings*, 2 J. BUS. ENTREPRENEURSHIP & L. 1 (2008); Justin Torres, *The Government Giveth, and the Government Taketh Away: Patents, Takings, and 28 U.S.C. § 1498*, 63 N.Y.U. ANN. SUR. AM. L. 315 (2007); Jesse S. Chui, *To What Extent Can Congress Change the Patent Right Without Effecting a Taking?*, 34 HASTINGS CONST. L.Q. 447 (2007); Shubha Ghosh, *Toward A Theory of Regulatory Takings for Intellectual Property: The Path Left Open After* College Savings v. Florida Prepaid, 37 SAN DIEGO L. REV. 637 (2000).

[210] 42 U.S.C. §§ 2181(a), 2187.

[211] TRIPS: Agreement on Trade-Related Aspects of Intellectual Property Rights, Apr. 15, 1994, Marrakesh Agreement Establishing the World Trade Organization, Annex 1C, 1869 U.N.T.S. 299 (1994), https://www.wto.org/english/docs_e/legal_e/27-trips_01_e.htm, at art. 27. For analysis of how the limits of TRIPS might apply to exclusions from patent protection or compulsory licensing in the COVID-19 pandemic, see CRS Legal Sidebar LSB10436, *COVID-19: International Trade and Access to Pharmaceutical Products*, by Nina M. Hart.

incentives to create and develop medical countermeasures against COVID-19.[212]

THE PREP ACT: LIABILITY AND COMPENSATION FOR COVID-19 VACCINE INJURIES

To encourage the expeditious development and deployment of medical countermeasures during a public health emergency, the PREP Act[213] authorizes the Secretary of HHS to limit legal liability for losses relating to the administration of medical countermeasures, including diagnostics, treatments, and vaccines.[214] In a declaration effective February 4, 2020 (the COVID-19 PREP Act Declaration), the Secretary of HHS invoked the PREP Act and declared COVID-19 to be a public health emergency warranting liability protections for covered countermeasures.[215] Under the COVID-19 PREP Act Declaration, covered persons are generally immune from legal liability for losses relating to the administration or use of covered countermeasures against COVID-19.[216] The sole exception to PREP Act immunity is for death or serious physical injury caused by "willful misconduct."[217] However, individuals who die or suffer serious injuries directly caused by the administration of covered countermeasures may be eligible to receive compensation through an HHS administrative

---

[212] *See, e.g.*, Fred Reinhart, *Exercising Bayh-Dole March-in Rights Would Handicap Covid-19 Innovation,* STAT (May 4, 2020), https://www.statnews.com/2020/05/04/bayh-dole-march-in-rights-handicap-covid-19-innovation/; James Edwards, *We Won't Stop Coronavirus Without IP*, IPWATCHDOG (Mar. 10, 2020), https://www.ipwatchdog.com/2020/03/10/wont-stop-coronavirus-without-ip/id=119735/.

[213] Pub. L. 109-148, div. C, 119 Stat. 2680, 2818-32 (2005) (codified as amended at 42 U.S.C. §§ 247d-6d, 247d-6e).

[214] 42 U.S.C. § 247d-6d(b)(1).

[215] Declaration Under the Public Readiness and Emergency Preparedness Act for Medical Countermeasures Against COVID-19, 85 Fed. Reg. 15,198 (Mar. 17, 2020) (effective Feb. 4, 2020) [hereinafter COVID-19 PREP Act Declaration].

[216] *Id.* at 15,201-02; 42 U.S.C. § 247d-6d(a)(1).

[217] 42 U.S.C. § 247d-6d(d)(1).

process called the Countermeasures Injury Compensation Program (CICP).[218]

Courts have characterized PREP Act immunity as "sweeping."[219] It applies to all types of legal claims under state and federal law.[220] For example, under state tort law, individuals who suffer injuries caused by the intentional or negligent acts or omissions of another person may generally sue that person to recover monetary compensation.[221] Thus, in the health care context, if a health care provider negligently administers a drug or device that causes a foreseeable injury to a patient, the injured person may be able to sue the provider for compensation.[222]

Federal laws such as the PREP Act may preempt state tort laws—as well as other state and federal laws—in certain contexts.[223] Preemptive federal legislation displaces state law to alter the usual liability rules or immunize certain individuals from liability.[224] In the PREP Act, Congress made the judgment that, in the context of a public health emergency, immunizing certain persons and entities from liability was necessary to ensure that potentially life-saving countermeasures will be efficiently developed, deployed, and administered.[225]

So long as the COVID-19 PREP Act Declaration remains in effect, COVID-19 vaccine manufacturers, distributors, and qualified health care providers are generally immune from legal liability for losses relating to

---

[218] *Id.* § 247d-6e; 42 C.F.R. pt. 110.

[219] *See* Parker v. St. Lawrence Cty. Pub. Health Dep't, 102 A.D.3d 140, 143 (N.Y. App. Div. 2012).

[220] 42 U.S.C. § 247d-6d(a)(1).

[221] *See generally* CRS In Focus IF11291, *Introduction to Tort Law*, by Kevin M. Lewis.

[222] *Id.* at 1.

[223] *See generally* CRS Report R45825, *Federal Preemption: A Legal Primer*, by Jay B. Sykes and Nicole Vanatko.

[224] *See, e.g.*, CRS Legal Sidebar LSB10461, *Federal Legislation Shielding Businesses and Individuals from Tort Liability: A Legal and Historical Overview*, by Kevin M. Lewis (summarizing federal statutes that either insulate particular entities from tort liability or otherwise displace state tort law).

[225] *See, e.g.*, 151 CONG. REC. H12264 (daily ed. Dec. 18, 2005) (statement of Rep. Deal) ("Unfortunately, there is no business model that would have vaccine manufacturers take on the tremendous liability risks to produce [a pandemic flu] vaccine. We must address this concern or we will have none. It's really that simple. …What the [PREP Act] does is provide authority to the Secretary[:] the ability to declare limited liability protection. The Secretary can use these declarations to make sure the vaccine gets developed and to make sure doctors are willing to give it when the time comes.").

the use or administration of that vaccine. Instead, individuals who are injured or die as a result of receiving a COVID-19 vaccine may seek compensation through CICP. This section explains the scope of this PREP Act immunity as it applies to COVID-19 countermeasures, including vaccines, as well as the contours and availability of CICP compensation.

The Public Readiness and Emergency Preparedness Act

Scope of Immunity from Liability

For the PREP Act to apply, the Secretary of HHS must determine that a disease or other threat to health constitutes a public health emergency, or that there is a credible risk of such an emergency.[226] The Secretary shall consider the desirability of encouraging the design, development, testing, manufacture, and use of countermeasures in determining whether to issue a PREP Act declaration.[227] The Secretary must publish the PREP Act declaration in the *Federal Register* and identify, for each countermeasure, the particular disease, time period, population, and geographical area that the declaration covers.[228]

If within the scope of the declaration, the PREP Act immunizes a covered person from legal liability for all claims for loss relating to the administration or use of a covered countermeasure.[229] The requirements for PREP Act immunity thus break down into four elements: (1) the individual or entity must be a "covered person"; (2) the legal claim must be for a "loss"; (3) the loss must have a "causal relationship" with the

---

[226] 42 U.S.C. § 247d-6d(b)(1).

[227] *Id.* § 247d-6d(b)(6). A PREP Act declaration is distinct from the Secretary's power to declare a public health emergency under Section 319 of the PHSA, which has a separate set of legal implications. *Id.* § 247d; *see generally* U.S. Dep't of Health and Human Servs., Office of the Assistant Sec. for Preparedness and Response, Public Health Emergency Declaration (Nov. 26, 2019) (describing powers of Secretary of HHS under Section 319). The Secretary of HHS made the Section 319 declaration for COVID-19 on January 31, 2020. Alex M. Azar II, Sec'y of the Dep't of Health and Human Servs., Determination that a Public Health Emergency Exists, https://www.phe.gov/emergency/news/healthactions/phe/Pages/2019-nCoV.aspx (Jan. 31, 2020).

[228] 42 U.S.C. § 247d-6d(b)(1)-(3).

[229] *Id.* § 247d-6d(a)(1).

administration or use of a covered countermeasure; and (4) the medical product that caused the loss must be a "covered countermeasure."

"Covered Persons"

The PREP Act defines covered persons to include (i) the United States; (ii) manufacturers and distributors of covered countermeasures; (iii) "program planners"; and (iv) "qualified persons" who prescribe, administer, or dispense covered countermeasures.[230] Program planners include Indian Tribes, state governments, and local governments who supervise programs that dispense, distribute, or administer covered countermeasures, or provide policy guidance, facilities, and scientific advice on the administration or use of such countermeasures.[231] Qualified persons include licensed health professionals and other individuals authorized to prescribe, administer, or dispense covered countermeasures under state law, as well as other categories of persons identified by the Secretary in a PREP Act declaration.[232] Employees and agents of all these persons and entities are also covered persons.[233]

Covered "Claims for Loss"

PREP Act immunity reaches "all claims for loss" under federal and state law.[234] Loss is broadly defined to mean "any type of loss," including (i) death; (ii) physical, mental, or emotional injury, illness, disability, or condition; (iii) fear of such injury, including medical monitoring costs; and (iv) loss of or damage to property, including business interruption loss.[235] This language would seem to include, at a minimum, most state law tort, medical malpractice, and wrongful death claims resulting from the administration of covered countermeasures.

---

[230] *Id.* § 247d-6d(i)(2).
[231] *Id.* § 247d-6d(i)(6).
[232] *Id.* § 247d-6d(i)(8).
[233] *Id.* § 247d-6d(i)(2)(B)(v).
[234] *Id.* § 247d-6d(a)(1).
[235] *Id.* § 247d-6d(a)(2)(A)(i)-(iv).

Causal Relationship between the Loss and the Countermeasure

To be preempted by the PREP Act, the claims for loss must have a causal relationship to the administration and use of a covered countermeasure.[236] As with the other elements, the PREP Act's causation language sweeps broadly. PREP Act immunity applies to any claim for loss that has "a causal relationship with the design, development, clinical testing or investigation, manufacture, labeling, distribution, formulation, packaging, marketing, promotion, sale, purchase, donation, dispensing, prescribing, administration, licensing, or use" of a covered countermeasure.[237]

"Covered Countermeasures"

Finally, the medical product at issue must be a covered countermeasure. The PREP Act specifies three general types of covered countermeasures: (i) a qualified "pandemic or epidemic product"; (ii) a "security countermeasure"; and (iii) a drug, biological product, or device that FDA has authorized for emergency use.[238] As discussed below, Congress recently added a fourth covered countermeasure category specifically for respiratory protective devices.[239]

A *pandemic or epidemic product* includes any drug, biological product, or device developed "to diagnose, mitigate, prevent, treat, or cure a pandemic or epidemic."[240] In addition, drugs, biological products, or devices uses to treat the side effects of a pandemic or epidemic product, or to enhance their effects, may themselves be covered countermeasures.[241] In either case, to be a covered countermeasure, the pandemic or epidemic

---

[236] *Id.* § 247d-6d(a)(1).

[237] *Id.* § 247d-6d(a)(2)(B).

[238] *Id.* § 247d-6d(i)(1)(A)-(C).

[239] *Id.* § 247d-6d(i)(1)(D); *see infra* "Recent Congressional Actions on COVID-19 Countermeasures Liability."

[240] 42 U.S.C. § 247d-6d(i)(7)(A)(i). The PREP Act incorporates the general definitions of "drug," "biological product," and "device" under the FD&C Act and PHSA. *See* 21 U.S.C. § 321(g)(1), (h); 42 U.S.C. § 262(i).

[241] 42 U.S.C. § 247d-6d(i)(7)(A)(ii)-(iii).

product must be approved, licensed, or authorized for emergency use by FDA.[242]

A *security countermeasure* refers to a drug, biological product, or device used "to diagnose, mitigate, prevent, or treat harm from any biological, chemical, radiological, or nuclear agent" identified by the Secretary of Homeland Security as a material threat to national security.[243]

The *emergency use* category of covered countermeasure includes drugs, biological products, and devices that FDA has authorized for use outside its ordinary regulatory process through an EUA.[244] FDA has made wide use of its emergency authorities in response to the COVID-19 pandemic, issuing EUAs for certain in vitro diagnostic products (i.e., tests for COVID-19), antibody tests, personal protective equipment (e.g., respirators and face shields), devices modified for use as ventilators, and therapeutic drugs.[245]

Thus, so long as FDA licensed or authorized a COVID-19 vaccine, it would be a covered countermeasure within the scope of the PREP Act, either as a "pandemic or epidemic product" or through the emergency use category in the case of authorization through an EUA. Prior to licensure or authorization of a COVID-19 vaccine, the PREP Act would also afford liability protections for injuries that may occur in the clinical testing process, if the vaccine is "the object of research for possible use" as a pandemic or epidemic product and subject to an investigational use exemption.[246]

---

[242] *Id.* § 247d-6d(i)(7)(B)(i), (iii).

[243] *Id.* §§ 247d-6b(c)(1)(B), 247d-6d(i)(1)(B).

[244] *Id.* § 247d-6d(i)(1)(C); *see supra* "Emergency Use Authorizations Before Approval."

[245] *Emergency Use Authorization: Coronavirus Disease 2019 (COVID-19) EUA Information*, U.S. FOOD & DRUG ADMIN., https://www.fda.gov/emergency-preparedness-and-response/mcm-legal-regulatory-and-policy-framework/emergency-use-authorization#covid19euas (last updated June 1, 2020) (listing FDA's current EUAs for COVID-19 diagnostics, antibody tests, personal protective equipment, therapeutics, and ventilators).

[246] 42 U.S.C. § 247d-6d(i)(7)(B)(ii).

The Willful Misconduct Exception

If a claim for loss is within the PREP Act's scope, a covered person is generally immune from legal liability.[247] The "sole exception" to immunity is when a covered person proximately causes death or serious physical injury to another person through willful misconduct.[248] A serious physical injury must be life threatening, permanently impair a body function, permanently damage a body structure, or require medical intervention to avoid such permanent impairment or damage.[249] Willful misconduct requires that the covered person acted (i) intentionally to achieve a wrongful purpose; (ii) knowingly without legal or factual justification; *and* (iii) in disregard of a known or obvious risk that is so great as to make it highly probable that the harm will outweigh the benefit.[250]

The process by which an injured person (or their representative) may prove willful misconduct under the PREP Act is limited in several ways. Before filing a suit claiming willful misconduct, the injured person must first seek compensation through CICP, and they cannot sue if they elect to receive that compensation.[251] If they choose to file a lawsuit, injured persons may sue only in the U.S. District Court for the District of Columbia.[252] Such lawsuits are assigned to a three-judge panel, must meet heightened standards for pleading and discovery, and are subject to procedural provisions generally favorable to defendants.[253] Injured persons must prove willful misconduct by clear and convincing evidence,[254] a higher standard of proof than a typical civil case. Recovery for noneconomic damages such as pain and suffering is limited.[255]

---

[247] *Id.* § 247d-6d(a)(1).

[248] *Id.* § 247d-6d(d)(1). In the case of actions by or against the United States, the PREP Act shall not "be construed to abrogate or limit any right, remedy, or authority that the United States or any agency thereof may possess under any other provision of law or to waive sovereign immunity or to abrogate or limit any defense or protection available to the United States or its agencies, instrumentalities, officers, or employees under any other law ..." *Id.* § 247d-6d(f).

[249] *Id.* § 247d-6d(i)(10).

[250] *Id.* § 247d-6d(c)(1)(A).

[251] *Id.* § 247d-6e(d)(1), (5).

[252] *Id.* § 247d-6d(e)(1).

[253] *See id.* § 247d-6d(e)(3)-(6), (10).

[254] *Id.* § 247d-6d(c)(3).

[255] *Id.* § 247d-6d(e)(7)-(8).

In addition to these procedural and substantive limitations, the PREP Act contains two statutory defenses to claims of willful misconduct. First, program planners and qualified persons cannot be found to have engaged in willful misconduct if they "acted consistent with applicable directions, guidelines, or recommendations by the Secretary regarding the administration or use of a covered countermeasure," and notify either the Secretary or a state or local health authority of the injury or death allegedly caused by the countermeasure within seven days.[256] Second, countermeasure manufacturers and distributors may rely on regulatory compliance as a complete defense to a "willful misconduct" allegation.[257] When the act or omission alleged to be willful misconduct is "subject to regulation" under the PHSA or the FD&C Act, an injured person cannot succeed on a willful misconduct claim unless the Secretary of HHS or the Attorney General has brought certain "enforcement actions" against the manufacturer or distributor that result in the imposition of particular penalties.[258]

The Countermeasures Injury Compensation Program

An individual seriously injured or killed by the administration of a covered countermeasure, whether or not as a result of willful misconduct, may seek compensation through CICP.[259] CICP is a regulatory process administered by HHS's Health Resources and Services Administration.[260]

---

[256] *Id.* § 247d-6d(c)(4).

[257] *Id.* § 247d-6d(c)(5).

[258] *Id.* § 247d-6d(c)(5)(A)(i)-(ii). The necessary "enforcement actions" include criminal prosecutions, civil monetary proceedings based on willful misconduct, mandatory product recalls, or revocations, suspensions or withdrawals, based on willful misconduct, of FDA approval, licensure, or authorization. *Id.* § 247d-6d(c)(5)(B)(i). Before a willful misconduct claim can proceed, the enforcement action must conclude with the imposition of a "covered remedy" such as a criminal conviction, an injunction, a civil monetary payment, a product recall, or a suspension or withdrawal of FDA approval or licensure. *Id.* § 247d-6d(c)(5)(B)(ii).

[259] *Id.* § 247d-6e(a)-(b).

[260] *See generally Countermeasure Injury Compensation Program*, HEALTH RESOURCES & SERVS. ADMIN., https://www.hrsa.gov/cicp/index.html (last visited May 28, 2020).

HHS regulations govern CICP's procedures and eligibility determinations.[261] In general, eligible individuals (or their survivors) who suffer death or serious physical injury directly caused by the administration of a covered countermeasure may receive reimbursement through CICP for reasonable medical expenses, loss of employment income, and survivor benefits in the case of death.[262] Serious physical injuries under CICP are generally limited to those that warrant hospitalization or lead to a significant loss of function or disability.[263] Congress funds CICP compensation through emergency appropriations to the Covered Countermeasure Process Fund.[264]

CICP is distinct from the National Vaccine Injury Compensation Program,[265] which provides compensation for injuries caused by most vaccines routinely administered in the United States, such as childhood vaccines (e.g., MMR, polio, hepatitis A) and nonpandemic seasonal influenza vaccines.[266] By contrast, CICP only applies to countermeasures covered by a PREP Act declaration of a public health emergency, such as those issued for COVID-19, pandemic influenza (e.g., the 2009 H1N1 "swine flu"), and the Ebola virus.[267]

The COVID-19 PREP Act Declaration

On March 10, 2020, the Secretary of HHS invoked the PREP Act and determined that COVID-19 constitutes a public health emergency.[268] The COVID-19 PREP Act Declaration therefore authorizes PREP Act

---

[261] *See* 42 C.F.R. pt. 110.

[262] 42 U.S.C. § 247d-6e(a), (b), (e)(3), (e)(5); 42 C.F.R. § 110.2(a).

[263] 42 C.F.R. § 110.3(z).

[264] 42 U.S.C. § 247d-6e(a).

[265] *See* 42 U.S.C. §§ 300aa-10 to 300aa-34; 42 C.F.R. pt. 100.

[266] *See National Vaccine Injury Compensation Program: Covered Vaccines*, HEALTH RESOURCES & SERVS. ADMIN, https://www.hrsa.gov/vaccine-compensation/covered-vaccines/index.html (last updated Mar. 2020).

[267] *See* HEALTH RESOURCES & SERVS. ADMIN, COUNTERMEASURES INJURY COMPENSATION PROGRAM: FACT SHEET (Oct. 2017), https://www.hrsa.gov/sites/default/files/hrsa/cicp/cicpfactsheet.pdf.

[268] COVID-19 PREP Act Declaration, 85 Fed. Reg. at 15,201.

immunity for the "manufacture, testing, development, distribution, administration, and use" of covered countermeasures.[269] This immunity applies to all covered persons as defined in the PREP Act, including any person authorized by state and local public health agencies (or an EUA) to "prescribe, administer, deliver, distribute or dispense" covered countermeasures.[270] Covered countermeasures include "any antiviral, any other drug, any biologic, any diagnostic, any other device, or any vaccine, used to treat, diagnose, cure, prevent, or mitigate COVID-19."[271] The "administration" of a covered countermeasure includes "physical provision of the countermeasures" to patients, as well as "activities and decisions directly relating to . . . delivery, distribution and dispensing of" the countermeasures.[272] The declaration provides PREP Act immunity "without geographic limitation," beginning on February 4, 2020, and ending as late as October 1, 2025.[273]

Recent Congressional Actions on COVID-19 Countermeasures Liability

Three recent congressional enactments in response to the COVID-19 pandemic, all now signed into law, relate to the scope of immunity for individuals engaged in the COVID-19 response.

Section 6005 of the Families First Coronavirus Response Act[274] and Section 3103 of the CARES Act[275] amend the PREP Act to clarify that certain "personal respiratory protective devices" (such as N95 respirators) are covered countermeasures. To be covered by the PREP Act, the respiratory protective device must be (i) approved by the National Institute for Occupational Safety and Health (NIOSH) under 42 C.F.R. Part 84; and

[269] *Id.*
[270] *Id.* at 15,201-02.
[271] *Id.* at 15,202.
[272] *Id.*
[273] *See id.*
[274] Pub. L. No. 116-127, § 6005, 134 Stat. 178, 207 (2020).
[275] Pub. L. No. 116-136, § 3103 (2020).

(ii) determined by the Secretary of HHS to be a priority for use during a public health emergency.[276]

Section 3215 of the CARES Act contains an independent immunization from liability for volunteer health care professionals responding to the COVID-19 pandemic. Under Section 3215, licensed health care professionals are generally immune from state or federal liability for harm they cause while providing health care services in response to the COVID-19 public health emergency as a volunteer, if they act within the scope of their license and in good faith.[277] There are two exceptions to this immunity: (1) if the volunteer health care professional's acts constituted willful or criminal misconduct, gross negligence, reckless misconduct, or a conscious flagrant indifference to the rights or safety of the individual harmed;[278] or (2) if the volunteer health care professional rendered health care services under the influence of drugs or alcohol.[279] Section 3215 immunity may overlap with PREP Act immunity, or extend beyond it in some cases (e.g., situations not involving a covered countermeasure).

Finally, both the CARES Act and CPRSA appropriate funding that HHS may use for the Covered Countermeasure Process Fund, upon which CICP relies. CPRSA appropriates $3.1 billion to the Secretary of HHS to respond to COVID-19, including the development and purchase of countermeasures and vaccines, while allowing these funds to "be transferred to, and merged with" the Covered Countermeasure Process Fund.[280] The CARES Act appropriates $27 billion to the Secretary of HHS for similar purposes, again providing that the Secretary may transfer these funds to the Covered Countermeasure Process Fund.[281]

---

[276] 42 U.S.C. § 247-6d(i)(1)(D). Prior to these amendments, FDA issued an EUA on March 2, 2020, for the use of NIOSH-approved filtering respirators intended for general use in health care settings, and expressed its view that the PREP Act covered these respirators prior to the amendment because of their medical use. *See* Letter from Denise M. Hinton, Chief Scientist, FDA, to Robert R. Redfield, Director Centers for Disease Control and Prevention (March 28, 2020), https://www.fda.gov/media/135763/download.

[277] Pub. L. No. 116-136, § 3215(a).

[278] *Id.* § 3215(b)(1).

[279] *Id.* § 3215(b)(2).

[280] Pub. L. No. 116-123, tit. III, 134 Stat. 146, 149 (2020).

[281] Pub. L. No. 116-136, tit. VIII.

In: Vaccines
Editor: Oliver Huerta

ISBN: 978-1-53619-059-5

Chapter 9

VACCINE SAFETY IN THE UNITED STATES: OVERVIEW AND CONSIDERATIONS FOR COVID-19 VACCINES*

Kavya Sekar and Agata Dabrowska

SUMMARY

Widespread immunization efforts have been linked to increased life expectancy and reduced illness. U.S. vaccination programs, headed by the Centers for Disease Control and Prevention (CDC) within the Department of Health and Human Services (HHS), have helped eradicate smallpox and nearly eradicate polio globally, and eliminate several infectious diseases domestically. With the Coronavirus Disease 2019 (COVID-19) pandemic now causing major health and economic impacts across the world, efforts are underway to make safe and effective vaccines available quickly to help curb spread of the virus.

* This is an edited, reformatted and augmented version of Congressional Research Service, Publication No. R46593, dated November 4, 2020.

Background

Federal regulation of vaccine safety began with the Biologics Control Act of 1902, which was the first federal law to require premarket review of pharmaceutical products. Since the 1902 law was enacted, federal vaccine safety activities have expanded, with the aim of minimizing the possibility of adverse events following vaccination and detecting new adverse events as quickly as possible. Today, as covered in this chapter, federal efforts to ensure vaccine safety include the following activities:

- Premarket requirements: Clinical trials, or testing of investigational vaccines in human subjects, and U.S. Food and Drug Administration (FDA) licensure or authorization.
- Clinical recommendations: Recommendations for the clinical use of vaccines by the Advisory Committee on Immunization Practices (ACIP), and CDC clinical guidance and resources.
- Postmarket safety: Manufacturing requirements and ongoing safety monitoring of vaccines administered to patients.
- Federal research on vaccine safety: Ongoing research to inform a better scientific understanding of vaccine safety and comprehensive scientific reviews on the safety of vaccines in use.
- Vaccine injury compensation: In nonemergency circumstances, the National Vaccine Injury Compensation Program (VICP) provides compensation to eligible individuals found to have been injured by a covered vaccine. In emergency circumstances, like COVID-19, a separate Countermeasures Injury Compensation Program (CICP) may be used.
- Vaccine distribution: Programs and requirements to ensure safety controls in vaccine distribution programs, led by CDC.

COVID-19 Vaccine Safety Considerations

Safety considerations for COVID-19 vaccines in development are unique in many ways. FDA has never licensed a vaccine for a coronavirus, and much remains unknown about potential safety issues related to COVID-19 vaccines. Under Operation Warp Speed (OWS)—the Trump Administration's major medical countermeasure development initiative—COVID-19 vaccines are under an expedited development timeline. FDA may initially make the vaccine available under an Emergency Use Authorization (EUA) instead of its standard biologics licensing process—a first for the agency for a previously unapproved vaccine. In light of reported concerns from the public surrounding the safety and effectiveness of COVID-19 vaccines developed on an expedited timeline, FDA officials have sought to clarify that any vaccine candidate "will be reviewed according to the established legal and regulatory standards for medical products." If made available within the next several months, available safety and effectiveness data would be based on months of data collection rather than on years of data collection typically used in vaccine development. In addition, efforts are underway with regard to (1) clinical guidance and prioritization of individuals to receive the likely limited initial supply of COVID-19 vaccines; (2) strengthening safety monitoring systems to collect ongoing safety surveillance data on vaccines administered to the population; and (3) preparing for safety controls in vaccine distribution and patient administration, in addition to other activities.

Congressional Considerations

Ever since the Biologics Control Act of 1902, Congress and the Administration (especially through FDA and CDC) have strived to ensure the safety of vaccines in the United States—from initial development to patient administration. Congress may consider how to best leverage existing requirements and programs to ensure that risk of harm from eventual COVID-19 vaccines is mitigated and minimized. OWS, FDA, CDC, and others are working to expedite the availability of COVID-19 vaccines and to prepare for a nationwide immunization campaign. Safety has been cited as a consideration in all of these efforts. Congress may consider how to best provide oversight and make legislative changes to ensure a safe and successful COVID-19 vaccination campaign. In addition, Congress may consider and evaluate the entire federal vaccine safety system and assess whether this system warrants any policy changes to help ensure ongoing safety of all recommended vaccines.

INTRODUCTION

Widespread immunization efforts have been linked to increased life expectancy and reduced illness.[1] In 1900, for every 1,000 babies born in the United States, 100 would die before their first birthday, often due to

[1] Walter A. Orenstein and Rafi Ahmed, "Simply Put: Vaccination Saves Lives," *Proceedings of the National Academy of Sciences*, vol. 114, no. 16 (April 10, 2017).

infectious diseases.[2] One study estimated that from 1993 to 2013, routine childhood immunization in the United States helped prevent 322 million illnesses, 21 million hospitalizations, and 732,000 premature deaths.[3] U.S. immunization programs, headed by the Centers for Disease Control and Prevention (CDC) within the Department of Health and Human Services (HHS), have helped eradicate smallpox and nearly eradicate polio globally.[4] U.S. immunization programs have also helped eliminate measles and rubella domestically, and have led to substantial reductions in hospitalizations linked to pneumococcus, rotavirus, and varicella (i.e., chickenpox).[5] With the Coronavirus Disease 2019 (COVID-19) pandemic now causing major health and economic impacts across the world, efforts are underway to make safe and effective vaccines available quickly to help curb spread of the virus.

Available evidence from thousands of scientific studies shows that currently recommended vaccines are largely safe. At a population level, widespread vaccination with recommended vaccines is safer than the spread of the infectious diseases they prevent.[6] Adverse health events for which available scientific evidence shows a causal relationship with currently recommended vaccines are rare—ranging from 1 case per million doses administered (e.g., encephalitis caused by the pertussis vaccine) to

---

[2] Institute of Medicine (now National Academy of Medicine), *Adverse Effects of Vaccines: Evidence and Causality*, Washington, DC, August 25, 2011, https://www.ncbi.nlm.nih.gov/books/NBK190024/.

[3] Cynthia G. Whitney, Fangjun Zhou, James Singleton, et al., "Benefits from Immunization during the Vaccines for Children Program Era—United States, 1994–2013," *Morbidity and Mortality Weekly Report*, vol. 63, no. 16 (April 25, 2014), pp. 352-355.

[4] Eric E. Mast, Stephen L. Cochi, Olen M. Kew et al., "Fifty Years of Global Immunization at CDC, 1966-2015," *Public Health Reports*, vol. 132, no. 1 (Jan-Feb 2017), pp. 18-26.

[5] Pneumococcus is the most common form of bacteria that causes severe pneumonia. Rotaviruses are a genus of viruses that cause a large portion of severe diarrhea cases. Varicella is the scientific name for "chickenpox" disease. See Amanda Cohn, Lance E. Rodewald, Walter A. Orenstein, et al., "Immunization in the United States," in *Plotkin's Vaccines*, ed. Stanley A. Plotkin, Walter A. Orenstein, and Paul A. Offit, 7th ed. (Elsevier, 2017), p. 1436.

[6] Margaret A. Maglione, Courtney Gidengil, Lopamudra Das, et al. "Safety of Vaccines Used for Routine Immunization in the United States," *Agency for Healthcare Research and Quality*, July 2014, https://effectivehealthcare.ahrq.gov/sites/default/files/pdf/vaccine-safety_research.pdf, and Institute of Medicine (now National Academy of Medicine), *Adverse Effects of Vaccines: Evidence and Causality*, Washington, DC, August 25, 2012, https://www.ncbi.nlm.nih.gov/books/NBK190010/#sec_0009.

333 cases per million doses (e.g., febrile seizures caused by the measles-mumps-rubella; MMR vaccine).[7]

Undervaccination linked to concerns about vaccine safety has been an issue in recent years. U.S. outbreaks of measles in 2019—the highest number of annual measles cases since 1992—were driven in part by geographic clusters with low vaccination rates for the MMR vaccine.[8] U.S. surveys show that concerns about vaccine safety are a top reason for vaccine delays or refusals.[9]

From a public health perspective, vaccines for infectious diseases often work by helping provide *herd immunity*, meaning that enough of the population has vaccine-induced immunity against the target disease to curb ongoing transmission and protect those who cannot receive vaccines (e.g., persons with compromised immune systems).[10] Widespread vaccination can help with achieving *elimination* or *eradication* of a given disease (see text box). To effectively prevent disease spread, many vaccines must be administered to a large segment of the population. Public health practice generally aims for near 100% vaccination rates among populations recommended to receive vaccines, though the level required for herd immunity is generally lower and can vary by vaccine and population (75%-95% of the population).[11] Nonetheless, widespread vaccination that does not meet target rates can aid in significantly curbing disease spread.[12]

---

[7] Frank DeStefano, Paul A. Offit, and Allison Fisher, Ch. 82, "Vaccine Safety," in *Vaccines*, ed. Stanley A. Plotkin, Walter A. Orenstein, Paul A. Offit et al. 67h ed. (Elsevier, 2017), pp. 1584-1600.

[8] CDC, "Measles Cases and Outbreaks," last updated August 2020, https://www.cdc.gov/measles/cases-outbreaks.html.

[9] CRS Insight IN11125, *Measles Outbreaks, Vaccine Hesitancy, and Federal Policy Options*, and Amanda Cohn, Lance E. Rodewald, Walter A. Orenstein, et al., "Immunization in the United States," in *Plotkin's Vaccines*, ed. Stanley A. Plotkin, Walter A. Orenstein, and Paul A. Offit, 7th ed. (Elsevier, 2017), p. 1432.

[10] Paul Fine, Ken Eames, and David L. Heymann, "''Herd Immunity'': A Rough Guide," *Vaccines*, vol. 52 (2011).

[11] Ibid., and Pedro Plans-Rubió, "Evaluation of the Establishment of Herd Immunity in the Population by Means of Serological Surveys and Vaccination Coverage," *Human Vaccines & Immunotherapeutics*. vol. 8, no. 2 (February 2012), pp. 184-88.

[12] Paul Fine, Ken Eames, and David L. Heymann, "''Herd Immunity'': A Rough Guide," *Vaccines*, vol. 52 (2011).

Definitions: Elimination and Eradication

The World Health Organization (WHO) defines disease elimination and eradication as follows:

Elimination (or interruption) of transmission: Reduction to zero of the incidence of infection caused by a specific pathogen in a defined geographical area, with minimal risk of reintroduction, as a result of deliberate efforts; continued actions to prevent reestablishment of transmission may be required.

Eradication: Permanent reduction to zero of a specific pathogen, as a result of deliberate efforts, with no more risk of reintroduction.

Source: WHO, "Generic Framework for the Control, Elimination, and Eradication of Neglected Tropical Diseases," 2015, https://www.who.int/ neglected_diseases/resources/ NTD_Generic_Framework_2015.pdf.

Vaccines are generally held to a higher safety standard than most other medical products for many reasons. For one, vaccines are often administered to healthy individuals to prevent disease; therefore, the expectation is that such individuals will remain healthy following vaccination. Moreover, drugs administered to healthy people are expected to have fewer side effects than drugs that treat disease, such as those for cancer or heart disease, mainly because the expected benefits differ. In addition, vaccines are often administered to vulnerable populations, including infants and pregnant women. Also, since vaccines are often mandated by state and sometimes federal law for certain groups (e.g., school children and military service members), the government has an interest in ensuring that vaccines are as safe as possible. Because vaccines are often administered to a large segment of the population, even a rare risk of adverse reactions to a vaccine could affect a sizeable number of people.[13]

---

[13] Frank DeStefano, Paul A. Offit, and Allison Fisher, "Vaccine Safety," in *Vaccines*, ed. Stanley A. Plotkin, Walter A. Orenstein, Paul A. Offit, et al. 67h ed. (Elsevier, 2017), pp. 1584-1600, and Matthew Z. Dudley, Daniel A. Salmon, Neal A. Halsey, et al., "Monitoring Vaccine Safety," in *The Clinician's Vaccine Safety Resource Guide* (Springer, Cham, 2018).

Scope of This Chapter

This chapter provides an overview of the federal government's role in ensuring safety of vaccines for infectious diseases. Specifically, this chapter

- describes federal statutory and regulatory requirements and administrative functions governing vaccine licensure (including pre- and post-licensure safety), development of clinical recommendations, and vaccine injury compensation;
- summarizes ongoing federal activities related to vaccine post-licensure safety (e.g., ongoing safety monitoring and research), as well as safety assurances in federal vaccine distribution programs; and
- discusses safety considerations in the context of developing and making available vaccine(s) for COVID-19.

This chapter does not provide a comprehensive scientific review on the safety of existing vaccines, nor does it specifically address vaccines for noninfectious diseases (e.g., cancer). A discussion of payment and coverage for vaccines and related health care services is outside the scope of this chapter.

What Is a Vaccine?

A vaccine is a biological preparation that contains small amounts of weak, dead, or modified disease-causing agents known as *antigens*, which can include viruses, bacteria, fractions of these agents, or the toxins they produce. Once introduced to the body, the antigen elicits a response by the immune system creating antibodies and immune memory cells that prevent future infection from the same disease. The immune response from a vaccine is similar to the immune response from acquiring an infectious disease naturally; however, since the antigen in the vaccine is weakened or dead, the vaccine usually does not cause disease. In the case of vaccines made with weakened live attenuated viruses or bacteria, the vaccine may cause a form of the disease that is usually much milder than the actual disease. In addition, the immune response triggered by any vaccine may cause some symptoms in some patients.[14]

Along with the antigen, vaccines contain other ingredients such as preservatives, stabilizers, and adjuvants. Preservatives, like thimerosal, can help keep the vaccine free of contamination by other germs (e.g., bacteria, fungi). Thimerosal is currently used only in multidose vials of vaccines, such as certain formulations of the influenza (flu) vaccine. Stabilizers, like sugar or gelatin, allow the vaccine to be stored for a period of time and help keep the antigen stable.

Adjuvants, such as aluminum salts, help trigger the immune response to the vaccine, particularly for vaccines made with fractions of disease-causing agents. Vaccines may also contain small amounts of residual material from the manufacturing process, such as egg proteins, formaldehyde, and antibiotics.[15]

Federal Vaccine Safety Regulation and Programs

Federal regulation of vaccine safety began with the Biologics Control Act of 1902, which was the first federal law to require premarket review of pharmaceutical products.[16] The Biologics Control Act was enacted in response to deaths (many of them children) from tetanus contamination of

[14] CDC, "Principles of Vaccination," in *Epidemiology and Prevention of Vaccine-Preventable Diseases*, ed. Jennifer Hamborsky, Andrew Kroger, and Charles Wolfe, 13th ed. (Washington, DC: Public Health Foundation, 2015).

[15] Department of Health and Human Services (HHS), "Vaccine Ingredients," *Vaccines.gov,* December 2017, https://www.vaccines.gov/basics/vaccine_ingredients; CDC, "What's in Vaccines?" August 2019, https://www.cdc.gov/vaccines/vac-gen/additives.htm; and the Food and Drug Administration (FDA), "Common Ingredients in U.S. Licensed Vaccines," https://www.fda.gov/vaccines-blood-biologics/safety-availability-biologics/common-ingredients-us-licensed-vaccines.

[16] P.L. 57-244, enacted July 1, 1902. David M. Dudzinski, "Reflections on Historical, Scientific, and Legal Issues Relevant to Designing Approval Pathways for Generic Versions of Recombinant Protein-Based Therapeutics and Monoclonal Antibodies," *Food & Drug Law Journal*, 2005, vol. 60, no. 2., p. 147.

smallpox vaccine and diphtheria antitoxin (a prophylaxis used for diphtheria at the time). The act imposed requirements on the manufacturing and labeling of biological products ("biologics") and required inspection of manufacturing facilities before a federal license was issued for marketing the products. The Biologics Control Act was revised and recodified when the Public Health Service Act (PHSA) was enacted in 1944. Biologics are now subject to regulation by the U.S. Food and Drug Administration (FDA) under the PHSA and the Federal Food, Drug, and Cosmetic Act (FFDCA).[17]

Since the 1902 law was enacted, federal vaccine safety activities have expanded to minimize the possibility of adverse events following vaccination (such as by vaccine contamination) and to detect new adverse events as quickly as possible, as discussed throughout this chapter. Major reforms to federal vaccine safety programs were enacted as a part of the National Childhood Vaccine Injury Act of 1986 (NCVIA; P.L. 99-660, Title III), which mandated reporting of adverse events caused by vaccines to FDA and CDC, established the National Vaccine Program Office (NVPO) within HHS to coordinate federal vaccine efforts, granted FDA mandatory recall authority for biological products, and established the National Vaccine Injury Compensation Program (VICP). NCVIA was enacted after a spate of lawsuits against vaccine manufacturers alleging safety issues. The lawsuits caused several vaccine manufacturers to exit the market, leading to concerns about the vaccine supply and possible reintroduction of certain diseases.[18]

---

[17] Until 1972, biologics, including vaccines, were regulated by the National Institutes of Health (NIH, or its precursors) under the Biologics Control Act of 1902. In 1972, regulatory responsibility over biologics was transferred from NIH to the U.S. Food and Drug Administration (FDA). See David M. Dudzinski, "Reflections on Historical, Scientific, and Legal Issues Relevant to Designing Approval Pathways for Generic Versions of Recombinant Protein-Based Therapeutics and Monoclonal Antibodies," *Food and Drug Law Journal*, 2005, vol. 60, no. 2, pp. 143-260. See also CRS Report R44620, *Biologics and Biosimilars: Background and Key Issues*.

[18] Geoffrey Evans, "Update on Vaccine Liability in the United States: Presentation at the National Vaccine Program Office on Strengthening the Supply of Routinely Recommended Vaccines in the United States, 12 February 2002," *Clinical Infectious Diseases*, vol. 42 (2006), pp. S130-7, and Nora Freeman Engstrom, "A Dose of Reality for Specialized Courts: Lessons from the VICP," *University of Pennsylvania Law Review*, vol. 163 (June 28, 2015), pp. 1655-1658.

Federal Agencies Involved in Vaccine Safety

Within the Department of Health and Human Services (HHS):

- FDA regulates the safety, effectiveness, and quality of vaccines through premarket review and postmarket requirements (e.g., adverse event reporting).
- CDC supports cross-cutting immunization programs that include, as relevant to vaccine safety: safety monitoring, clinical guidance for vaccines, vaccine safety research, and efforts to ensure safety in public vaccine distribution.
- The National Institutes of Health (NIH) is the primary federal agency that supports medical and health research, including vaccine research.
- The Centers for Medicare & Medicaid Services (CMS) monitors vaccine safety among the Medicare population.
- The Agency for Healthcare Research and Quality (AHRQ) conducts vaccine safety reviews.
- The Health Resources and Services Administration (HRSA) administers the VICP.

The Department of Veterans Affairs (VA) conducts some vaccine research and monitors vaccine safety among veterans who receive care in the VA system.

The Department of Defense (DOD) conducts some vaccine research and has a database for monitoring adverse events from vaccination among military service members and their families.

As covered in this chapter, efforts to ensure vaccine safety include several federal activities:

- *Premarket requirements:* Clinical trials and FDA licensure or authorization.
- *Clinical recommendations:* Recommendations for the safe and appropriate clinical use of vaccines by the Advisory Committee on Immunization Practices (ACIP), and CDC clinical guidance and resources.

- *Postmarket safety:* Manufacturing requirements and ongoing safety monitoring of vaccines administered to patients.
- *Federal research on vaccine safety:* Ongoing research to inform a better scientific understanding of vaccine safety, and comprehensive scientific reviews on the safety of vaccines.
- *Vaccine injury compensation:* In nonemergency circumstances, the VICP can provide compensation to eligible individuals found to have been injured by a covered vaccine.
- *Vaccine distribution:* Programs and requirements to ensure safety controls in vaccine distribution programs, led by CDC.

Vaccine Safety Basics

As defined by FDA regulations, safety is "the relative freedom from harmful effect to persons affected, directly or indirectly, by a product when prudently administered, taking into consideration the character of the product in relation to the condition of the recipient at the time."[19] Vaccine safety is distinct from efficacy and effectiveness; however, it is useful to consider vaccine safety in the context of efficacy and effectiveness, which are defined as follows:

- Vaccine *efficacy* is defined as the reduction in disease incidence in a vaccinated group compared with an unvaccinated group under optimal conditions (i.e., healthy individuals and proper administration).
- Vaccine *effectiveness* is defined as the reduction in disease incidence in a vaccinated group compared with an unvaccinated group under real-world conditions.[20]

---

[19] 21 C.F.R. §600.3(p).

[20] Vaccine efficacy and effectiveness definitions are based on Shelly McNeil, *Overview of Vaccine Efficacy and Vaccine Effectiveness*, Canadian Center for Vaccinology, Presentation to the World Health Organization, https://www.who.int/influenza_vaccines_plan/resources/Session4_VEfficacy_VEffectiveness.PDF, and Centers for Disease Control and

Like all pharmaceutical products, vaccines are not 100% safe for all patients. Vaccine safety programs continually assess the benefits and risks of vaccination. Adverse events following vaccination can be classified in many ways:[21]

- Frequency—is the adverse event common or rare?
- Severity—is the adverse event mild, such as minor pain or swelling, or severe, such as leading to hospitalization, disability, or death?
- Causality—can a causal relationship be established with the vaccine with clinical, laboratory, or epidemiologic evidence? (see text box below)
- Preventability—is the adverse event intrinsic to the vaccine (i.e., provoked by the immune response caused by the vaccine), or related to faulty production or administration of the vaccine?

Some adverse events following vaccination may be linked directly to the antigen in the vaccine, such as paralytic poliomyelitis (i.e., paralysis), which is rarely caused by the live oral polio vaccine. Other adverse events are precipitated by the vaccine, such as febrile seizures that occur following a vaccine-induced fever. Some adverse events can be linked to improper vaccine administration; for example, a vaccine administered too high on the arm of an adult can cause deltoid bursitis (inflammation of the shoulder joint).[22] In the past, improper vaccine manufacturing has been tied to large-scale adverse health events. In 1955, one polio vaccine manufacturer failed to completely inactivate the poliovirus in the

---

Prevention (CDC), "How Flu Vaccine Effectiveness and Efficacy Is Measured," 2016, https://www.cdc.gov/flu/vaccines-work/effectivenessqa.htm.

[21] CDC, "Vaccine Safety," in *Epidemiology and Prevention of Vaccine-Preventable Diseases*, ed. Jennifer Hamborsky, Andrew Kroger, and Charles Wolfe, 13th ed. (Washington, DC: Public Health Foundation, 2015).

[22] CDC, "Vaccine Safety," in *Epidemiology and Prevention of Vaccine-Preventable Diseases*, ed. Jennifer Hamborsky, Andrew Kroger, and Charles Wolfe, 13th ed. (Washington, DC: Public Health Foundation, 2015).

manufacturing process. As a result, 40,000 people developed mild polio from the vaccine, 200 became paralyzed, and 10 died.[23]

In some cases, establishing a causal connection between a vaccine and an adverse event is difficult. Vaccination may *co-occur* with an adverse health event. For example, early childhood— a time when several recommended pediatric vaccines are typically administered—coincides with the same period when signs and symptoms of developmental disorders, such as autism, may begin to appear.[24] Available evidence rejects a causal relationship between childhood vaccines and autism.[25] To determine causality between a vaccine and a given health event, scientists and public health experts evaluate many kinds of evidence, including the time period between vaccination and the event; the biologic plausibility that the health event was caused by vaccination; clinical or laboratory evidence that supports causation by the vaccine; and population-based epidemiological analyses that assess whether vaccinated individuals are more likely to develop a certain health outcome within a certain time period following vaccination compared to individuals who did not receive the vaccine in that time period.[26] Several of the programs covered in this chapter generate data or other evidence that can allow for causality assessments to link certain adverse events with vaccination (see text box).

---

[23] Frank DeStefano, Paul A. Offit, and Allison Fisher, "Vaccine Safety," in *Plotkin's Vaccines*, ed. Stanley A. Plotkin, Walter A. Orenstein, and Paul A. Offit, 7th ed. (Elsevier, 2017), p. 1584.

[24] Frank DeStefano, Paul A. Offit, and Allison Fisher, "Vaccine Safety," in *Plotkin's Vaccines*, ed. Stanley A. Plotkin, Walter A. Orenstein, and Paul A. Offit, 7th ed. (Elsevier, 2017), p. 1593.

[25] Frank DeStefano, Heather Monk Bodenstab, and Paul A. Offit, "Principal Controversies in Vaccine Safety in the United States," *Clinical Infectious Diseases*, vol. 69 (August 15, 2019), pp. 726-31.

[26] CDC, "Vaccine Safety," in *Epidemiology and Prevention of Vaccine-Preventable Diseases*, ed. Jennifer Hamborsky, Andrew Kroger, and Charles Wolfe, 13th ed. (Washington, DC: Public Health Foundation, 2015).

What Is a Causality Assessment?

Immune systems are arguably among the most complex biological systems—therefore, studying vaccines and their effect on the human body can be difficult. Individual studies may provide suggestive evidence of adverse health effects linked to vaccines. For example, an analysis of health data on a population of thousands of individuals could find that vaccination with a certain vaccine is statistically associated with higher rates of a certain adverse health event that occurred following vaccination. Yet, another similar study could conduct a similar analysis among a different population and find no such evidence. In addition, further evidence based on the research in the laboratory, such as with animals or human tissue samples, might find that a certain adverse event following vaccination is or is not likely based on an understanding of biological systems. Therefore, in order to determine if all the available evidence favors a *causal* relationship between a vaccine and a subsequent adverse health event, researchers will combine evidence across many types of studies as a part of a causality assessment. Good quality systematic causality assessments usually include the following attributes:

- Search methods to identify all possible studies of interest within all relevant areas of research.
- A selection process to determine which studies are actually relevant and used rigorous scientific methods that provide quality evidence based on defined criteria.
- A review process to compare evidence across studies, considering differences such as study populations, study design, and the quality of each study.
- Methods to weigh different types of evidence and combine evidence across studies in order to determine whether all the evidence, in total, supports or does not support a causal relationship between vaccination with a specific vaccine and a subsequent adverse event, or yields inconclusive results.

For a further discussion, see the "Federal Research on Vaccine Safety" section. Causality assessments may also be conducted on an ongoing basis using data and information from postmarket monitoring systems (see the "Postmarket Safety" section).

For examples of causality assessments on the safety of vaccines, see Institute of Medicine (now National Academy of Medicine, "Adverse Effects of Vaccines: Evidence and Causality," 2012, https://www.nap.edu/catalog/13164/adverse-effects-of-vaccines-evidence-and-causality; and Margaret A. Maglione, Courtney Gidengil, Lopamudra Das, et al. "Safety of Vaccines Used for Routine Immunization in the United States," *Agency for Healthcare Research and Quality*, July 2014, https://effectivehealthcare.ahrq.gov/sites/default/files/pdf/vaccine-safety_research.pdf. Also, for an overview of causality assessments for vaccines, see Frank DeStefano, Paul A. Offit, and Allison Fisher, "Ch. 82:

Vaccine Safety," in *Plotkin's Vaccines*, ed. Stanley A. Plotkin, Walter A. Orenstein, and Paul A. Offit, 7th ed. (Elsevier, 2017), p. 1589.

PREMARKET SAFETY

Vaccines generally follow the same clinical development and approval process as drugs and other biologics (i.e., therapeutics derived from living organisms).[27] To be marketed in the United States, a new vaccine must first receive licensure (i.e., approval) from FDA. Licensure is based on a determination by FDA that the vaccine and the facility in which it is manufactured, processed, packed, or held meet standards to ensure that the product is safe, pure, and potent (effective).[28] Except under very limited circumstances, FDA requires data from clinical trials—formally designed, conducted, and analyzed studies of human subjects—to provide evidence of a vaccine's safety and effectiveness. These requirements apply to all

[27] Biological products include vaccines, monoclonal antibodies, and cytokines, among other examples. For additional information about biologics, see CRS Report R44620, *Biologics and Biosimilars: Background and Key Issues*.

[28] PHSA §351(a)(2)(C) [42 U.S.C. §262(a)(2)(C)]. FDA approves drugs that are *safe and effective*; the equivalent terminology for biologics is *safe, pure, and potent*. FDA has interpreted *potency* to include effectiveness. See the FDA Guidance for Industry, *Scientific Considerations in Demonstrating Biosimilarity to a Reference Product*, https://www.fda.gov/media/82647/download.

vaccines marketed in the United States, regardless of whether the manufacturing facility is located domestically or in a foreign country.

Clinical Trials

Vaccines are typically tested in several stages of human clinical trials. Before beginning clinical testing, a vaccine's sponsor must file an investigational new drug (IND) application, which is a request for FDA authorization to administer an investigational biologic (or drug) to humans.[29] The IND must include information about the proposed clinical study design, completed animal test data, and the lead investigator's qualifications.[30] The investigator also must provide assurance that an Institutional Review Board (IRB) will provide initial and continuous review and approval of each of the studies in the clinical investigation to ensure that participants are aware of the drug's investigational status, and that any risk of harm will be necessary, explained, and minimized.[31] FDA has 30 days to review an IND, after which a manufacturer may begin clinical testing if FDA has not objected and imposed a clinical hold.

Clinical trials for an IND may be sponsored by the drug company seeking to commercially market the vaccine, a university or nonprofit organization, a government agency, or a combination or partnership of all the above. The funder(s) may differ for each stage of testing. In typical circumstances, the public sector (e.g., federal agencies, nonprofit organizations) generally finances more of the earlier stages of clinical trials, such as Phase 1 clinical trials. Later-stage testing, such as Phase 3 clinical trials, are typically funded more so by drug companies than government agencies.[32]

---

[29] FFDCA §505(i) [21 U.S.C. §355(i)], PHSA §351(a)(3) [42 U.S.C. §262(a)(3)], 21 C.F.R. Part 312.

[30] 21 C.F.R. 312 Subpart B.

[31] 21 C.F.R. §312.23(a)(1)(iv) and 21 C.F.R. Part 56.

[32] Stuart O. Schweitzer and Z. John Lu, "The Pharmaceutical Industry," in *Pharmaceutical Economics and Policy: Perspectives, Promises, and Problems* (New York, NY: Oxford University Press, 2018), pp. 37-40, and Gillian K. Gresham, Stephan Erhardt, Jill L. Meinert, et al., "Characteristics and Trends of Clinical Trials Funded by the National

The sponsor of the trial is responsible for selecting qualified investigators, maintaining an effective IND, and ensuring proper monitoring of the investigations, including that they are conducted in accordance with the IND. In certain cases, the sponsor may establish an independent Data and Safety Monitoring Board (DSMB) of relevant experts with no relevant financial or other ties to the sponsor to oversee the investigations.[33] The DSMB often advises the sponsor on the ongoing safety of trial subjects and the continuing validity and scientific merit of the trial. One DSMB may be responsible for overseeing multiple clinical trials.

In general, vaccine clinical trials occur in three sequential phases:

- Phase 1 trials are the first in-human studies of a vaccine candidate, and they assess safety and immunogenicity[34] in a small number of volunteers.
- Phase 2 trials assess side effects and the dosing at which the investigational vaccine may have a protective effect and may enroll hundreds of volunteers.
- Phase 3 trials assess effectiveness and continue to monitor safety and typically enroll thousands of volunteers.[35]

Most clinical trials for vaccines include a control group, such as a placebo or alternative vaccine, to compare outcomes for those who received the target vaccine compared with those who did not. Phase 3 clinical trial data are typically needed to fully assess the safety and effectiveness of an investigational vaccine. Typically, only the Phase 3 clinical trials are large enough to allow for robust scientific evidence on the

Institutes of Health Between 2005 and 2015," *Clinical Trials*, vol. 15, no. 1 (September 7, 2017), pp. 65-74.

[33] FDA, "Guidance for Clinical Trial Sponsors Establishment and Operation of Clinical Trial Data Monitoring Committees," March 2006, https://www.fda.gov/media/75398/download.

[34] *Immunogenicity* refers to the extent to which a substance is able to stimulate an immune response. An immune response to a pharmaceutical product may affect its safety and effectiveness. See Jonathan Law and Elizabeth Martin, ed., *Concise Medical Dictionary* (Oxford University Press).

[35] 21 C.F.R. 312.21. FDA, "Vaccine Product Approval Process," https://www.fda.gov/vaccines-blood-biologics/ development-approval-process-cber/vaccine-product-approval-process.

safety and effectiveness of the investigational vaccine among different population segments (e.g., children, older adults).[36] Under typical circumstances, a vaccine candidate moves through each phase of clinical testing upon successful completion of the prior phase.

Phase 3 clinical trials are typically longer (usually at least a year) than the other phases in order to fully assess the safety and effectiveness of the investigational vaccine. Adequate time is often needed to give trial participants a chance to be exposed to the target disease in the community and to assess if infection rates vary between the vaccine recipient and control groups. In some cases, an experimental vaccine that showed promise in Phase 1 and Phase 2 clinical trials was found to be ineffective in Phase 3 trials. For example, an experimental vaccine for herpes simplex virus type 2 (HSV-2) showed safety and preliminary evidence of an immune response to the virus in Phase 2 clinical trials (i.e., HSV-2 antibodies in the bloodstream). However, during the Phase 3 clinical trials, by a year after vaccination, there was no difference in rates of acquired HSV-2 infections between the recipient and control groups, despite vaccine recipients showing a preliminary immune response.[37]

In addition to providing insights into the effectiveness of investigational vaccines, long-term Phase 3 studies can uncover important safety data. For example, three years of safety data on the vaccine for dengue virus produced by Sanofi Pasteur (Dengvaxia) found an issue of *antibody-mediated enhancement* of infections, where the antibodies raised in response to vaccination could worsen the severity of dengue for those without a prior dengue infection. Data on the vaccine showed a higher rate of hospitalizations for dengue three years after vaccination in young children compared with children who were unvaccinated.[38]

---

[36] Frank DeStefano, Paul A. Offit, and Allison Fisher, "Vaccine Safety," in *Plotkin's Vaccines*, ed. Stanley A. Plotkin, Walter A. Orenstein, and Paul A. Offit, 7th ed. (Elsevier, 2017), pp. 1584.

[37] FDA, *22 Case Studies Where Phase 2 and Phase 3 Trials had Divergent Results*, January 2017.

[38] S.R. Hadinegoro, J.L. Arredondo-Garcia, and M.R. Capeding, et al., "Efficacy and Long-Term Safety of a Dengue Vaccine in Regions of Endemic Disease," *The New England Journal of Medicine*, vol. 373, no. 13 (September 24, 2015). Helen Branswell, "Caution on New Dengue Vaccine: In Some Countries, Harm Outweighs Benefit," *STAT*, September 1, 2016.

For some vaccines, Phase 3 clinical trials are very large to detect rare adverse events. For instance, two second-generation rotavirus vaccines (RotaTeq and RotaRix) were subject to Phase 3 clinical trials involving over 60,000 infants in order to ascertain the risk of intussusception (intestinal obstruction) following vaccine administration (estimated to be about 1 in 10,000 in the first-generation vaccine).[39] However, such large trials involve higher costs and increased time to licensure.

Biologics License Application (BLA) and Licensure Requirements

After completing clinical trials, a sponsor may submit a Biologics License Application (BLA) to FDA's Center for Biologics Evaluation and Research (CBER). A BLA is a request for permission to market the vaccine and must contain certain information, including data from nonclinical laboratory and clinical studies demonstrating that the product meets requirements of safety, purity, and potency.[40] For each nonclinical laboratory study, the BLA must include either (1) a statement that the study was conducted in compliance with FDA regulations governing Good Laboratory Practice (GLP) for nonclinical laboratory studies[41] or (2) if the study was not conducted in compliance with GLP regulations, a brief statement explaining the reason for noncompliance. In addition, for each clinical investigation involving human subjects, the BLA must contain statements that each clinical investigation either was conducted in compliance with the requirements for institutional review set forth in FDA regulations,[42] or that it was not subject to such requirements and was conducted in compliance with requirements for informed consent.[43] The

---

[39] Frank DeStefano, Paul A. Offit, and Allison Fisher, "Vaccine Safety," in *Plotkin's Vaccines*, ed. Stanley A. Plotkin, Walter A. Orenstein, and Paul A. Offit, 7th ed. (Elsevier, 2017), pp. 1584.

[40] FDA regulations at 21 C.F.R. §601.2(a) specify the required contents of a BLA.

[41] 21 C.F.R. Part 58 "Good Laboratory Practice for Nonclinical Laboratory Studies."

[42] 21 C.F.R. Part 56 "Institutional Review Boards."

[43] 21 C.F.R. Part 50 "Protection of Human Subjects."

BLA also must contain "a full description of manufacturing methods; data establishing stability of the product through the dating period; sample(s) representative of the product for introduction or delivery for introduction into interstate commerce; summaries of results of tests performed on the lot(s) represented by the submitted sample(s); specimens of the labels, enclosures, and containers;" and the address of each location involved in the manufacture of the vaccine. If applicable, a BLA must contain any medication guide proposed to be used for the product. Finally, the BLA must include a financial certification or disclosure statement(s) or both for clinical investigators.

As noted above, a vaccine manufacturer must submit proposed vaccine labeling as part of a BLA. FDA reviews the proposed labeling to determine whether it is scientifically accurate and that it conforms to regulatory requirements. As for prescription drugs and other biologics, vaccine labeling must include warnings and precautions, contraindications, dosage and administration, storage and handling conditions, and adverse reactions, among other information.[44] Labeling for vaccines must specifically contain a statement describing how suspected adverse reactions can be reported.[45] In addition, the labels affixed to each container or package of a vaccine must include the name of the manufacturer, the lot number or other lot identification,[46] and the recommended individual dose (for multiple dose containers), among other information.[47] Vaccines require special processing and handling, such as refrigeration and proper storage, and information about storage temperature and other handling instructions must be on the label affixed to each package containing a vaccine.[48]

FDA regulations also provide for biological product manufacturing establishment standards. Such standards cover personnel, the physical establishment in which a product is manufactured, records maintenance, retention of samples, reporting of product deviations, and product

[44] 21 C.F.R. §§201.56 and 201.57.

[45] 21 C.F.R. §201.57(a)(11)(iii).

[46] "Lot" refers to "that quantity of uniform material identified by the manufacturer as having been thoroughly mixed in a single vessel." 21 C.F.R. § 600.3(x).

[47] 21 C.F.R. §§610.60 and 610.61.

[48] 21 C.F.R. §610.61.

temperature during shipment.[49] Most of these requirements apply broadly to biologics, but several provisions are vaccine-specific, including requirements for live vaccine work areas[50] and live vaccine processing,[51] as well as product-specific maintenance temperatures.[52] In addition, FDA regulations establish requirements for testing product potency, sterility, purity, and identity, as well as requirements for constituent materials used in licensed products, including preservatives, diluents, and adjuvants.[53] Vaccines, like other biological products, are subject to lot release requirements, which provide that "[n]o lot of any licensed product shall be released by the manufacturer prior to the completion of tests for conformity with standards applicable to such product."[54] FDA may require that samples of any lot of any licensed product and the protocols and applicable test results be submitted to CBER. In such case, a manufacturer may not distribute a lot of a vaccine until it is released by FDA.[55]

Expedited Pathways and Access to Unapproved Vaccines

Because clinical testing and the FDA review process typically take several years, FDA and Congress have established mechanisms to expedite the premarket development and review processes for pharmaceutical products, including vaccines, coming onto the market, as well as to expand access to products that are still under investigation. Historically, certain FDA expedited pathways such as Emergency Use Authorization (EUA) have been used infrequently for vaccines. However, a public health emergency, such as a pandemic, may affect the risk assessment in making a vaccine available before full long-term safety data are available.

---

[49] 21 C.F.R. Part 600.
[50] 21 C.F.R. §600.10(c)(4).
[51] 21 C.F.R. §600.11(c)(4).
[52] 21 C.F.R. §600.15.
[53] 21 C.F.R. Part 610.
[54] 21 C.F.R. §610.1.
[55] 21 C.F.R. §610.2.

Expedited Development and Review

To address unmet medical needs in the treatment or prevention of serious or life-threatening diseases or conditions, FDA can expedite the development and review processes for drugs and biologics, including vaccines, through four programs:

- fast track product designation,
- breakthrough therapy designation,
- accelerated approval, and
- priority review.[56]

Vaccines may be designated to more than one program. Fast track product designation and breakthrough therapy are both intended to streamline the clinical development process, but the qualifying criteria and features of these programs differ.

To qualify for *fast track product designation*, a vaccine must be intended for a serious condition, and nonclinical or clinical data must demonstrate its potential to address an unmet medical need.[57] The sponsor of a fast track-designated product is eligible for frequent interactions with the FDA review team, priority review, and rolling review (in which FDA reviews portions of a BLA before a complete application is submitted).[58]

To qualify for *breakthrough designation*, a vaccine must be intended for a serious condition, and preliminary clinical evidence must indicate that it demonstrates potential substantial improvement on a clinically significant endpoint(s) over available therapies. Features of breakthrough therapy designation include rolling review; intensive FDA guidance on designing an efficient drug development program; involvement of "senior managers and experienced review and regulatory health project management staff in a proactive, collaborative, cross-disciplinary review"

[56] FFDCA §506 [21 U.S.C. §356]. FDA, "Guidance for Industry Expedited Programs for Serious Conditions–Drugs and Biologics," May 2014, https://www.fda.gov/media/86377/download.
[57] FFDCA §506(b) [21 U.S.C. §356(b)].
[58] FFDCA §506(a) [21 U.S.C. §356(a)].

to expedite the development and review of a breakthrough therapy; and eligibility for other expedited programs.

Interested sponsors must submit to FDA a request for fast track product designation or breakthrough therapy designation. The request may be submitted with either the IND or any time after,[59] as further specified in FDA guidance.[60]

The *accelerated approval* pathway allows a vaccine to be licensed based on its effect on a surrogate endpoint (e.g., a laboratory measurement such as development of neutralizing antibodies) that predicts effectiveness, or on a clinical endpoint that can be measured earlier than irreversible morbidity or mortality. To qualify for accelerated approval, a vaccine must (1) be intended for a serious condition, (2) generally provide a meaningful advantage over available therapies, and (3) demonstrate an effect on an endpoint that is reasonably likely to predict clinical benefit. Postmarketing confirmatory studies generally must be completed to demonstrate actual effectiveness.[61] Because surrogate endpoints for vaccines are often difficult to characterize, owing to the complexity of protective immune responses, accelerated approval may not be a relevant licensure pathway for many vaccines.[62]

A *priority review* designation signifies that FDA's goal is to take action on an application within 6 months of its filing, compared with 10 months for standard review. A BLA may qualify for priority review designation if, for example, it is for a vaccine intended for a serious condition and, if approved, would provide a significant improvement in safety or effectiveness. A BLA also may qualify for priority review if submitted with a priority review voucher.[63]

---

[59] FFDCA §506(a)(2) & (b)(2) [21 U.S.C. §356(a)(2) & (b)(2)].

[60] FDA, "Guidance for Industry Expedited Programs for Serious Conditions–Drugs and Biologics," May 2014, https://www.fda.gov/media/86377/download.

[61] FFDCA §506(c) [21 U.S.C. §356(c)].

[62] Stanley A. Plotkin, "Updates on Immunologic Correlates of Vaccine-Induced Protection," *Vaccine*, vol. 38 (November 22, 2019).

[63] Three priority review voucher programs are currently authorized in the FFDCA: (1) the tropical disease priority review program, (2) the rare pediatric disease priority review program, and (3) the material threat MCM priority review voucher program. Under each of these programs, the sponsor of an NDA or BLA that meets the statutory requirements of the specific program is eligible to receive, upon approval, a transferable voucher, and the

Animal Rule

As mentioned above, FDA typically requires substantial evidence of effectiveness from adequate and well-controlled trials conducted in humans prior to licensing a vaccine. However, in certain cases, evaluating a vaccine's efficacy or effectiveness through human trials is not possible. For example, it would not be ethical to expose human subjects to lethal toxic substances in order to test an investigational vaccine.

Under the Animal Rule, if human efficacy studies are not ethical, and if field trials (i.e., trials conducted outside of the clinical setting) are not feasible, FDA may license a vaccine based on adequate and well-controlled animal efficacy studies if those studies establish that the vaccine is likely to produce clinical benefit in humans.[64] The Animal Rule is intended for drugs and biologics that would treat or prevent serious or life-threatening conditions caused by chemical, biological, radiological, or nuclear substances (e.g., nerve agents, emerging infectious pathogens, snake venom, and industrial chemicals). For FDA to rely on evidence from animal studies to provide evidence of effectiveness, four criteria must be met:

> There is a reasonably well-understood pathophysiological mechanism of the toxicity of the substance and its prevention or substantial reduction by the product;
>
> The effect is demonstrated in more than one animal species expected to react with response predictive for humans, unless the effect is demonstrated in a single animal species that represents a sufficiently well-characterized animal model for predicting the response in humans;
>
> The animal study endpoint is clearly related to the desired benefit in humans, generally the enhancement of survival or prevention of major morbidity; and

---

sponsor may either use that voucher for the priority review of another application or sell it to another sponsor to use.

[64] 21 C.F.R. §601.90 through §601.95 for biologics, including vaccines. See also FDA Guidance for Industry, "Product Development under the Animal Rule," October 2015, https://www.fda.gov/media/88625/download.

> The data or information on the kinetics and pharmacodynamics of the product or other relevant data or information, in animals and humans, allows selection of an effective dose in humans.[65]

Drugs and vaccines evaluated for efficacy under the Animal Rule are evaluated for safety under the existing requirements for drugs and biologics. Postmarketing studies, such as field studies, must be conducted once feasible, and the sponsor of the vaccine must prepare certain patient-specific information explaining that the approval was based on efficacy studies conducted in animals alone. FDA also may impose postmarketing restrictions on distribution of the product if necessary to ensure safety (e.g., restricting distribution to certain facilities or practitioners with special training or experience).[66] To date, FDA has licensed one vaccine under the Animal Rule: BioThrax (Anthrax Vaccine Adsorbed [injection]). Specifically, in 2015, the Animal Rule was used to approve a new use—post-exposure prophylaxis of disease—of a previously licensed anthrax vaccine.[67]

Emergency Use Authorization (EUA)

In general, a vaccine may be provided to patients only if FDA has licensed its marketing under a BLA or authorized its use in a clinical trial under an IND. In certain circumstances, however, FDA may allow patients to access investigational vaccines outside this framework, including through emergency use authorization (EUA).

FDA may enable access to an unapproved vaccine by granting an EUA, if the HHS Secretary declares that circumstances exist to justify the emergency use of an unapproved product or an unapproved use of an

---

[65] 21 C.F.R. §601.91. FDA Guidance for Industry, "Product Development under the Animal Rule," October 2015, https://www.fda.gov/media/88625/download.

[66] 21 C.F.R. §601.91.

[67] FDA, "CBER Regulated Biologic Animal Rule Approvals," https://www.fda.gov/media/107839/download. FDA, "FDA approves vaccine for use after known or suspected anthrax exposure," November 23, 2015, http://wayback.archive-it.org/7993/20171114165441/https://www.fda.gov/NewsEvents/Newsroom/PressAnnouncements/ucm474027.htm.

approved medical product.[68] The HHS Secretary's declaration must be based on one of four determinations; for example, a determination that an actual or significant potential exists for a public health emergency that affects or has significant potential to affect national security or the health and security of U.S. citizens living abroad.[69] Following the HHS Secretary's declaration, FDA, in consultation with the Assistant Secretary for Preparedness and Response (ASPR), the National Institutes of Health (NIH), and CDC, may issue an EUA authorizing the emergency use of a vaccine, provided that the following criteria are met:

- the agent that is the subject of the EUA can cause a serious or life-threatening disease or condition;
- based on the totality of the available scientific evidence, it is reasonable to believe that the product may be effective in diagnosing, treating, or preventing such disease or condition, and that the known and potential benefits of the product outweigh its known and potential risks; and
- there is no adequate, approved, or available alternative to the product.[70]

The standard of evidence for an EUA is different than that for approval. EUA issuance, as noted above, is based on FDA's determination that the totality of the available scientific evidence suggests that a product *may be effective* in diagnosing, treating, or preventing a disease or condition, and that the known and potential benefits of the product outweigh its known and potential risks. This standard of evidence is different from the one required for full FDA approval or licensure, which

---

[68] FFDCA §564 [21 U.S.C. §360bbb-3]. For additional information, see CRS In Focus IF10745, *Emergency Use Authorization and FDA's Related Authorities*.

[69] FFDCA §564(b)(1) [21 U.S.C. §360bbb-3(b)(1)].

[70] FFDCA §564(c) [21 U.S.C. §360bbb-3(c)]. These criteria are explained in more detail in the FDA guidance Emergency Use Authorization of Medical Products and Related Authorities, January 2017, p. 7, https://www.fda.gov/ media/97321/download.

is based on *substantial evidence* of effectiveness derived from adequate and well-controlled studies.[71]

FDA must impose certain conditions as part of an EUA to the extent practicable (e.g., distributing certain information to health care providers and patients) and may impose additional discretionary conditions where appropriate.[72] FDA may waive or limit current good manufacturing practices (e.g., storage and handling) and prescription dispensing requirements for products authorized under an EUA. In addition, FDA may establish conditions on advertisements and other promotional printed matter that relates to the emergency use of a product. An EUA remains in effect for the duration of the emergency declaration made by the HHS Secretary under FFDCA Section 564, unless revoked at an earlier date.

To date, FDA has not granted an EUA for an unapproved (i.e., unlicensed) vaccine. However, in 2005, FDA had issued an EUA for the *unapproved use* of a previously licensed vaccine.[73]

Advisory Committee Consultation

FDA consults with a federal advisory committee on various vaccine-related matters. Specifically, the Vaccines and Related Biological Products Advisory Committee (VRBPAC) is made up of non-FDA medical and scientific experts who inform FDA's regulation of vaccines and related biological products. The committee "reviews and evaluates data concerning the safety, effectiveness, and appropriate use of vaccines and related biological products" and "considers the quality and relevance of FDA's research program which provides scientific support for the regulation of these products and makes appropriate recommendations" to

[71] FFDCA §505(d) [21 U.S.C. §355(d)].

[72] FFDCA §564(e) [21 U.S.C. §360bbb-3(e)].

[73] Authorization of Emergency Use of Anthrax Vaccine Adsorbed for Prevention of Inhalation Anthrax by Individuals at Heightened Risk of Exposure Due to Attack With Anthrax, 70 *Federal Register* 5452, February 2, 2005.

the FDA Commissioner.[74] VRBPAC may, for example, meet to discuss approaches for demonstrating effectiveness of a particular vaccine in a specific population.[75] VRBPAC is subject to the requirements of the Federal Advisory Committee Act.[76]

CLINICAL RECOMMENDATIONS

Official HHS/CDC clinical recommendations for vaccination—such as the age and population groups recommended to receive each vaccine, as well as the number of doses and interval between doses—are informed by the Advisory Committee on Immunization Practices (ACIP), a federal advisory committee composed of medical and public health experts who make policy recommendations for the use of licensed vaccines and related agents for the control of vaccine- preventable diseases in the civilian population of the United States.[77] ACIP may also develop guidance for use of unlicensed vaccines "if circumstances warrant." ACIP was established by the U.S. Surgeon General in 1964, under authority provided by Public Health Service Act (PHSA) Section 222.[78]

After FDA licenses a new vaccine or licenses an existing vaccine for a new indication, ACIP typically makes one of two types of clinical recommendations:

---

[74] Vaccines and Related Biological Products Advisory Committee, https://www.fda.gov/advisory-committees/blood-vaccines-and-other-biologics/vaccines-and-related-biological-products-advisory-committee.

[75] FDA, "2018 Meeting Materials, Vaccines and Related Biological Products Advisory Committee," https://www.fda.gov/advisory-committees/vaccines-and-related-biological-products-advisory-committee/2018-meeting-materials-vaccines-and-related-biological-products-advisory-committee.

[76] For additional information about the Federal Advisory Committee Act (FACA) and FACA committees, see CRS Report R44253, *Federal Advisory Committees: An Introduction and Overview*.

[77] Amanda Cohn, Lance E. Rodewald, Walter A. Orenstein, et al., "Immunization in the United States," in *Plotkin's Vaccines*, ed. Stanley A. Plotkin, Walter A. Orenstein, and Paul A. Offit, 7th ed. (Elsevier, 2017), p. 1421.

[78] CDC, "ACIP Charter," June 5, 2018, https://www.cdc.gov/vaccines/acip/committee/charter.html.

- *Full recommendation:* The vaccine is recommended for all people in an age- or risk-based group, except for those with a *contraindication* (i.e., a condition that would make the vaccine harmful, such as a condition that compromises the immune system). For example, ACIP has issued a full recommendation for two doses of the measles-mumps-rubella (MMR) vaccine routinely for children, with the first dose administered at 12-15 months and the second dose administered before school entry at four to six years of age.[79]
- *Clinical Decisionmaking:* The vaccine is recommended for certain subpopulations, and its use is based on clinical decisionmaking.[80] For example, ACIP recommends the two Serogroup B Meningococcal vaccines for persons 10 years of age or older who have certain health conditions or are at increased risk of exposure to the disease, as specified.[81]

To make its vaccine recommendations, ACIP considers disease epidemiology and burden of disease,[82] vaccine efficacy and effectiveness, the quality of evidence reviewed, economic analyses, and implementation issues. Recommendations made by ACIP are reviewed by the CDC Director and, if adopted, published as official CDC/HHS

---

[79] Huong Q. McLean, Amy Parker Fibelkorn, Jonathan L. Temte, et al., "Prevention of Measles, Rubella, Congenital Rubella Syndrome, and Mumps, 2013: Summary Recommendations of the Advisory Committee on Immunization Practices (ACIP)," *Morbidity and Mortality Weekly Report (MMWR)*, vol. 62, no. RR04 (June 14, 2013), pp. 1-34.

[80] Richard Hughes, Reed Maxim, and Alessandra Fix, "Vague Vaccine Recommendations May Be Leading to Lack of Provider Clarity, Confusion Over Coverage," *Health Affairs*, May 7, 2019; and Larry K. Pickering, Walter A. Orenstein, and Wellington Sun, et al., "FDA Licensure of and ACIP Recommendations for Vaccines," *Vaccine*, vol. 35 (2017), p. 5027–5036.

[81] Monica E. Patton, David Stephens, and Kelly Moore, "Updated Recommendations for Use of MenB-FHbp Serogroup B Meningococcal Vaccine—Advisory Committee on Immunization Practices, 2016," *Morbidity and Mortality Weekly Report (MMWR)*, vol. 66, no. 19 (May 19, 2017), pp. 509-513.

[82] Burden of disease is a standardized measure for comparing the health impacts of different diseases based on cumulative disability, loss of full health, and premature mortality caused by each disease. See World Health Organization (WHO), "About the Global Burden of Diseases (GBD) Project," https://www.who.int/healthinfo/global_burden_disease/about/en/.

recommendations.[83] ACIP recommendations inform which vaccines are provided through the CDC's Vaccines for Children program,[84] as well as which vaccines must be covered by private health care insurance plans subject to the preventive health services requirement as added by the Patient Protection and Affordable Care Act (ACA).[85]

ACIP recommendations are used to establish the CDC-recommended child and adult immunization schedules (for children, birth to 18 years of age; for adults, 19 years of age and older), which are used by health care providers, parents, and others to understand which vaccines should be administered at various ages. The immunization schedules distinguish between vaccines recommended to all people in a certain age group and vaccines recommended only for certain high-risk groups. As a part of the immunization schedules, CDC also publishes a specific table of vaccine recommendations by common contraindications, such as persons with HIV, immunocompromised individuals, and pregnant individuals. The table includes when recommended vaccines should *not* be administered to individuals with these contraindications.[86]

Once clinical recommendations are made, CDC develops and provides resources and training for health care providers on current vaccine recommendations, best practices for vaccine administration, and patient education.[87] CDC develops Vaccination Information Statements (VIS) on the risks and benefits of vaccinations; these statements are required to be given to vaccine recipients and their parents or legal guardians whenever vaccines recommended for routine use among children and pregnant women are administered.[88] VISs are developed by CDC in consultation

---

[83] CDC, "ACIP Charter," June 5, 2018, https://www.cdc.gov/vaccines/acip/committee/charter.html.

[84] Vaccines for Children is a Medicaid-financed program administered by CDC that provides vaccines at no cost to eligible children 18 years or younger, including those who are American Indian or Alaska Native, Medicaid-eligible, uninsured, or underinsured (as defined). See https://www.cdc.gov/features/vfcprogram/index.html.

[85] ACA, P.L. 111-148, as amended, which established PHSA §2713.

[86] CDC, "Immunization Schedules," https://www.cdc.gov/vaccines/schedules/index.html.

[87] CDC, "Vaccines-Healthcare Providers," 2018, https://www.cdc.gov/vaccines/hcp/index.html.

[88] Requirement established by the National Childhood Vaccine Injury Act, P.L. 99-660; PHSA §2126 [42 U.S.C. §300aa-26].

with the Advisory Commission on Childhood Vaccines (ACCV; a committee of health care professionals, attorneys, and parents of vaccine-injured children), health care providers, and FDA, and are published in the *Federal Register* for public comment.[89]

POSTMARKET SAFETY

Although pre-licensure clinical trials and research are designed to identify common safety risks associated with a vaccine, such trials may not identify all long-term or rare adverse effects (similar to all pharmaceutical products). As such, vaccines may be subject to additional postmarket study requirements, called Phase 4 studies, or other safety monitoring to provide additional information about a vaccine's risks, benefits, and optimal use.[90] FDA may require a vaccine manufacturer to conduct a postapproval study or clinical trial to assess a known serious risk or signals of serious risk related to use of the vaccine, or to identify an unexpected serious risk when available data indicate the potential for a serious risk.[91] In addition, because vaccines require special manufacturing processes to avoid contamination, post-licensure safety programs are designed to ensure safety in vaccine manufacturing. Post-licensure safety requirements and programs are also intended to identify long-term or rare adverse health events that result from vaccination, and FDA may require vaccine manufacturers to revise vaccine product labeling if new information becomes available after licensure.[92]

---

[89] P.L. 99-660; PHSA §2126 [42 U.S.C. §300aa-26].

[90] 21 C.F.R. §312.85. See also FDA, "Vaccine Product Approval Process," https://www.fda.gov/vaccines-blood-biologics/development-approval-process-cber/vaccine-product-approval-process.

[91] PHSA §351(a)(2)(D) [42 U.S.C. §262(a)(2)(D)] and FFDCA §505(o)(3) [21 U.S.C. §355(o)(3)].

[92] PHSA §351(a)(2)(D) [42 U.S.C. §262(a)(2)(D)] and FFDCA §505(o)(4) [21 U.S.C. §355(o)(4)].

Manufacturing Safety

FDA continues to inspect vaccine manufacturing facilities post-licensure.[93] The HHS Secretary may authorize any HHS officer, agent, or employee to "during all reasonable hours enter and inspect any establishment for the propagation or manufacture and preparation of any biological product [e.g., vaccine]."[94] If FDA determines that a batch, lot, or other quantity of a vaccine "presents an imminent or substantial hazard to the public health," the agency must issue an order immediately recalling the batch, lot, or other quantity of the vaccine.[95]

Manufacturers of vaccines listed in the Vaccine Injury Table (see the "National Vaccine Injury Compensation" section) or mandated to be state-administered must maintain records related to the safety and quality of each batch of vaccines produced, and must report any identified public health hazards to FDA.[96] Specifically, vaccine manufacturers are required to maintain records documenting the manufacturing, processing, testing, and reworking of each batch, lot, or other quantity of a vaccine, including whether any significant problems were identified during these processes, and to report if any safety test on such batch, lot, or other quantity indicates a potential imminent or substantial public health hazard.[97]

In addition, vaccine manufacturers are required to report adverse events to FDA. This includes the submission of 15-day alert reports and periodic safety reports. A 15-day alert report is required for each serious and unexpected adverse experience and must be submitted to FDA as soon as possible but no later than 15 days from initial receipt of the information by the manufacturer.[98] The manufacturer must "promptly investigate" such adverse event and submit follow-up reports within 15 days of receiving

---

[93] FDA, "Ensuring the Safety of Vaccines in the United States," last updated July 2011, https://www.fda.gov/media/ 83528/download.

[94] PHSA §351(c) [42 U.S.C. §262(c)].

[95] PHSA §351(d)(1) [42 U.S.C. §262(d)(1)].

[96] PHSA §2128 [42 U.S.C. §300aa–28]. This authority has been delegated from the HHS Secretary to the FDA Commissioner, per the FDA Staff Manual Guide 1410.10, item 31, effective date August 26, 2016, https://www.fda.gov/media/81983/download.

[97] PHSA §2128(a) [42 U.S.C. §300aa–28(a)].

[98] 21 C.F.R §600.80(c).

new information or as requested by FDA. Periodic safety reports are required for each adverse experience not reported in a 15-day alert report and must be submitted to FDA at quarterly intervals for three years from the date of issuance of the vaccine's license, and at annual intervals thereafter. Individual case safety reports for vaccines submitted to FDA must include specified information about the patient who is the subject of the report (e.g., name, age, gender) and the vaccine (e.g., manufacturer, lot number).[99] If a vaccine manufacturer fails to establish and maintain records or report adverse events, FDA can take enforcement action, including revocation of the BLA for that vaccine.[100]

Surveillance

CDC and FDA are the primary federal agencies that conduct surveillance (i.e., data monitoring) activities on the safety of administered vaccines. Other federal agencies such as the Department of Defense (DOD) and the Centers for Medicare & Medicaid Services (CMS) also operate databases on vaccine safety events among their covered populations.[101] The NVPO within the HHS Office of Infectious Disease and HIV/AIDS Policy (OIDP) is tasked with coordinating vaccine safety monitoring across federal agencies.[102]

FDA and CDC monitor and conduct research on vaccine safety through various mechanisms. As discussed below, each of the programs or systems has strengths and limitations, but together they provide various ways of assessing vaccines to ensure their safety. Each of the systems allows for monitoring of adverse events linked to specific lots of manufactured vaccines. This lot-specific monitoring enables distinctions

---

99 21 C.F.R §600.80(g).

100 21 C.F.R §600.80(l).

101 Matthew Z. Dudley, Daniel A. Salmon, Neal A. Halsey, et al., "Monitoring Vaccine Safety," in *The Clinician's Vaccine Safety Resource Guide* (Springer, Cham, 2018).

102 National Vaccine Advisory Committee (NVAC), *White Paper on the United States Vaccine Safety System*, September 2011, p. 21, https://www.hhs.gov/sites/default/files/nvpo/nvac/nvac_vswp.pdf.

between adverse events linked to improper manufacturing, compared with adverse events linked to a particular type of vaccine.[103]

> **Key Terms: Passive and Active Surveillance**
>
> Public health surveillance, or ongoing data monitoring, can be passive or active. A *passive surveillance system* relies on reports, often from health care providers or patients. In an *active surveillance system*, data are collected proactively—either through active analysis of electronic health data (such as for the monitoring systems covered here), or where data are collected directly by contacting health care organizations or obtaining records.
>
> Source: CDC, "Introduction to Public Health Surveillance," https://www.cdc.gov/publichealth101/surveillance.html.

Vaccine Adverse Event Reporting System (VAERS)

VAERS, established in 1990 and operated jointly by FDA and CDC, is a monitoring system for adverse events related to vaccines. Using the VAERS system, anyone, including physicians, nurses, and the general public, can submit an online report of an adverse event following vaccination. Pursuant to PHSA Section 2125, health care providers and vaccine manufacturers are required to report the occurrence of any adverse event in the Vaccine Injury Table (see the "National Vaccine Injury Compensation" section), the occurrence of a contraindicating reaction specified on the vaccine label, and other serious and unexpected events as required through regulations.[104] Scientists at CDC and FDA monitor VAERS reports and use the information to conduct further investigations

---

[103] HHS, *Comprehensive Review of Federal Vaccine Safety Programs and Public Health Activities*, December 2008, https://www.hsdl.org/?abstract&did=6793; and Meghan A. Baker, Michael Nguyen, and David V. Cole, "Post- Licensure Rapid Immunization Safety Monitoring Program (PRISM) Data Characterization," *Vaccine*, vol. 31S (2013), pp. K98-K112.

[104] PHSA §2125 [42 U.S.C. §300aa-25]; 21 C.F.R. Part 600.

on the reported cases.[105] Consolidated data on reported adverse events in the VAERS system are publicly available online.[106]

VAERS is a passive reporting system. Its data represent reports of adverse health events related to vaccines, rather than validated cases. In addition, data in the system lack information on total vaccines administered in the covered populations. Therefore, VAERS data are often inadequate for epidemiological analyses of adverse health events at a population level.[107] VAERS is useful, however, for helping identify new and unusual clusters of cases of adverse health events linked to vaccination. VAERS also can provide some of the first postmarket safety data on newly introduced vaccines. In addition, VAERS can help identify extremely rare and unusual adverse health events that occur following vaccination. Researchers can use VAERS reports to generate hypotheses about vaccine safety and then use other sources of data (such as from the databases discussed below) and clinical evidence to assess their hypotheses.[108]

Vaccine Safety Datalink (VSD)

VSD, established in 1990 and operated by CDC, is an active surveillance system that allows for population-level scientific analyses of adverse events that follow vaccination. VSD is a collaborative project for conducting studies on vaccine safety between CDC and eight integrated health care organizations (i.e., combined payer and provider organizations) around the country. VSD uses electronic patient and medical records from participating sites, which allows for large- scale and controlled analyses of medical events (e.g., hospitalizations, diagnoses) that occur after

---

105 CDC, "Understanding the Vaccine Adverse Event Reporting System (VAERS)," https://www.cdc.gov/vaccines/hcp/patient-ed/conversations/downloads/vacsafe-vaers-color-office.pdf.

106 VAERS, "VAERS data," https://vaers.hhs.gov/data.html.

107 CDC, "Vaccine Safety Datalink (VSD)," https://www.cdc.gov/vaccinesafety/ensuring safety/monitoring/vsd/; and Frank DeStefano, Paul A. Offit, and Allison Fisher, "Vaccine Safety," in *Plotkin's Vaccines*, ed. Stanley Plotkin, Walter Orenstein, Paul Offit, Kathryn M. Edwards, 7th ed. (Elsevier, 2018), pp. 1586.

108 Frank DeStefano, Paul A. Offit, and Allison Fisher, "Vaccine Safety," in *Plotkin's Vaccines*, ed. Stanley A. Plotkin, Walter A. Orenstein, and Paul A. Offit, 7th ed. (Elsevier, 2017), pp. 1586-1587.

vaccination to identify associated risks.[109] VSD studies may supplement these records with other sources of information, such as patient surveys, medical charts, and pharmacy, laboratory, and radiology data, to validate vaccination data and outcomes. Health data on about 9 million people are included annually in VSD.[110]

VSD allows for near real-time detection of large-scale adverse events linked to vaccination. Researchers have developed methods to use VSD data to study the health effects of vaccines, such as whether the measles-mumps-rubella (MMR) vaccine is associated with autism (studies have found no such association). Among its limitations, the population represented by VSD, while large, is not completely representative of the entire U.S. population in terms of geography, race, socioeconomic status, and other factors, particularly because the participating organizations are private health plans which generally over-represent people of higher socioeconomic status and non-minority groups.[111] In addition, VSD's population size may not be adequate for detecting extremely rare adverse events linked to vaccination.[112]

Sentinel Initiative

FDA established the Sentinel Initiative in 2008, fulfilling a statutory directive to collaborate with public, academic, and private entities to develop methods for obtaining access to disparate data sources and to validate means of linking and analyzing safety data from multiple

---

109 CDC, "Vaccine Safety Datalink (VSD)," https://www.cdc.gov/vaccinesafety/ensuring safety/monitoring/vsd/.

110 Frank DeStefano, Paul A. Offit, and Allison Fisher, "Vaccine Safety," in *Plotkin's Vaccines*, ed. Stanley A. Plotkin, Walter A. Orenstein, and Paul A. Offit, 7th ed. (Elsevier, 2017), pp. 1587.

111 CDC, "Vaccine Safety Datalink (VSD)," https://www.cdc.gov/vaccinesafety/ensuringsafety/monitoring/vsd/; and Frank DeStefano, Paul A. Offit, and Allison Fisher, "Vaccine Safety," in *Plotkin's Vaccines*, ed. Stanley Plotkin, Walter Orenstein, Paul Offit, Kathryn M. Edwards, 7th ed. (Elsevier, 2018), pp. 1584-1600.

112 Michael Nguyen, Robert Ball, Karen Midthun, et al., "The Food and Drug Administration's Post-Licensure Rapid Immunization Safety Monitoring Program: Strengthening the Vaccine Safety Enterprise,"*Pharmacoepidemiology and Drug Safety*, vol. 21, no. S1 (2012), pp. 291-97.

sources.[113] As part of the Sentinel Initiative, FDA has established two programs that address vaccines: (1) the Post-Licensure Rapid Immunization Safety Monitoring (PRISM) program, and (2) the Biologics Effectiveness and Safety (BEST) system.

PRISM is an active surveillance program that uses electronic health records from insurance providers and state immunization registries to monitor adverse events following vaccination. It was established in 2009 and deployed during the H1N1 influenza pandemic.[114] PRISM has been the largest linked database for monitoring vaccine safety in the United States, involving data on over 100 million people.[115] PRISM, similar to the CDC VSD program, can allow for population-level scientific analyses of adverse events following vaccination. Because of the larger population covered, PRISM can detect rarer adverse events than VSD and enable stratified analyses of vaccine-linked adverse events by subpopulation (e.g., by race/ethnicity).[116] As of 2012, VSD allowed for more rapid analyses than PRISM due to data-sharing agreements between the participating health organizations and CDC that allow for near real-time data collection.[117]

PRISM has been used to inform FDA-required postmarket labeling changes.[118] For example, after some studies found an association between risk of intussusception (i.e., intestinal blockage) and administration of two rotavirus vaccines (RotaTeq and Rotarix), FDA launched a study in

---

[113] The Sentinel system was implemented as an "Active Post-Market Risk Identification and Analysis program" under FFDCA §505(k)(3), as amended by §905 of the FDA Amendments Act, P.L. 110-85.

[114] PRISM is the vaccine component of FDA's Sentinel Initiative.

[115] FDA, "Advances in the Science, Surveillance, and Safety of Vaccines," 2013, https://www.hhs.gov/vaccines/ national-vaccine-plan/annual-report-2013/goal-2/advances-in-science-surveillance-safety-of-vaccines/index.html; and Matthew Z. Dudley, Daniel A. Salmon, Neal A. Halsey, et al., "Monitoring Vaccine Safety," in *The Clinician's Vaccine Safety Resource Guide* (Springer, Cham, 2018).

[116] Michael Nguyen, Robert Ball, Karen Midthun, et al., "The Food and Drug Administration's Post-Licensure Rapid Immunization Safety Monitoring Program: Strengthening the Vaccine Safety Enterprise," *Pharmacoepidemiology and Drug Safety*, vol. 21, no. S1 (2012), pp. 291-97.

[117] Matthew Z. Dudley, Daniel A. Salmon, Neal A. Halsey, et al., "Monitoring Vaccine Safety," in *The Clinician's Vaccine Safety Resource Guide* (Springer, Cham, 2018).

[118] FDA CBER, "Post-licensure Rapid Immunization Safety Monitoring (PRISM) Public Workshop," December 7, 2016, Bethesda, MD, https://www.fda.gov/media/103876/download.

PRISM to assess whether infants faced a similar risk.[119] The PRISM study identified an increased, but rare, risk of intussusception with RotaTeq among infants, which led to FDA-required labeling changes for the licensed vaccine.[120]

In 2017, CBER initiated the BEST system as part of Sentinel to assure the safety and effectiveness of vaccines and other biologics. It is broader than PRISM in that it also covers blood and blood products, tissue products, and other advanced therapeutic biologics.[121] The goal of BEST is to "leverage high-quality data, analytics and innovation to enhance surveillance, real-world evidence generation, and clinical practice that benefits patients." Like other Sentinel components, BEST uses electronic health record, administrative, and claims-based data for active surveillance and research. BEST fulfills the FDAAA requirements for an active postmarket risk and analysis system covering at least 100 million persons.[122]

Other Safety Monitoring Systems

As mentioned above, federal agencies other than FDA and CDC conduct vaccine safety monitoring. CMS has a database for vaccine safety among the Medicare population; the database represents vaccines administered to persons aged 65 and older. DOD has a database for monitoring adverse events from vaccination among military service

[119] FDA, "RotaTeq (Rotavirus Vaccine) Questions and Answers," https://www.fda.gov/vaccines-blood-biologics/ vaccines/rotateq-rotavirus-vaccine-questions-and-answers.

[120] According to FDA, "The Mini-Sentinel PRISM study is the largest study of intussusception after rotavirus vaccines to date and identified an increased risk of intussusception in the 21 day time period after the first dose of RotaTeq, with most cases occurring in the first 7 days after vaccination. No increased risk was found after the second or third doses. These findings translate into 1 to 1.5 additional cases of intussusception per 100,000 first doses of RotaTeq." See "FDA Safety Communication: FDA Approves Required Revised Labeling for RotaTeq Based Final Study Results of a Mini- Sentinel Postlicensure Observational Study of Rotavirus Vaccines and Intussusception," July 22, 2013, https://www.sentinelinitiative.org/communications/fda-safety-communications/fda-safety-communication-fda- approves-required-revised.

[121] Sentinel, "Vaccines, Blood, & Biologics Assessments," https://www.sentinelinitiative.org/assessments/vaccines- blood-biologics.

[122] FDA, "CBER Biologics Effectiveness and Safety (BEST) System," https://www.fda.gov/vaccines-blood-biologics/ safety-availability-biologics/cber-biologics-effectiveness-and-safety-best-system.

members and their families, and the Department of Veterans Affairs (VA) has a database for veterans who receive care in the VA system. In addition, the Indian Health Service (IHS) operates a database for vaccine safety monitoring among the IHS-covered population.[123]

Safety Monitoring Using Multiple Surveillance Systems: A Case Study

Researchers have used information from multiple vaccine safety monitoring systems to draw associations between vaccines and subsequent adverse health events. For example, during the 2010-2011 influenza season, VAERS received an increased number of reports of febrile seizures following vaccination with Fluzone.™ FDA then initiated a PRISM study to investigate febrile seizures after vaccination with Fluzone™ and other trivalent inactivated influenza vaccines (TIVs). The study found no statistically significant association between TIVs and increased risk of febrile seizures.

Source: FDA, "Update: FDA Postlicensure Rapid Immunization Safety Monitoring (PRISM) study demonstrates no statistically significant association between Trivalent Inactivated Influenza Vaccine and Febrile Seizures in Children during the 2010-2011 influenza season," May 16, 2014, https://www.sentinelinitiative.org/communications/fda-safety-communications/update-fda-postlicensure-rapid-immunization-safety.

Clinical Assessment

The Clinical Immunization Safety Assessment (CISA), a CDC program established in 2001, is a network of clinical scientists who conduct clinical studies (i.e., studies with patients) on vaccine safety. Scientists in the network can conduct studies on complex individual patient cases of possible adverse health events that followed vaccination.[124] Using

---

123 Matthew Z. Dudley, Daniel A. Salmon, Neal A. Halsey, et al., "Monitoring Vaccine Safety," in *The Clinician's Vaccine Safety Resource Guide* (Springer, Cham, 2018).

124 CDC, "Clinical Immunization Safety Assessment (CISA) Project," https://www.cdc.gov/vaccinesafety/ ensuringsafety/monitoring/cisa/index.html.

CISA, scientists can assess the biological mechanisms that cause adverse health events after vaccination.[125] In addition, CISA manages a repository of biospecimen samples from patients who experience unusual adverse events following vaccination.[126] These samples can be systemically analyzed to inform a mechanistic understanding of such adverse events.

FEDERAL RESEARCH ON VACCINE SAFETY

Postmarket surveillance systems and clinical assessments provide important data and evidence on potential adverse events following vaccination. To further understand and determine whether vaccines cause or could plausibly cause certain adverse health events, scientists conduct various types of research that inform a scientific understanding of vaccine safety (separate from the clinical trials under an IND). Such activities are supported primarily by HHS agencies, mainly CDC and the National Institutes of Health (NIH). In addition, FDA supports regulatory research related to methods for evaluating vaccine safety. Major areas of research related to vaccines can include the following:[127]

- *Biological research:* Research often with animals, cell cultures, or biological specimens (e.g., human tissue samples) to explore the mechanisms by which vaccines act in biological systems, informing an understanding of how adverse events may occur. (Also referred to as basic biomedical research).
- *Epidemiological research:* A form of statistical research involving health data collected among defined human populations (such as postmarket surveillance data) to explore whether statistical

[125] Frank DeStefano, Paul A. Offit, and Allison Fisher, "Vaccine Safety," in *Plotkin's Vaccines*, ed. Stanley Plotkin, Walter Orenstein, Paul Offit, Kathryn M. Edwards, 7th ed. (Elsevier, 2018), pp. 1588.

[126] NVAC, *White Paper on the United States Vaccine Safety System*, September 2011, p. 16, https://www.hhs.gov/sites/ default/files/nvpo/nvac/nvac_vswp.pdf.

[127] NVAC, *White Paper on the United States Vaccine Safety System*, September 2011, p. 16, https://www.hhs.gov/sites/ default/files/nvpo/nvac/nvac_vswp.pdf.

associations exist between vaccination and subsequent adverse events, and any related risk factors for those events among those populations.

- *Clinical research:* Research with patients to understand the clinical features of adverse health events among patients that are hypothesized to be connected to vaccination.

Research can also explore the underlying methodologies used to assess vaccine safety through any of these forms of research.

CDC Research

CDC conducts and supports many types of research on vaccine safety, including epidemiological and clinical studies. Many of CDC's research publications rely on data and findings from its safety monitoring systems, as listed above, including VAERS, VSD, and CISA. CDC research often focuses on the use of specific vaccines in specific populations, as well as hypothesized side effects and adverse events potentially attributable to vaccination.[128] For example, a recent CDC study published in 2020 explored probability-based methods of determining which vaccine or combination of vaccines were linked to an adverse event following vaccination (in this case, a seizure) when multiple vaccines were administered at once.[129]

NIH Research

In addition to CDC research, biological research related to immunology or infectious disease supported by NIH informs an

---

[128] CDC, "Vaccine Safety Publications," https://www.cdc.gov/vaccinesafety/research/publications/index.html.

[129] Shirley V. Wang, Kristina Stefanini, Edwin Lewis, et al., "Determining Which of Several Simultaneously Administered Vaccines Increase Risk of an Adverse Event," *Drug Safety*, vol. 43 (July 1, 2020), pp. 1057-65.

understanding of vaccine safety. NIH tends to support more biological research than CDC, in that NIH research focuses on the fundamental biological mechanisms underlying vaccine safety, as well as research methodologies for examining it. For the past several years, NIH, in collaboration with CDC and NVPO, has issued annual funding opportunity announcements for "Research on Vaccine Safety." Research projects can include scientific investigations into physiological and immunological responses to vaccines; explorations of how genetic variations affect responses to vaccines; investigations into risk factors for adverse responses to vaccination; exploration and validation of statistical methods for analyzing data on vaccine safety; and the application of genomic and molecular technologies to assess vaccine safety.[130]

The National Institute of Allergy and Infectious Diseases (NIAID, which is one of 27 NIH Institutes and Centers) also supports the Human Immunology Project Consortium (HIPC), a program established in 2010 that collects in-depth biological data over time on the immune systems of a diverse cohort of patients. The program consolidates data on the cohort into centralized databases for use by researchers.[131] Researchers are using HIPC to study certain aspects of vaccine safety, such as whether a relationship exists between short-term adverse events caused by vaccination and long-term health effects.[132] When combined with postmarket surveillance data and studies, NIH-supported research can contribute to robust evaluations on the safety of vaccines.

---

130 NIH, "Research to Advance Vaccine Safety (R01)," July 24, 2018, https://grants.nih.gov/grants/guide/pa-files/PA- 18-873.html.

131 NIH, "Human Immunology Project Consortium," https://www.immuneprofiling.org/hipc/page/showPage?pg=about.

132 National Academy of Medicine, *The Childhood Immunization Schedule and Safety: Stakeholder Concerns, Scientific Evidence, and Future Studies*, Washington, DC, January 16, 2013, http://nationalacademies.org/HMD/ Reports/2013/The-Childhood-Immunization-Schedule-and-Safety.aspx.

FDA Research

FDA conducts regulatory science research to facilitate its evaluation of vaccine safety and effectiveness, and to support the development of new vaccines. For example, CBER scientists have published studies on the agency's effort to develop and evaluate assays and animal models for studying the safety and efficacy of vaccines against specific pathogens, as well as to characterize biomarkers of vaccine safety and efficacy.[133] In addition, FDA has studied certain adjuvants and preservatives added to vaccines, including thimerosal and the impact of aluminum in vaccines on infants.[134] FDA research efforts have also focused on vaccine availability, specifically on influenza vaccine production and ensuring a sufficient supply of a safe vaccine.[135]

Other Federal Research

Other federal agencies conduct or support research related to vaccine safety. For example, the NVPO has issued Funding Opportunity Announcements (FOA) for grants to support vaccine safety research.[136] The Agency for Healthcare Research and Quality (AHRQ) has conducted vaccine safety reviews. The Department of Defense (DOD) and the Department of Veterans Affairs (VA) also support some vaccine safety research.[137]

---

[133] FDA, Vaccines Research, current as of August 14, 2020, https://www.fda.gov/vaccines-blood-biologics/biologics- research-projects/vaccines-research.

[134] L. K. Ball, R. Ball, R. D. Pratt, "An assessment of thimerosal use in childhood vaccines," *Pediatrics*, 2001, vol. 107 no. 5, pp. 1147-1154. The study was required by the FDA Modernization Act (FDAMA, P.L. 105-115). FDA, "Study Reports Aluminum in Vaccines Poses Extremely Low Risk to Infants," https://wayback.archive-it.org/7993/20170405003134/https:/www.fda.gov/BiologicsBloodVaccines/ScienceResearch/ucm284520.htm.

[135] FDA, "Facilitating Influenza Virus Vaccine Production by Optimizing Vaccine Strains," https://www.fda.gov/vaccines-blood-biologics/biologics-research-projects/facilitating-influenza-virus-vaccine-production-optimizing- vaccine-strains.

[136] See, for example, BetaSam.gov, "Research, Monitoring and Outcomes Definitions for Vaccine Safety," https://beta.sam.gov/fal/c8125303527f478981f6b7395c528788/view.

[137] Vaccines.gov, "Vaccine Safety," https://www.vaccines.gov/basics/safety.

Periodically, federal agencies (particularly HHS) conduct or commission comprehensive scientific reviews on the safety of recommended vaccines. As described in the text box on page 6, these reviews often evaluate and combine evidence from a large number of studies and a range of research types to make assessments about the safety of vaccines that are as conclusive as possible. For example, in 2011, under HHS contract, the National Academy of Medicine (NAM)[138] conducted a comprehensive review of the scientific evidence regarding the safety of eight pediatric vaccines. The resulting NAM report, *Adverse Effects of Vaccines: Evidence and Causality*, was used to inform an update of the Vaccine Injury Table for the National Vaccine Injury Compensation Program (see the "National Vaccine Injury Compensation" section).[139] This review was subsequently updated in 2014 with additional research by AHRQ, supported by the NVPO; AHRQ is currently in the process of updating this review.[140]

Challenges of Vaccine Safety Reviews

As discussed earlier, causality assessments that combine evidence across many studies allow for researchers to assess if all the available evidence favors a causal relationship between a vaccine and a subsequent adverse health event. In general, establishing true causal linkages between a vaccine and certain subsequent adverse health events can be challenging; however, researchers draw conclusions using multiple forms of evidence. The clinical trials required for vaccine licensure are well-controlled scientific experiments that allow researchers to draw conclusions about the safety of products. Postmarket safety studies, on the other hand, can face a variety of methodological challenges. For one, the population of

---

[138] NAM was named the Institute of Medicine when the Immunization Safety Review Committee was formed.

[139] Institute of Medicine, *Adverse Effects of Vaccines: Evidence and Causality*, August 25, 2011.

[140] Margaret A. Maglione, Courtney Gidengil, Lopamudra Das, et al. "Safety of Vaccines Used for Routine Immunization in the United States," *Agency for Healthcare Research and Quality*, July 2014, https://effectivehealthcare.ahrq.gov/sites/default/files/pdf/vaccine-safety_research.pdf, and AHRQ, "Safety of Vaccines Used for Routine Immunization in the United States: Research Protocol," April 2020, https://effectivehealthcare.ahrq.gov/products/safety-vaccines/protocol.

vaccinated individuals is often much larger than and demographically different from the population of unvaccinated individuals, making it difficult to draw comparisons in health outcomes between the two groups. Researchers therefore often rely on time intervals between vaccination and an adverse health event—assessing whether a certain adverse health event is more likely to occur within a defined time interval after vaccination compared with other time periods. While this approach can work for short-term health effects caused by vaccines, it can be less effective for hypothesized long-term effects of vaccines or adverse health events that are otherwise common in the population. Statistical *association* between vaccination and an adverse health event is often necessary but not sufficient to establish *causality*. As discussed earlier, to make a causality assessment about whether a particular vaccine causes an adverse health event, experts use evidence and results from many scientific studies, including epidemiological evidence, clinical evidence, and biological laboratory evidence, usually with methods to weigh, compare, and combine evidence across studies.[141] Such causality assessments may be conducted as a part of a comprehensive scientific review by federal or academic scientists, or by independent scientific advisory bodies, such as the NAM.

National Vaccine Injury Compensation

The National Vaccine Injury Compensation Program (VICP) provides compensation to individuals who file a petition and are found to have been injured by a covered vaccine. VICP is based in the Health Resources and Services Administration (HRSA) and was established by the National Childhood Vaccine Injury Act of 1986 (P.L. 99-660).[142] VICP publishes a "Vaccine Injury Table" that lists vaccines covered by the program and the

---

[141] Frank DeStefano, Paul A. Offit, and Allison Fisher, "Vaccine Safety," in *Plotkin's Vaccines*, ed. Stanley A. Plotkin, Walter A. Orenstein, and Paul A. Offit, 7th ed. (Elsevier, 2017), pp. 1589.

[142] HRSA, "National Vaccine Injury Compensation," https://www.hrsa.gov/vaccine-compensation/index.html.

injuries associated with those vaccines for which claims may be filed, developed based on the causality assessments conducted by IOM and AHRQ. Claimants may submit claims for injuries that are not listed on the table, but they must present evidence that the vaccine caused the injury.[143] In addition to HHS/HRSA, VICP involves the Department of Justice (DOJ) and the U.S. Court of Federal Claims.[144] The Advisory Committee on Childhood Vaccines (ACCV) also provides oversight of VICP by making recommendations to the HHS Secretary, including those related to the Vaccine Injury Table.

ACCV is a nine-member federal advisory committee made up of health and legal representatives, as well as parents or legal representatives of children who have been injured by vaccines.[145]

VICP is funded by the Vaccine Compensation Trust Fund, which is funded by an excise tax on vaccines paid by manufacturers. VICP was established in response to vaccine shortages that occurred after hundreds of injury lawsuits were filed against vaccine manufacturers in the 1980s, leading to halts in vaccine production and creating instability in the vaccine market. VICP is a no- fault system to compensate individuals who were injured as a result of vaccination. It serves to protect manufacturers from injury lawsuits. As of October 1, 2020, over 22,272 petitions have been filed with VICP, and 7,611 were determined to be compensable, with total compensation paid of about $4.4 billion since the program was established in 1988.[146]

---

[143] HRSA, "National Vaccine Injury Compensation Program—Covered Vaccines," June 2019, https://www.hrsa.gov/ vaccine-compensation/covered-vaccines/index.html.

[144] HRSA, "About the National Vaccine Injury Compensation Program," June 2019, https://www.hrsa.gov/vaccine- compensation/about/index.html.

[145] HHS, "Charter-Advisory Commission on Childhood Vaccines," https://www.hrsa.gov/sites/default/files/hrsa/advisory-committees/vaccines/accvcharter.pdf. For the parents or legal representatives of children who have suffered a vaccine-related injury or death, HRSA specifies that to be considered for appointment, "there must have been a finding (i.e., a decision) by the U.S. Court of Federal Claims or a civil court that a VICP-covered vaccine caused, or was presumed to have caused, the represented child's injury or death." From HRSA, "Advisory Commission on Vaccines: Frequently Asked Questions," 2018, https://www.hrsa.gov/sites/default/files/hrsa/vaccine-compensation/job-opportunities/ACCV-FAQs.pdf.

[146] HRSA, "Data & Statistics," https://www.hrsa.gov/sites/default/files/hrsa/vaccine-compensation/data/data-statistics- report.pdf.

During an emergency situation such as the COVID-19 pandemic, vaccines may be covered under a different injury compensation program—the Countermeasures Injury Compensation Program (CICP), as discussed in the "Injury Compensation and Patient Safety Information" section.[147]

Safety in Vaccine Distribution

Managing vaccine supply and distribution requires temperature control, safety controls, and regular monitoring of expiry dates due to the limited shelf life of products.[148] Given that public dollars (federal and state) pay for over 50% of vaccines (by volume) in the United States, federal agencies play a role in the supply and distribution of vaccines.[149] CDC, in particular, conducts activities to help improve management of the vaccine supply chain. Vaccine storage practices especially have implications for a vaccine's potency (i.e., effectiveness).[150]

Vaccines are distributed through a decentralized network of health care providers, health centers, pharmacies, and health departments. State requirements vary regarding the types of entities that can be licensed or authorized to administer various vaccines. In the CDC's Vaccines for Children (VFC) program, health care providers can apply to receive and provide VFC-covered vaccines through state or local coordinators, who ensure that the provider meets program requirements (e.g., ability to properly store and handle vaccines).[151] Any provider that is licensed or otherwise authorized to administer pediatric vaccines can apply to

---

[147] CRS Legal Sidebar LSB10443, *The PREP Act and COVID-19: Limiting Liability for Medical Countermeasures*.

[148] Judith R. Kaufmann, Roger Miller, and James Cheyne, "Vaccine Supply Chains Need To Be Better Funded And Strengthened, Or Lives Will Be At Risk," *Health Affairs*, vol. 30, no. 6 (2011), pp. 1113-1121.

[149] Matthew J. Robbins and Sheldon H. Jacobson, "Analytics for Vaccine Economics and Pricing: Insights and Observations," *Expert Review of Vaccines*, vol. 14, no. 4 (December 1, 2014), pp. 606-616.

[150] CDC, "Vaccine Storage and Handling Toolkit," January 2019, https://www.cdc.gov/ vaccines/hcp/admin/storage/ toolkit/storage-handling-toolkit.pdf.

[151] CDC, "Why Join and How to Become a VFC Provider," https://www.cdc.gov/ vaccines/programs/vfc/providers/ questions/qa-join.html.

participate in a state's VFC program and receive and administer a supply of vaccine.[152]

Vaccine programs are expected to make vaccines widely available, while ensuring that they are safely stored, properly administered, and used or discarded before their expiry date. However, this requirement is a challenge for many vaccine programs. A 2012 HHS Inspector General report found that many VFC providers did not meet vaccine management requirements, either by exposing vaccines to improper temperatures, storing expired and nonexpired vaccines together, or failing to maintain documentation. CDC agreed with the report recommendations and committed to improving management among providers.[153] Following the report, CDC changed VFC program requirements and issued recommendations to providers and immunization program managers.[154]

CDC's immunization programs include several efforts among state and local partners to improve the vaccine supply chain and vaccine distribution:

- The *Vaccine Management Business Improvement Project* (VMBIP) is an effort among CDC and state and local partners to improve the management of the vaccine supply chain, particularly for vaccines distributed through VFC. Since the project began in 2003, it has changed funding mechanisms, forecasting for supply needs, provider distribution, and inventory tracking among vaccine providers.[155]
- The *Vaccine Tracking System* (VTrckS) is an information technology platform for managing the publicly funded vaccine

---

[152] Social Security Act §1928(c); 42 U.S.C. §1396s(c).

[153] HHS Office of Inspector General, *Vaccines for Children Program: Vulnerabilities in Vaccine Management*, June 2012, https://oig.hhs.gov/oei/reports/oei-04-10-00430.pdf.

[154] Association of Immunization Managers, *AIM Statement on Vaccine Storage and Management*, February 7, 2017, https://cdn.ymaws.com/www.immunizationmanagers.org/resource/resmgr/policy/ AIM_Statement_on_Vaccine_Sto.pdf.

[155] CDC, "Vaccine Management Business Improvement Project," https://www.cdc.gov/vaccines/programs/vtrcks/ vmbip.html.

supply chain available to CDC, state and local health departments, and providers.[156]

SAFETY CONSIDERATIONS FOR COVID-19 VACCINES

The COVID-19 vaccine development, approval, and distribution planning situation is evolving. Readers should note the date of this publication and be aware that this chapter may not reflect events or actions that occurred after that date.

Much remains unknown about potential safety issues related to COVID-19 vaccines. FDA has never licensed a vaccine for a coronavirus. Several COVID-19 vaccines in development use novel vaccine technologies, some of which have never before been used in licensed FDA vaccines.[157] Among the few mass emergency vaccination efforts in the past century, there have been some unexpected safety issues. For example, in 1976, the federal government attempted a rapid mass influenza (flu) vaccination campaign in response to a novel swine flu strain. The vaccines were later found to lead to higher rates of Guillain-Barre Syndrome (a neurological disorder) among those vaccinated, ending the campaign.[158]

U.S. vaccine development efforts have been supported and coordinated by Operation Warp Speed (OWS), the nation's major COVID-19 vaccine, therapeutic, and diagnostic (medical countermeasures) development initiative. OWS has chosen to support 14 potential COVID-19 vaccine candidates from a pool of 93, with the stated goal of reducing the number of candidates to 7 as additional results from clinical trials and research

---

[156] CDC, "Vaccine Tracking System," https://www.cdc.gov/vaccines/programs/vtrcks/index.html.

[157] CRS Report R46427, *Development and Regulation of Medical Countermeasures for COVID-19 (Vaccines, Diagnostics, and Treatments): Frequently Asked Questions*.

[158] Lawrence O. Gostin and Lindsay F. Wiley, "Chapter 11: Public Health Emergency Preparedness: Terrorism, Pandemics, and Disasters," in *Public Health Law: Duty, Power, Restraint* (University of California Press, 2016), pp. 4[illegible]0-12.

become available.[159] As of October 29, 2020, eight investigational vaccines were supported within OWS's portfolio.[160] OWS and CDC are planning for a federally coordinated nationwide COVID-19 vaccine distribution campaign.[161]

Making safe and effective COVID-19 vaccines available within a year represents an unprecedented scientific and public health effort. The safety considerations and applicability of the requirements, processes, and programs described in this chapter will likely differ when applied to COVID-19 vaccines in several key ways, particularly with respect to (1) vaccine development, (2) FDA marketing authorization, (3) clinical recommendations and prioritization, (4) surveillance and safety monitoring, (5) injury compensation and patient safety information, and (6) vaccine distribution. Each of these is described in more detail below.

Vaccine Development and Current Status

Typically, the vaccine development and testing process is linear, with an investigational vaccine progressing through each phase of clinical testing upon completion of the prior phase. As mentioned above, the first stage is basic research, and if laboratory and animal test data indicate that a vaccine candidate appears safe and effective against a pathogen, then a first-in-human Phase 1 trial generally follows. If the Phase 1 trial indicates that the vaccine is safe in humans, then Phase 2 testing commences, further examining safety and at what dosage the vaccine has an effect. Finally, if

---

159 Department of Health and Human Services (HHS), "Fact Sheet: Explaining Operation Warp Speed," press release, updated August 7, 2020, https://www.hhs.gov/about/news/2020/06/16/fact-sheet-explaining-operation-warp-speed.html.

160 Moncef Slaoui and Matthew Hepburn, "Developing Safe and Effective Covid Vaccines—Operation Warp Speed's Strategy and Approach," *New England Journal of Medicine*, October 29, 2020.

161 Operation Warp Speed, "From the Factory to the Frontlines The Operation Warp Speed Strategy for Distributing a COVID-19 Vaccine," https://www.hhs.gov/sites/default/files/strategy-for-distributing-covid-19-vaccine.pdf?source= email, and CDC, *COVID-19 Vaccination Program: Interim Playbook for Jurisdiction Operations*, September 16, 2020, https://www.cdc.gov/vaccines/imz-managers/downloads/COVID-19-Vaccination-Program-Interim_Playbook.pdf.

those studies are successful, then a large, placebo-controlled Phase 3 trial follows. This sequential process helps minimize potential health risks to study participants and financial risks to the company sponsoring the investigations. The OWS COVID-19 vaccine development process is not following this phased approach. Instead, it is conducting some of these steps simultaneously to generate safety and effectiveness data in a shorter period.[162]

Several COVID-19 vaccines are currently in Phase 3 clinical trials, and initial results are available from several vaccines that have completed Phase 2 clinical trials.[163] Federal officials have indicated that OWS expects to have initial results from Phase 3 clinical trials in late 2020 and early 2021.[164] Results from several Phase 1 and Phase 2 clinical trials of COVID-19 candidate vaccines have demonstrated short-term safety and some evidence of efficacy. Initial safety data on vaccines supported by Moderna, Pfizer/BioNTech, AstraZeneca, and Johnson & Johnson found no serious safety issues, although more participants who received the vaccine in the trials experienced mild or moderate side effects (e.g., fatigue, fever) compared with the control groups. In addition, all four vaccines show initial evidence of immunogenicity, including antibodies (immune proteins) and other blood cells that neutralized the virus in blood samples of those who received the candidate vaccines.[165] Much remains unknown about COVID-19 immunity, and these results are considered preliminary.

As covered in this chapter, critical data related to the safety and efficacy of vaccines are generally collected in Phase 3 clinical trials. Given

---

162 FDA, "FDA Insight: Vaccines for COVID-19, Part 2," July 28, 2020, https://www.fda.gov/news-events/fda-insight/ fda-insight-vaccines-covid-19-part-2.

163 STAT, "COVID-19 Drugs and Vaccine Tracker," https://www.statnews.com/ feature/coronavirus/drugs-vaccines- tracker/.

164 Moncef Slaoui and Matthew Hepburn, "Developing Safe and Effective Covid Vaccines—Operation Warp Speed's Strategy and Approach," *New England Journal of Medicine*, October 29, 2020.

165 Pedro M. Folegatti, Katie J.Ewer, Parvinder K. Alley, et al., "Safety and Immunogenicity of the ChAdOx1 nCoV-19 Vaccine Against SARS-CoV-2: a Preliminary Report of a Phase 1/2, Single-Blind, Randomised Controlled Trial," *The Lancet*, July 20, 2020, and Sara Oliver, *COVID-19 Vaccines: Work Group Interpretations*, Advisory Committee on Immunization Practices, August 26, 2020, https://www.cdc.gov/vaccines/acip/ meetings/downloads/slides-2020-08/ COVID-07-Oliver.pdf.

that no vaccine for a coronavirus has been previously tested in Phase 3 clinical trials, much remains unknown about the safety issues that may arise. In particular, experts are concerned about the potential for *vaccine enhanced disease*, in which vaccination could worsen the health effects of COVID-19 infections, as seen with the dengue and other vaccines. Animal studies of other coronavirus vaccines have found some potential for vaccine enhanced disease, and experts recommend rigorous monitoring in clinical trials to detect this safety issue.[166] One scientific review noted that the scientific and clinical evidence with COVID-19, thus far, provides limited evidence with respect to the issue of enhanced disease.

Along with other evidence, the authors explore evidence from treatment of COVID-19 patients with convalescent plasma (a treatment involving antibodies) and note that distinguishing antibody enhanced disease from worsening of symptoms is difficult, and therefore the potential for this issue should be studied further.[167]

OWS reports that it is providing scientific support for COVID-19 vaccine clinical trials, in collaboration with other federal agencies like NIH. According to a medical journal publication authored by OWS leaders, OWS is coordinating many components of the vaccine development process. With regard to efficacy data, "OWS will maximize the size of phase 3 trials (30,000 to 50,000 participants each) and optimize trial-site location by consulting daily epidemiologic and disease-forecasting models to ensure the fastest path to an efficacy readout." Phase 3 trial endpoints have been coordinated between the trials, in collaboration with NIAID.[168] NIH has leveraged some of its existing clinical trials networks for testing certain COVID-19 vaccines participating in Operation Warp Speed, named the COVID-19 Prevention Trials Network (COVPN)

---

[166] Paul-Henri Lambert, Donna M Ambrosino, and Svein R Andersen, "Consensus Summary Report for CEPI/BC March 12-13, 2020 Meeting: Assessment of Risk of Disease Enhancement with COVID-19 Vaccines," *Vaccine*, vol. 31 (June 26, 2020), pp. 4783-4791.

[167] Ann M. Arvin, Katja Fink, and Michael A. Schmid, "A Perspective on Potential Antibody-Dependent Enhancement of SARS-CoV-2," *Nature*, vol. 584 (August 20, 2020), pp. 353-363.

[168] Moncef Slaoui and Matthew Hepburn, "Developing Safe and Effective Covid Vaccines—Operation Warp Speed's Strategy and Approach," *New England Journal of Medicine*, August 26, 2020.

that, among other things, works to harmonize clinical endpoints for the trials and recruit study participants.[169]

All of the COVID-19 vaccines supported by OWS that are in Phase 3 clinical trials have a Data and Safety Monitoring Board (DSMB) that independently reviews safety and effectiveness data on the investigational vaccine to determine if the trial should continue, be modified, be terminated, or be considered for FDA marketing authorization (see the "FDA Marketing Authorization" section).[170] Three Phase 3 clinical trials of candidate vaccines supported by OWS—those of Moderna, AstraZeneca, and Johnson & Johnson—are overseen by a common DSMB developed in consultation with NIH's Accelerating COVID-19 Therapeutic Interventions and Vaccines partnership as a part of the COVPN.[171] The Pfizer/BioNTech vaccine has a separate DSMB.[172]

On September 8, 2020, it was reported that AstraZeneca paused its Phase 3 clinical trial in response to a potential safety issue; such pauses are not uncommon in any drug or biologic development effort.[173] On October 12, 2020, it was reported that Johnson & Johnson paused its Phase 3 trial due to "an unexplained illness in a study participant" and that a DSMB has been convened to review the case.[174] As of October 23, 2020, these trials have resumed.[175] In response to calls for transparency, several vaccine

---

[169] National Institutes of Health (NIH), "NIH Launches Clinical Trials Network to Test COVID-19 Vaccines and Other Prevention Tools," press release, July 8, 2020.

[170] U.S. Congress, Senate Committee on Health, Education, Labor, and Pensions, *Senate Health, Education, Labor and Pensions Committee Holds Hearing on the Role of Vaccines in Preventing Outbreaks*, 116th Cong., 2nd sess., September 9, 2020.

[171] National Institutes of Health, "Fourth Large-Scale COVID-19 Vaccine Trial Begins in the United States," press release, September 23, 2020, https://www.nih.gov/news-events/news-releases/fourth-large-scale-covid-19-vaccine- trial-begins-united-states.

[172] Matthew Harper, "A Layperson's Guide to How—and When—a Covid-19 Vaccine Could be Authorized," *STAT*, September 28, 2020.

[173] Rebecca Robbins, Adam Feuerstein, and Helen Branswell, "AstraZeneca Covid-19 Vaccine Study Put on Hold Due to Suspected Adverse Reaction in Participant in the U.K.," *STAT*, September 8, 2020, https://www.statnews.com/2020/ 09/08/astrazeneca-covid-19-vaccine-study-put-on-hold-due-to-suspected-adverse-reaction-in-participant-in-the-u-k/.

[174] Matthew Herper, "Johnson & Johnson Covid-19 Vaccine Study Paused Due to Unexplained Illness in Participant," *STAT*, October 12, 2020, https://www.statnews.com/ 2020/10/12/johnson-johnson-covid-19-vaccine-study-paused-due-to-unexplained-illness-in-participant/.

[175] Katherine J. Wu, Carl Zimmer, and Sharon LaFraniere, et al., "Two Companies Restart Virus Trials in U.S. After Safety Pauses," *The New York Times*, October 23, 2020,

developers, including Moderna, Pfizer/BioNTech, AstraZeneca, and Johnson & Johnson, have made their Phase 3 clinical trial protocols for COVID-19 vaccines publicly available.[176]

As shown in the protocols, the trials are using an event-driven design, meaning that efficacy of the vaccines are to be evaluated once a certain number of "events" occur among the study population—in this context, COVID-19 cases with symptoms. Once a certain number of COVID- 19 cases are detected, the DSMB is to evaluate the data and conduct a statistical analysis to determine if the difference in cases between the vaccine recipient group and the control group meet the FDA's standard for effectiveness for a COVID-19 vaccine. For example, Moderna has determined that 151 COVID-19 cases among its study population would provide enough statistical power to determine whether the vaccine is 60% effective, with interim analyses of the data by the DSMB planned at 35% and 70% of the total target cases. The DSMB may recommend that the vaccine companies end the trials if interim analyses indicate safety issues or do not show adequate evidence of effectiveness.[177] Vaccine expert groups, such as the Coalition for Epidemic Preparedness, have advocated for the event-driven approach to COVID-19 vaccine trials in order to

---

https://www.nytimes.com/2020/10/23/health/covid-vaccine-astrazeneca-johnson-and-johnson.html.

[176] Pfizer, "A Phase 1/2/3 Study to Evaluate the Safety, Tolerability, Immunogenicity, and Efficacy of RNA Vaccine Candidates Against COVID-19 in Healthy Individuals," https://pfe-pfizercom-d8-prod.s3.amazonaws.com/2020-09/C4591001_Clinical_Protocol_0.pdf. Moderna, "A Phase 3, Randomized, Stratified, Observer-Blind, Placebo- Controlled Study to Evaluate the Efficacy, Safety, and Immunogenicity of mRNA-1273 SARS-CoV-2 Vaccine in Adults Aged 18 Years and Older," https://www.modernatx.com/sites/default/files/mRNA-1273-P301-Protocol.pdf. Janssen Vaccines & Prevention B.V.*, Clinical Protocol "A Randomized, Double-blind, Placebo-controlled Phase 3 Study to Assess the Efficacy and Safety of Ad26.COV2.S for the Prevention of SARS-CoV-2-mediated COVID-19 in Adults Aged 18 Years and Older," https://www.jnj.com/coronavirus/covid-19-phase-3-study-clinical-protocol.
AstraZeneca, Clinical Study Protocol, "A Phase III Randomized, Double-blind, Placebo-controlled Multicenter Study in Adults to Determine the Safety, Efficacy, and Immunogenicity of AZD1222, a Non-replicating ChAdOx1 Vector Vaccine, for the Prevention of COVID-19," https://s3.amazonaws.com/ctr-med-7111/D8110C00001/52bec400-80f6-4c1b-8791-0483923d0867/c8070a4e-6a9d-46f9-8c32-cece903592b9/D8110C00001_CSP-v2.pdf.

[177] Moderna, "Clinical Study Protocol," last amended August 20, 2020, https://www.modernatx.com/sites/default/files/mRNA-1273-P301-Protocol.pdf.

expedite vaccine availability without compromising scientific rigor.[178] Other vaccine experts have voiced concerns about this approach, arguing that it "may make statistical sense, but it defies common sense." These experts argue that the vaccines should be assessed for whether they protect against moderate and severe forms of COVID-19 and that the trials should be fully completed to generate adequate data.[179]

FDA Marketing Authorization

The development and testing process for a COVID-19 vaccine is designed to be significantly shorter compared with the usual timeline for vaccine development. This shortened process may make it difficult to detect potential unexpected adverse events that may not manifest right away. Moreover, because the review process is to be shorter than the typical 6 to 10 months needed for a Biologics License Application (BLA) review, FDA scientists would have had less time to review the safety and effectiveness data. Although FDA uses various formal mechanisms to expedite the development and review of medical products intended to address unmet medical need, FDA has not yet granted Emergency Use Authorization (EUA) for a previously unapproved (i.e., unlicensed) vaccine. Thus, if a COVID-19 vaccine is first made available under an EUA rather than a BLA, it will be a first for the agency.

In light of reported concerns from the public surrounding the safety and effectiveness of COVID- 19 vaccines developed on an expedited timeline, FDA officials have sought to clarify that any vaccine candidate "will be reviewed according to the established legal and regulatory standards for medical products."[180] In addition, FDA officials have indicated that the amount of safety and effectiveness data needed to

---

[178] Eddie Loeliger and Bob Small, *Vaccine Efficacy Assessment for COVID-19*, Coalition for Epidemic Preparedness COVID-19 Clinical Working Group, May 7, 2020, https://media.tghn.org/articles/Vaccine_Efficacy_V1.0_7_May_20.pdf.

[179] Peter Doshi and Eric Topol, "These Coronavirus Trials Don't Answer the One Question We Need to Know," *The New York Times*, September 22, 2020.

[180] Anand Shah, Peter Marks, and Jim Hahn, "Unwavering Regulatory Safeguards for COVID-19 Vaccines," *JAMA*, August 2020, vol. 324, no. 10, pp. 931–932.

support EUA issuance will be similar to the data that would be appropriate for a BLA.[181] As mentioned above, the level of evidence required by statute for EUA issuance is different from licensure, although both require the submission of safety and effectiveness data to FDA. For licensure under a BLA, a vaccine would need to be proven safe and have *substantial evidence of effectiveness* to receive full licensure under a BLA. In the case that a vaccine is first made available under an EUA, substantial evidence of effectiveness would not be required by statute. Rather, the totality of the available scientific evidence would need to indicate that the vaccine *may be effective* in preventing COVID-19, and that the known and potential benefits of the vaccine outweigh its known and potential risks.

To help companies develop a vaccine to prevent COVID-19, and to increase transparency regarding the FDA's expectations for safety and effectiveness data, the agency has issued two guidance documents. The first guidance, issued in June 2020, aims to clarify FDA's expectations regarding the data and information necessary to support licensure under a BLA.[182] The guidance notes, among other things, that with respect to effectiveness, FDA expects a COVID-19 vaccine to prevent disease or decrease disease severity in at least 50% of people who are vaccinated. On October 6, 2020, FDA issued a second guidance, which focuses on the agency's expectations for the data and information needed to support an EUA for a COVID-19 vaccine.[183] The recommendations outlined in the October 2020 guidance have been characterized as more stringent than what typically may be required for an EUA.[184] For example, the guidance indicates that data from Phase 3 trials submitted to the agency should include a median follow-up duration of at least two months after

---

[181] Duke Margolis Center for Health Policy, "Safe and Effective COVID-19 Vaccination: The Path from Here," September 10, 2020, meeting. Michael Mezher, "Marks, Hahn Confirm COVID Vaccine EUA Guidance Coming," September 11, 2020, https://www.raps.org/news-and-articles/news-articles/2020/9/marks-hahn-confirm-covid-vaccine-eua-guidance-comi.

[182] FDA, "Development and Licensure of Vaccines to Prevent COVID-19," Guidance for Industry, June 2020, https://www.fda.gov/media/139638/download.

[183] FDA, "Emergency Use Authorization for Vaccines to Prevent COVID-19," Guidance for Industry, October 2020, https://www.fda.gov/media/142749/download.

[184] Michael Erman and Manas Mishra, "U.S. FDA safety guidelines likely to push COVID-19 vaccine authorization past election," October 6, 2020, *Reuters*.

completion of the full vaccination regimen to help provide adequate information to assess a vaccine's benefit-risk profile. FDA also expects clinical testing of an EUA-authorized vaccine to continue to support eventual licensure under a BLA. As such, the guidance recommends that sponsors submit, as part of the EUA request, strategies that will be implemented to (1) address loss of follow-up information for participants who choose to withdraw from the study to receive the vaccine under an EUA, and (2) ensure that ongoing clinical trials of the vaccine are able to assess long-term safety and effectiveness (e.g., evaluating for vaccine-associated ERD, decreased effectiveness over time) in sufficient numbers to support vaccine licensure.

The FDA Vaccines and Related Biological Products Advisory Committee (VRBPAC) met on October 22, 2020, to discuss generally the development, authorization, and licensure of vaccines to prevent COVID-19.[185] The VRBPAC discussed, among other things, FDA's approach to safety and effectiveness as outlined in the agency's guidance documents; expectations for the data that must be submitted for licensure or EUA, including information about the manufacturing process; and plans for postmarket surveillance, including use of existing systems such as VAERS and BEST. FDA also is reportedly developing master protocols to guide its safety and effectiveness oversight, to be made publicly available on its website.[186] To further provide transparency, FDA has indicated it will convene additional VRBPAC meetings to discuss specific vaccine candidates ready for an EUA or licensure.[187]

---

[185] FDA, "Vaccines and Related Biological Products Advisory Committee October 22, 2020 Meeting Announcement," October 22, 2020, https://www.fda.gov/advisory-committees/advisory-committee-calendar/vaccines-and-related-biological-products-advisory-committee-october-22-2020-meeting-announcement.

[186] Kari Oakes, "FDA plans master protocols to monitor COVID vaccine safety, efficacy," *RAPS*, October 22, 2020, https://www.raps.org/news-and-articles/news-articles/2020/10/fda-plans-master-protocols-to-monitor-covid-vaccin.

[187] Matthew Harper, "A Layperson's Guide to How—and When—a Covid-19 Vaccine Could be Authorized," *STAT*, September 28, 2020. U.S. Congress, Senate Committee on Health, Education, Labor, and Pensions, *COVID-19: An Update on the Federal Response*, 116th Cong., 2nd sess., September 24, 2020, p. 35.

Clinical Recommendations and Prioritization

ACIP has begun to weigh considerations related to COVID-19 vaccine clinical recommendations and prioritization, and has made information available for its public meetings in June, July, August, and September 2020. Many of these deliberations note unknowns with regard to COVID-19 vaccines, in particular, as related to clinical trial data on the safety and efficacy of vaccines.[188]

In addition, at the direction of NIH and CDC, the National Academies of Science, Engineering, and Medicine (NASEM) set up an ad hoc committee to develop a framework for equitably allocating COVID-19 vaccines, both domestically and globally.[189] NASEM published its draft framework on September 1 and published its final report with recommendations on October 2. The framework establishes a prioritization methodology that recommends who should be the first to receive COVID-19 vaccines when they become available. Recommended recipients include high-risk workers in health care facilities, first responders, older adults, people with underlying conditions known to be associated with severe outcomes, critical risk workers (workers who are in essential industries and are at substantially higher risk of exposure), and teachers and school staff (see Figure 1).[190]

As of September 2020, ACIP has begun to publicly weigh NASEM's recommendations and compare them to the recommendations from other groups, in particular, from the WHO Strategy Advisory Group of Experts (SAGE) and from the Johns Hopkins Bloomberg School of Public Health. ACIP is considering these recommendations in the context of its own proposed ethical principles of (1) maximizing benefits and minimizing

---

[188] CDC ACIP, "Advisory Committee on Immunization Practices (ACIP)," August 3, 2020.

[189] National Academy of Sciences, Engineering, and Medicine (NASEM), "A Framework for Equitable Allocation of Vaccine for the Novel Coronavirus," https://www.nationalacademies.org/our-work/a-framework-for-equitable-allocation-of-vaccine-for-the-novel-coronavirus.

[190] National Academy of Sciences, Engineering, and Medicine, *Discussion Draft of the Preliminary Framework for Equitable Allocation of COVID-19 Vaccine*, September 1, 2020.

harm, (2) equity, (3) justice, (4) fairness, and (5) transparency.[191] In addition, ACIP has considered how to prioritize vaccine allocation within groups recommended for Phase 1 allocation, should limited vaccine supply require such choices.[192] According to media reporting, these discussions continued at a public meeting in late October (meeting materials are not yet available on ACIP's website).[193]

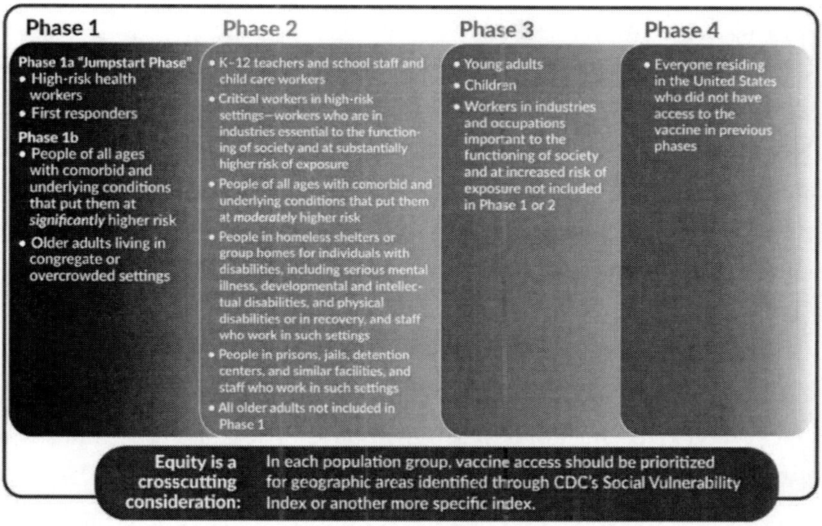

Source: National Academy of Sciences, Engineering, and Medicine, *Framework for Equitable Allocation of COVID-19 Vaccine*, October 2, 2020.

Figure 1. NASEM-Recommended Phased Approach to COVID-19 Vaccine Allocation.

Both the ACIP and NASEM groups are advisory; they do not establish binding policy. Although HHS has historically followed ACIP's recommendations and often considers NASEM recommendations, it is unclear whether and to what extent these recommendations will inform

[191] ACIP COVID-19 Vaccines Work Group, "Overview of Vaccine Equity and Prioritization Frameworks," September 22, 2020, https://www.cdc.gov/vaccines/acip/meetings/downloads/slides-2020-09/COVID-06-Oliver.pdf.

[192] ACIP COVID-19 Vaccines Work Group, "Phase 1 Allocation COVID-19 Vaccine: Work Group Considerations," September 22, 2020, https://www.cdc.gov/vaccines/acip/meetings/downloads/slides-2020-09/COVID-07-Dooling.pdf.

[193] Joe Neel and Pien Huang, "Advisers To CDC Debate How COVID-19 Vaccine Should Be Rolled Out," *National Public Radio*, October 30, 2020.

HHS's COVID-19 vaccine prioritization policies. A report to Congress from Operation Warp Speed on September 16, 2020 noted the NASEM and ACIP roles in prioritizing eventual vaccines but stated that final decisions about prioritization will not be made until closer to implementation.[194]

Safety in Vaccine Distribution

CDC has begun to establish requirements for vaccine management, including requirements related to storage and transportation. As announced on August 14, McKesson Corporation is to act as a central distributor for the COVID-19 vaccine campaign—the same distributor that managed the federally coordinated H1N1 influenza pandemic vaccine campaign.[195] States, localities, territories, and tribes (hereinafter, jurisdictions) are to have much of the responsibility for tracking vaccines provided and for local transportation of vaccines within the jurisdiction.

COVID-19 vaccines in development have different temperature control requirements: some must be refrigerated (2 to 8 degrees Celsius), some must be stored frozen (-15 to -25 degrees Celsius) and some must be kept ultra-cold (-60 to -80 degrees Celsius). CDC's planning guidance to jurisdictions takes these different temperature requirements into account and seeks to minimize potential breaks in the cold chain during vaccine distribution. According to CDC, "certain COVID-19 vaccine products, such as those with ultra-cold temperature requirements, will be shipped directly from the manufacturer to the vaccination provider site," while others will be distributed by CDC's distributor directly to the provider sites or secondary depots for distribution (e.g., chain drug store's central

---

[194] Operation Warp Speed, "From the Factory to the Frontlines: The Operation Warp Speed Strategy for Distributing a COVID-19 Vaccine," https://www.hhs.gov/sites/default/files/strategy-for-distributing-covid-19-vaccine.pdf?source= email.

[195] HHS, "Trump Administration Collaborates with McKesson for COVID-19 Vaccine Distribution," press release, August 14, 2020, https://www.hhs.gov/about/news/2020/08/14/trump-administration-collaborates-mckesson-covid-19-vaccine-distribution.html, and CRS Report R40554, *The 2009 Influenza Pandemic: An Overview.*

distribution). The guidance then further explains how these vaccines should be stored onsite until usage.[196]

CDC, in collaboration with jurisdictions, is planning trainings for newly registered providers regarding safe storage, handling and administration of the vaccines. Providers who seek to participate in the COVID-19 vaccination program must be credentialed/licensed in the jurisdiction where vaccination takes place, and sign and agree to the conditions in the *CDC COVID-19 Vaccination Program Provider Agreement*. Jurisdictions' immunization programs and health care providers administering COVID-19 vaccines are to be responsible for many aspects of vaccine tracking, storage, and handling to ensure that vaccine safety and effectiveness are maintained, as outlined in CDC's preliminary guidance.[197] This guidance is likely to evolve as more information is available regarding the vaccines.

Surveillance and Safety Monitoring

Given the condensed nature of the COVID-19 development programs, FDA may require additional clinical studies to be conducted post-licensure to allow for continued monitoring of adverse events.[198] In guidance, FDA further recommends that at the time of a BLA submission for a COVID-19 vaccine, a Pharmacovigilance Plan (PVP) be submitted to address known and potential risks of the vaccine. FDA may recommend that a PVP include expedited or more frequent adverse event reporting or the establishment of a pregnancy exposure registry to collect information on associated pregnancy and infant outcomes. As mentioned above, manufacturers of BLA-licensed vaccines typically must report adverse

---

196 CDC, *COVID-19 Vaccination Program: Interim Playbook for Jurisdiction Operations*, October 29, 2020, https://www.cdc.gov/vaccines/imz-managers/downloads/COVID-19-Vaccination-Program-Interim_Playbook.pdf.

197 CDC, *COVID-19 Vaccination Program: Interim Playbook for Jurisdiction Operations*, October 29, 2020, https://www.cdc.gov/vaccines/imz-managers/downloads/COVID-19-Vaccination-Program-Interim_Playbook.pdf, pp 21-22.

198 FDA, "Development and Licensure of Vaccines to Prevent COVID-19," Guidance for Industry, June 2020, p. 17, https://www.fda.gov/media/139638/download.

events to FDA within 15 days of becoming aware of them. In the event that a COVID-19 vaccine is first made available under an EUA rather than a BLA, FDA is expected to impose, as a condition of an EUA, requirements for health care providers and vaccine manufacturers to report and track any adverse events associated with administration of the vaccine.[199]

Several federal vaccine safety databases are to be used to monitor postmarket safety for COVID- 19 vaccines. A CDC presentation from the August ACIP meeting identifies that CMS, VA, DOD, IHS, FDA, and CDC databases will be leveraged to provide ongoing monitoring of COVID-19 vaccine safety. It was also reported that “FDA plans to develop new electronic data sources through [electronic health record] EHR partners.”[200]

CDC has reported several efforts to enhance its safety monitoring systems in anticipation of the COVID-19 vaccination program. For health care providers participating in the COVID-19 vaccination program, per the *CDC COVID-19 Vaccination Program Provider Agreement*, providers are required to report adverse events following vaccination through VAERS and are advised to report such events even if the providers are not sure that vaccination caused the adverse event.[201] A preliminary list of “adverse events of special interest” has been developed for monitoring attention in VAERS reports.[202] As communicated to CRS, CDC is strengthening its existing safety monitoring systems in several ways, including by adding additional clinicians to the CISA network, by adding staff to the VAERS network, and by preparing these systems to provide rapid analyses on

---

[199] CDC, *COVID-19 Vaccination Program: Interim Playbook for Jurisdiction Operations*, October 29, 2020, p. 47, https://www.cdc.gov/vaccines/imz-managers/downloads/COVID-19-Vaccination-Program-Interim_Playbook.pdf.

[200] Tom Shimabukuro, “COVID-19 Vaccine Safety Monitoring,” CDC COVID-19 Vaccine Planning Unit, Presented at Advisory Committee on Immunization Practices meeting, August 26, 2020, https://www.cdc.gov/vaccines/acip/ meetings/downloads/slides-2020-08/COVID-04-Shimabukuro.pdf.

[201] CDC, *COVID-19 Vaccination Program: Interim Playbook for Jurisdiction Operations*, October 29, 2020, p. 47, https://www.cdc.gov/vaccines/imz-managers/downloads/COVID-19-Vaccination-Program-Interim_Playbook.pdf.

[202] Tom Shimabukuro, “COVID-19 Vaccine Safety Monitoring,” CDC COVID-19 Vaccine Planning Unit, Presented at Advisory Committee on Immunization Practices meeting, September 22, 2020, https://www.cdc.gov/vaccines/acip/ meetings/downloads/slides-2020-09/COVID-03-Shimabukuro.pdf.

COVID-19 vaccine safety data. CDC plans to implement smartphone-based active vaccine safety monitoring of early recipients of COVID-19 vaccines, called Vaccine Safety Assessment for Essential Workers, or v-safe.[203] This process would involve text, text-to- web survey, and email-to-web survey monitoring of healthcare workers and essential workers who might be prioritized to receive early doses of vaccine when it becomes available (see Figure 2).[204]

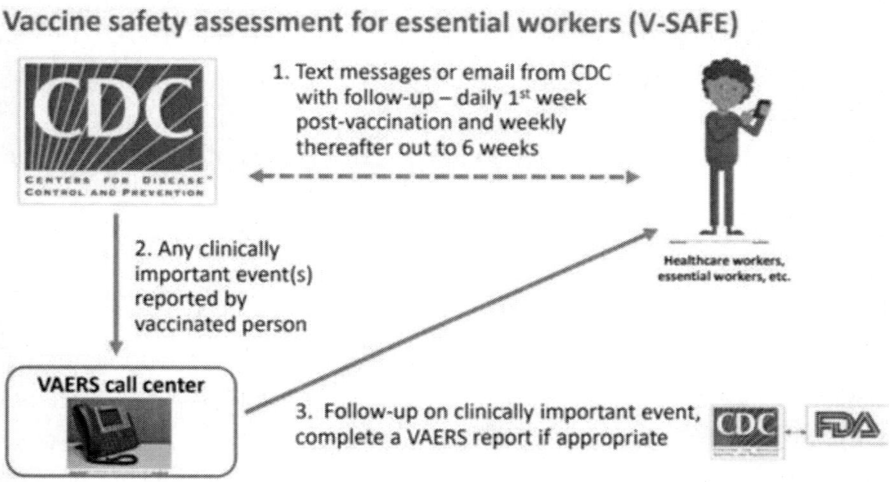

Source: Tom Shimabukuro, "COVID-19 Vaccine Safety Monitoring," CDC COVID-19 Vaccine Planning Unit, Presented at Advisory Committee on Immunization Practices meeting, September 22, 2020, https://www.cdc.gov/vaccines/acip/meetings/downloads/slides-2020-09/COVID-03-Shimabukuro.pdf.

Figure 2. Graphical Presentation of Vaccine Safety Assessment for Essential Workers; Presented at Advisory Committee on Immunization Practices meeting, September 22, 2020.

---

[203] Tom Shimabukuro, "COVID-19 Vaccine Safety Monitoring," CDC COVID-19 Vaccine Planning Unit, presented at Advisory Committee on Immunization Practices meeting, September 22, 2020, https://www.cdc.gov/vaccines/acip/ meetings/downloads/slides-2020-09/COVID-03-Shimabukuro.pdf.

[204] CDC communication with CRS, September 9, 2020, and CDC, *COVID-19 Vaccination Program: Interim Playbook for Jurisdiction Operations*, October 29, 2020, p. 48-49, https://www.cdc.gov/vaccines/imz-managers/downloads/ COVID-19-Vaccination-Program-Interim_Playbook.pdf.

Injury Compensation and Patient Safety Information

Vaccine injury compensation for COVID-19 vaccines will likely differ from usual injury compensation under VICP. The Public Readiness and Emergency Preparedness Act (PREP Act) declaration issued on March 10, 2020, established certain immunity from legal liability related to the "manufacture, testing, development, distribution, administration, and use" of covered countermeasures as part of the public health response to COVID-19. Persons who suffer serious injury or death from a covered countermeasure may seek compensation through the Covered Countermeasure Process Fund as a part of the Countermeasures Injury Compensation Program (CICP). The HHS Secretary may transfer funds available in the Public Health and Social Services Emergency Fund (PHSSEF) in several coronavirus supplemental appropriations acts to this fund.[205]

Because COVID-19 vaccines will likely not be added to the Vaccine Injury Table used for VICP (at least initially), CDC is not required to develop Vaccine Information Statements (VIS) for COVID-19 vaccines. CDC may choose to do so. Separately, if a vaccine is made available under an EUA, FDA has stated it will make fact sheets available for vaccine recipients (or their parents/legal guardians) and vaccine providers.[206] CDC and vaccine manufacturers are also developing other educational material regarding the vaccines.[207]

Congressional Considerations

Since enactment of the Biologics Control Act of 1902, Congress and the Administration (especially through FDA and CDC) have strived to

[205] CRS Legal Sidebar LSB10443, *The PREP Act and COVID-19: Limiting Liability for Medical Countermeasures*.

[206] CDC, *COVID-19 Vaccination Program: Interim Playbook for Jurisdiction Operations*, October 29, 2020, p. 46, https://www.cdc.gov/vaccines/imz-managers/downloads/COVID-19-Vaccination-Program-Interim_Playbook.pdf.

[207] Ibid., p. 23.

ensure the safety of vaccines in the United States—from initial development to patient administration. With the COVID-19 pandemic causing considerable health and economic consequences, there is significant interest in developing safe and effective vaccines to help curb transmission of the disease. Congress may consider how to best leverage existing requirements and programs to ensure that risk of harm from eventual COVID-19 vaccines is mitigated and minimized. Several efforts are underway through OWS, FDA, and CDC to expedite the availability of COVID-19 vaccines and to prepare for a nationwide immunization campaign. Safety has been cited as a primary concern in all of these efforts. Congress may consider how to best provide oversight and make legislative changes to ensure a safe and successful COVID-19 vaccination campaign. In addition, Congress may consider and evaluate the entire federal vaccine safety system and assess whether this system warrants any policy changes to help ensure the safety of all recommended vaccines.

In: Vaccines
Editor: Oliver Huerta
ISBN: 978-1-53619-059-5

Chapter 10

VACCINE SAFETY

Centers for Disease Control and Prevention (CDC)

Vaccines are safe and effective. Because vaccines are given to millions of healthy people — including children — to prevent serious diseases, they're held to very high safety standards.

In this section, you'll learn more about vaccine safety — and get answers to common questions about vaccine side effects.

HOW ARE VACCINES TESTED FOR SAFETY?

Every licensed and recommended vaccine goes through years of safety testing including:

- Testing and evaluation of the vaccine before it's licensed by the Food and Drug Administration (FDA) and recommended for use by the Centers for Disease Control and Prevention (CDC)
- Monitoring the vaccine's safety after it is recommended for infants, children, or adults

Vaccines Are Tested Before They're Recommended for Use

Before a vaccine is ever recommended for use, it's tested in labs. This process can take several years. FDA uses the information from these tests to decide whether to test the vaccine with people.

During a clinical trial, a vaccine is tested on people who volunteer to get vaccinated. Clinical trials start with 20 to 100 volunteers, but eventually include thousands of volunteers. These tests take several years and answer important questions like:

- Is the vaccine safe?
- What dose (amount) works best?
- How does the immune system react to it?

Throughout the process, FDA works closely with the company producing the vaccine to evaluate the vaccine's safety and effectiveness. All safety concerns must be addressed before FDA licenses a vaccine.

Every Batch of Vaccines Is Tested for Quality and Safety

Once a vaccine is approved, it continues to be tested. The company that makes the vaccine tests batches to make sure the vaccine is:

- Potent (It works like it's supposed to)
- Pure (Certain ingredients used during production have been removed)
- Sterile (It doesn't have any outside germs)

FDA reviews the results of these tests and inspects the factories where the vaccine is made. This helps make sure the vaccines meet standards for both quality and safety.

Vaccines Are Monitored After They're Recommended to the Public

Once a vaccine is licensed and recommended for use, FDA, CDC, and other federal agencies continue to monitor its safety.

Check out this infographic for details on how vaccines are developed, approved, and monitored.

There Are Many Different Parts of the National Vaccine Monitoring System

The United States has one of the most advanced systems in the world for tracking vaccine safety. Each of the systems below supplies a different type of data for researchers to analyze. Together, they help provide a full picture of vaccine safety.

- Vaccine Adverse Events Reporting System (VAERS): VAERS is an early warning system managed by CDC and FDA that is designed to find possible vaccine safety issues. Patients, health care professionals, vaccine companies, and others can use VAERS to report side effects that happen after a patient received a vaccine. Some side effects might be related to vaccination while others might be a coincidence (happen by chance). VAERS helps track unusual or unexpected patterns of reporting that could mean there's a possible vaccine safety issue that needs further evaluation.

- The Vaccine Safety Datalink (VSD): VSD is a collaboration between CDC and several health care organizations across the nation. VSD uses databases of medical records to track vaccine safety and do research in large populations. By using medical records instead of self-reports, VSD can quickly study and compare data to find out if reported side effects are linked to a vaccine.
- Post-licensure Rapid Immunization Safety Monitoring System (PRISM): PRISM is part of the Sentinel Initiative, which is FDA's national system for monitoring medical products after they're licensed for use. PRISM focuses on vaccine safety — it uses a database of health insurance claims to identify and evaluate possible safety issues for licensed vaccines.
- Clinical Immunization Safety Assessment Project (CISA): CISA is a collaboration between CDC and a national network of vaccine safety experts from medical research centers. CISA does clinical vaccine safety research and — at the request of providers — evaluates complex cases of possible vaccine side effects in specific patients.
- Additional research and testing: The Department of Defense (DoD) and U.S. Department of Veterans Affairs (VA) have systems to monitor vaccine safety and do vaccine safety research. The National Institutes of Health (NIH) and the Office of Infectious Disease and HIV/AIDS Policy (OIDP) also support ongoing research on vaccines and vaccine safety.

In: Vaccines
Editor: Oliver Huerta

ISBN: 978-1-53619-059-5

Chapter 11

GLOBAL VACCINATION: TRENDS AND U.S. ROLE*

Sara M. Tharakan

SUMMARY

For more than 50 years, the United States has taken an interest in the eradication of vaccine-preventable diseases (VPDs) in children worldwide, as well as vaccine research and development, particularly since playing a vital role in the global campaign to eradicate smallpox in the 1960s. Since then, vaccinating children against VPDs has been a major U.S. foreign policy effort.

Vaccinations are one of the most cost-effective ways to prevent infectious disease and associated morbidity and mortality. According to UNICEF, immunizations save around 3 million lives per year. As of 2019, VPDs continue to cause high levels of morbidity (illness) and mortality (death), and the World Health Organization (WHO) notes that the adoption of new vaccines by low- and middle-income countries (which often have the highest disease burdens) has been slower than in high-income countries.

* This is an edited, reformatted and augmented version of Congressional Research Service Publication No. R45975, dated October 18, 2019.

Receiving a vaccination during childhood can protect the recipient from VPDs, decrease the spread of related diseases, and improve child survival prospects (as children, particularly those under five years old, are more likely than adults to die from VPDs).

Recently, a global resurgence of certain VPDs has caused concern among public health officials and drawn attention to the challenges of vaccine hesitancy and stigma. For example, polio continues to elude global eradication and remains endemic in three countries. In 2019 measles has seen a resurgence in some middle- and high-income countries due to a variety of factors, including reluctance among some individuals and religious communities to vaccinate their children. In April 2019, the WHO reported an increase in global measles cases compared to the same period in 2018, with the greatest surges in cases in the Americas, the Middle East, and Europe. A number of European countries are at risk of or have lost their measles eradication certificate from the WHO, raising questions about global consensus on the use of vaccines, participation in and support for the Global Alliance for Vaccines and Immunization (GAVI, now called GAVI, the Vaccine Alliance) and other global immunization efforts. Prompted in part by this global resurgence, the WHO has listed "vaccine hesitancy" as one of the 10 biggest global public health threats.

The U.S. government is the second-leading government donor to global vaccination campaigns. Through annual appropriations to the Department of Health and Human Services (HHS) and the Department of State, Congress funds global immunization activities through the Centers for Disease Control and Prevention (CDC), the United States Agency for International Development (USAID), and GAVI. In recent years, annual appropriations by Congress for multilateral immunizations campaigns led by GAVI have averaged $290 million and $226 million for bilateral campaigns led by CDC. USAID works to support routine immunization overseas through health systems strengthening, and Global Polio Eradication Initiative Activities. The authorization, appropriation, and oversight of U.S. funding for global child vaccination is thus an ongoing area of concern for many in Congress. Other key issues for Congress include the extent of donor coordination and burden-sharing for such efforts, and the extent to which global child vaccination promotes U.S. foreign policy, development, and domestic health security (i.e., pandemic preparedness) goals.

INTRODUCTION

Beginning with the campaign to eradicate smallpox in the 1960s, the United States has been interested in the eradication of vaccine-preventable diseases (VPDs) in children worldwide, as well as vaccine research and development. The success of the smallpox eradication campaign led to the establishment of the World Health Organization's Expanded Programme on Immunization in 1974.[1] Since then, global vaccination campaigns have been broadened and garnered near universal international support.

Today, the U.S. government is a leading donor to global vaccination campaigns (*Figure 3*).[2] In FY2019, Congress appropriated $290 million in foreign aid for the Global Alliance for Vaccines and Immunization (GAVI, now called GAVI, the Vaccine Alliance) and $226 million for Department of Health and Human Services (HHS) to support child vaccine campaigns abroad. The authorization, appropriation, and oversight of U.S. funding for global child vaccination is thus an ongoing area of concern for many in Congress, as is the extent of donor coordination and burden-sharing for such efforts. Additional potential issues include the extent to which global child vaccination promotes U.S. foreign policy, development, and domestic health security (i.e., pandemic preparedness) goals.

Donor-backed child vaccination campaigns have reduced mortality in poor countries, though occasionally they have faced setbacks. In the early 1990s, U.S. foreign assistance for large-scale vaccination campaigns led by the World Health Organization (WHO) and the United Nations Children's Fund (UNICEF), and with significant U.S. funding and technical support, contributed to an approximately 80% immunization rate for three doses of the diphtheria, tetanus, and pertussis vaccine (DTP3).[3] Progress, as

---

[1] J.M. Okwo-Bele and T. Cherian, "The expanded programme on immunization: a lasting legacy of smallpox eradication.," *Vaccine*, vol. 29 (December 30, 2011).

[2] See *Figure 3*. Since 2000, the United States has contributed nearly 12% of GAVI's total funding (roughly $2.5 billion), following the United Kingdom (24%), and the Bill and Melinda Gates Foundation (20%).

[3] DTP3 coverage is used as a proxy for vaccination coverage of a population for all recommended vaccines. After smallpox, the pertussis, diphtheria, and tetanus vaccines are the oldest vaccines (developed in 1914, 1926, and 1938 respectively and combined into the DTP vaccine in 1948).

measured by vaccination rates, stalled on certain vaccines—notably the diphtheria, tetanus, pertussis, and measles vaccines—in the late-1990s for a variety of reasons, including management of vaccine stocks, effective vaccine delivery, and cost of vaccinations.[4]

What Is a Vaccine-Preventable Disease?

A vaccine-preventable disease (VPD) is an infectious disease for which an effective preventive vaccine exists. Examples include measles and polio. If a person acquires a VPD and dies from it, the death is considered a vaccine-preventable death.

A population achieves "herd immunity," whereby a sufficient proportion of the population is immunized in order to prevent disease spread, when 93% to 95% of individuals in a community are vaccinated.

Recommended childhood vaccines are listed in *Figure 3*.

Source: Centers for Disease Control and Prevention (CDC), Vaccines and Preventable Diseases, https://www.cdc.gov/vaccines/vpd/index.html.

In 2000, a public-private partnership, the Global Alliance for Vaccines and Immunization (GAVI) was launched to address both declining global momentum for child immunization campaigns and declining funding for these programs. Since its inception, GAVI has supported the immunization of 700 million children.[5] As a founding member of GAVI, the United States holds a rotating seat on GAVI's board and provides it with funding (see "U.S. Role and Funding").

Vaccinations are considered one of the most cost-effective ways to prevent infectious disease and associated morbidity and mortality. WHO recommends that all children receive 10 vaccines (*Table 1*).[6] Receiving the

---

[4] Beth Jarosz and Reshma Naik, *Progress Stalls on Vaccine-Preventable Diseases*, Population Reference Bureau, June 25, 2015, https://www.prb.org/vaccine-preventable-disease-progress/. Beth Jarosz and Reshma Naik, *Solutions to Reducing Vaccine-Preventable Childhood Diseases*, Population Reference Bureau, June 24, 2015, https://www.prb.org/vaccine-preventable-childhood-disease/.

[5] GAVI, Facts and Figures, 2019.

[6] The WHO recommends children receive these vaccinations prior to 23 months of age, with the exception of the HPV vaccine, which is recommended for children by age 12 years.

recommended childhood vaccinations can protect the recipient from illness and death associated with VPDs, and can reduce infectious disease spread. According to UNICEF, these immunizations save around 3 million lives per year.[7] Globally, coverage of recommended childhood vaccines vary, with VPDs causing high levels of morbidity (illness) and mortality (death), primarily in certain low- and middle-income countries that have had limited success in achieving universal coverage.[8] Recently, some high-income countries, for example France and the United States, have seen exponential increases in cases of VPDs, due primarily to vaccine hesitancy.[9]

Global Vaccine Coverage

According to GAVI, from 2000 through 2018, more than 760 million children worldwide were immunized against VPDs, including 66 million children in 2018. Approximately 100 million children are immunized each year. At the end of 2018, 20 million infants and children worldwide had not received the full schedule of recommended vaccines.[10] According to GAVI, full vaccination coverage could prevent one in seven deaths in under-5 children.[11] Over 1.5 million children die every year from VPDs.[12] Nearly 60% of these children live in 10 countries: Angola, Brazil, DRC, Ethiopia, India, Indonesia, Nigeria, Pakistan, the Philippines, and Vietnam.[13]

---

[7] UNICEF, *Immunization programme*, 2019, https://www.unicef.org/immunization.

[8] F. Bustreo, J-M Okwo-Bele, and L. Kamara, World Health Organization perspectives on the contribution of GAVI on reducing child mortality, World Health Organization, October 14, 2014.

[9] "Vaccine hesitancy: a generation at risk," The Lancet Child & Adolescent Health, vol. 3, no. 5 (May 2019).

[10] WHO, *Immunization*, July 18, 2019, https://www.who.int/news-room/facts-in-pictures/detail/immunization.

[11] GAVI, *About GAVI, the Vaccine Alliance*, Geneva, Switzerland, 2019, https://www.gavi.org/about/.

[12] UNICEF, *The State of the World's Children 2016: A fair chance for every child*, 2016

[13] WHO, *Immunization*, July 18, 2019, https://www.who.int/news-room/facts-in-pictures/detail/immunization.

Table 1. WHO recommended immunizations for children

Recommended Vaccine	Number of Doses and Disease Protection
Bacilus Calmette Guerin (BCG)	1 dose, protects against tuberculosis.
Diphtheria, Tetanus and Pertussis vaccine (commonly referred to as DTP3, DTPcv3 or DTaP)	3 doses, protects against diphtheria, tetanus, and pertussis (whooping cough)
Hepatitis B vaccine	3-4 doses, protects against hepatitis B disease, which can cause liver failure, and cancer.
Haemophilus Influenzae Type b (Hib) Vaccine	3 doses, protects against Hib disease, which can cause bacterial meningitis, and pneumonia.
Pneumococcal (PCV-3)	3 doses, protects against pneumonia.
Poliomyelitis vaccine (IPV-1)	3 doses, protects against poliovirus, which can cause paralysis and meningitis.
Rotavirus vaccine	3-4 doses, protects against severe diarrhea, vomiting, and stomach pain caused by rotavirus.
Measles vaccine (commonly referred to as MMR, or MCV)	2 doses, protects against measles, often administered in combination with mumps and rubella vaccines.
Rubella (commonly referred to as MMR or MCV)	1 dose, protects against rubella disease.
Human Papillomavirus (HPV) vaccine	2 doses, protects against HPV types 16 and 18, which can cause cervical cancer.

Source: WHO, Recommended Routine Immunizations for Children, April 2019. CDC, Vaccine Information Statements, 2019.

From 1990 to 2017, overall child deaths fell from 12.7 million to 5.8 million, largely due to gains made by global immunization campaigns and expanded national immunization programs.[14] For example, from 2000 to 2017, scaled-up measles vaccination coverage averted an estimated 15.6 million deaths from the disease.[15]

Global coverage for several recommended vaccines has continued to climb over the past decade (see *Figure 1*); however, progress in expanding the number of children vaccinated with DTP3 (a three-dose diphtheria, tetanus and pertussis vaccine) has stagnated in recent years, though its coverage remains higher than coverage for other required vaccinations (see *Figure 2*). GAVI reports recent stagnation in coverage is due to "acute problems that a small number of previously high performing countries

[14] UNICEF, *Under-five mortality*, March 2018.
[15] Ibid.

have faced."[16] Diphtheria, tetanus and pertussis are particularly fatal to neonates, new mothers, and pregnant women. Maternal and neonatal tetanus (MNTE) has been almost eliminated globally, and since 2000 there has been an 85% reduction in newborn deaths from tetanus.[17] As of March 2019, MNTE remains present in 14 countries.[18] In 2018, 86% of children under the age of one received all three doses of the DTP3 vaccine.

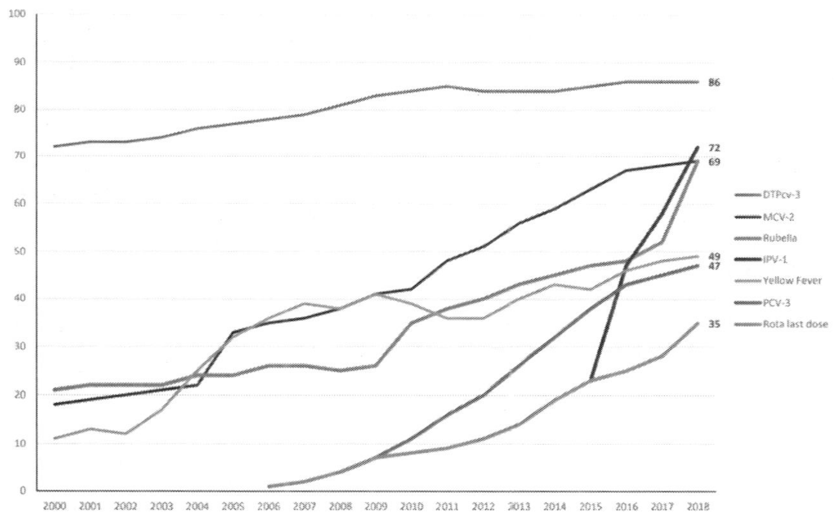

Source: WHO, Progress and Challenges with Achieving Universal Immunization Coverage, July 2019.

Notes: DTPcv-3 is coverage of the three recommended doses of the diptheria, tetanus, and pertussis vaccine. MCV-2 is coverage of the two recommended doses of the measles-containing vaccine. IPV-1 refers to the inactivated poliovirus vaccine. PCV-3 is the pneumococcal conjugate vaccine used to protect against pneumonia and other diseases caused by the streptococcus pneumoniae bacteria. The rubella vaccine protects against rubella and may be given in combination with other vaccines (i.e., as the MMRV vaccine) to protect against measles, mumps, rubella, and varicella (commonly known as chickenpox).

Figure 1. Global Coverage for SelectedVaccines, 2000-2018.

---

[16] GAVI, Annual Progress Report: 2018, 2019.

[17] WHO, Maternal and Neonatal Tetanus Elimination, June 2019.

[18] MNTE persists in Afghanistan, Angola, Central African Republic, Chad, Democratic Republic of Congo, Guinea, Mali, Nigeria, Pakistan, Papua New Guinea, Somalia, Sudan, South Sudan and Yemen. Pakistan and Nigeria have partially eliminated MNTE. WHO, *Protecting All Against Tetanus*, January 2019.

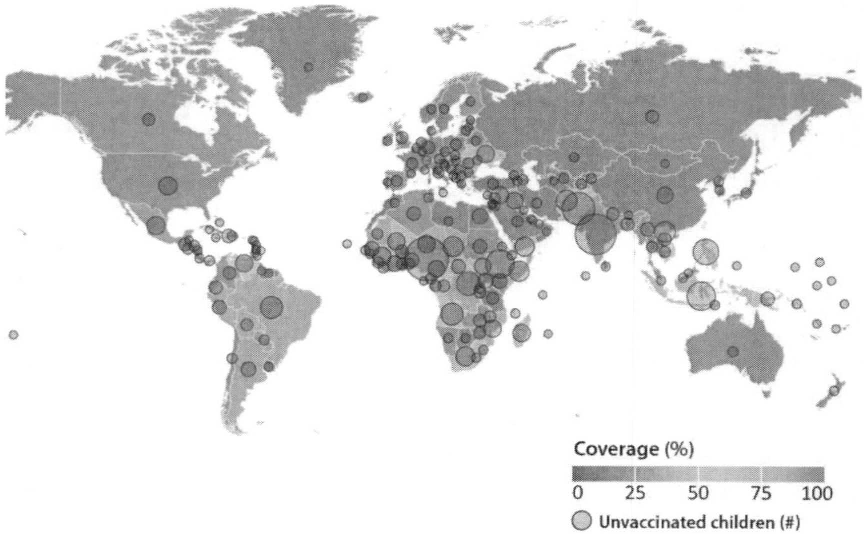

Source: WHO/UNICEF estimates of national immunization coverage (WUENIC), as of 2019, available at https://unicef.shinyapps.io/wuenic_analytics/; and UNDP World Population Prospects, 2019.

Notes: Estimates of immunization coverage stem from UNICEF/WHO member states, survey reports, and data from academic literature. Values may not sum to total due to rounding. Regional estimates of the number of unvaccinated children reflect the entire target population, whether or not a country has introduced the vaccination of interest.

Figure 2. Estimated Immunization Coverage and Number of Unvaccinated Children (DTP3), 2018.

As global uptake of childhood vaccines improves, an increasing proportion of child deaths are concentrated in sub-Saharan Africa and Southern Asia: four out of every five under-5 child deaths occur in these regions.[19] *Figure 2* displays geographical immunization coverage for three doses of the DTP3 vaccine. DTP3 immunization coverage is used as a proxy indicator to estimate the proportion of children vaccinated within their first year of life.[20]

[19] Ibid.

[20] WHO/UNICEF estimates of national immunization coverage, WUENIC Analytics, https:// unicef.shinyapps.io/ wuenic_analytics/.

Global Efforts to Decrease VPDs Among Children

In 2015, U.N. member states adopted the Sustainable Development Goals (SDG) as a common agenda to help alleviate global poverty, improve health and education, reduce inequality, and spur economic growth by 2030.[21] SDG Goal 3 is to end preventable deaths of newborns and under-5 children by 2030, with a targeted reduction of under-5 mortality to 25 per 1,000 live births in every country.[22] (According to 2018 figures, 80 countries worldwide have under-5 mortality rates that are higher than 25 per 1,000 live births.)[23] International efforts to decrease vaccine- preventable deaths among children younger than five years are led by international organizations such as WHO, UNICEF, and GAVI, with significant U.S. support (detailed in the section on U.S. role and funding). Several multilateral initiatives and commitments frame these efforts.

UNICEF

UNICEF supports immunization programs globally and is the biggest single global purchaser of vaccines. The organization focuses on providing vaccinations, monitoring and improving vaccine supply and quality (e.g., ensuring that vaccines are consistently stored at an appropriate temperature, known as "the cold chain"), vaccine innovation (e.g., research and development), and disease eradication and elimination programs. UNICEF has a permanent seat on GAVI's board and procures all vaccines for GAVI-supported programs to ensure a reliable supply of high-quality and affordable vaccines.[24] UNICEF's immunization goals align with WHO targets outlined in the Global Vaccine Action Plan (GVAP) 2011-2020; to

---

[21] See U.N. Sustainable Development Goals, at https://sustainabledevelopment.un.org/?menu=1300.

[22] United Nations, *Goal 3: Ensure healthy lives and promote well-being for all at all ages*, Sustainable Development Goals, 2015, https://www.un.org/sustainabledevelopment/health/.

[23] The World Bank, *Data: Mortality rate, under-5 (per 1,000 live births)*, 2018.

[24] GAVI, *Gavi's partnership model: UNICEF*, 2019, https://www.gavi.org/about/partners/unicef/.

reach 90% of children under the age of one with routine immunization, and achieve 80% immunization coverage for every country district by 2020.[25]

WHO

The WHO launched its first 10-year strategic framework on vaccines in 2005. The Global Immunization Vision and Strategy Immunization was intended to extend immunization achievements and to continue encouraging governments to maintain a commitment to protect their populations from VPDs. The GVAP for 2011-2020 was released in 2010 to build on the 2005 strategic framework. The GVAP aligns with the WHO's 2015-2030 strategic goals, which include promoting the development of new vaccines and vaccine delivery technologies to meet public health priorities, establishing norms and standards for vaccines and vaccine delivery technology, and ensuring quality.[26]

The WHO also develops evidence-based immunization policy recommendations for member states through an independent advisory group, the Strategic Advisory Group of Experts on Immunization (SAGE).[27] SAGE meets biannually to develop recommendations based on available evidence on immunization and vaccines. It also convenes on an emergency basis to discuss disease outbreaks and vaccine-related concerns (e.g., experimental Ebola vaccines).

GAVI, the Vaccine Alliance

GAVI is a multilaterally funded public-private partnership. It was founded in 2000 by the United States, the WHO, the United Nations, the World Bank, and the Bill and Melinda Gates Foundation to expand global access to vaccines and prevent deaths from VPDs. GAVI is guided by five year strategic plans, the Phase IV strategy for 2015-2020 aligns with the goals outlined in the GVAP. In 2019, GAVI set the overall goal to immunize 300 million children by 2025, and save 5-6 million lives in the

[25] A goal of 80% immunization coverage for every country district differs from a national 80% coverage rate because it does not mask differences in districts within a country (e.g., rural and urban gaps or gaps between poor and rich districts).

[26] WHO, From Vaccine Development to Policy: A Brief Review of WHO Vaccine-Related Activities and Advisory Processes, 2017.

[27] WHO, Strategic Advisory Group of Experts on Immunization, March 2019.

long term.[28] For more information on GAVI, see the section under U.S. Funding for Multilateral Initiatives.

Factors Affecting Immunization Coverage

Various factors affect global immunization coverage, including vaccine hesitancy and stigma, geographic location, inadequate country capacity, and poverty and socioeconomic status.

Vaccine Hesitancy and Stigma

Recently, a resurgence of certain VPDs has caused concern among public health officials and drawn attention to the challenges of vaccine hesitancy and stigma. For example, polio continues to elude global eradication, and in 2019 some middle- and high-income countries experienced a resurgence of measles, due to a variety of factors, including reluctance among some individuals and religious communities to vaccinate their children. In April 2019, the WHO reported a 300% increase in global measles cases compared to the same period in 2018, with the greatest surges in cases in the Americas, the Middle East, and Europe.[29]

Prompted in part by this resurgence, the WHO listed "vaccine hesitancy" as one of the 10 biggest global public health threats.[30] Corruption, authoritarian governance, and social or political discrimination can fuel vaccine hesitancy by undermining citizens' trust in authority figures (including government officials and health workers involved in vaccine campaigns). For example, Nigeria was close to eliminating polio for many years but did not do so until recently. Vaccination campaign efforts were hampered in part by conspiracy theories, "vaccine stigma," as well as by ethical concerns about government regulations and

---

[28] GAVI, Gavi's Strategy, 2019.

[29] WHO, Global Measles and Rubella Update, August 2019.

[30] The WHO defines "vaccine hesitancy" as "a delay in acceptance or refusal of vaccines despite availability of vaccine services." WHO, *Ten Threats to Global Health in 2019*, 2019, https://www.who.int/emergencies/ten-threats-to-global- health-in-2019.

pharmaceutical industry practices. Vaccine stigma, for its part, arises when a community normalizes vaccine denial.[31]

VPD Eradication Campaigns and U.S. National Security Actions[32]

Health practitioners can face a range of obstacles in administering vaccines, including security conditions in or near conflict zones and resistance from local populations rooted in cultural, religious, or political views. Real or perceived associations between vaccination efforts and foreign government interests may further limit the willingness of populations to participate and may contribute to security risks for health workers. In Pakistan, for example, some observers attribute a backlash against polio vaccination efforts to revelations that U.S. government entities used a hepatitis B vaccination program to covertly gather information confirming the whereabouts of Osama bin Laden in 2011.[33] A Pakistani doctor, Shakil Afridi, had been engaged in hepatitis B vaccination efforts that were indirectly used to confirm Bin Laden's whereabouts in 2011. Following Afridi's imprisonment and revelations from his trial, the expulsion of some foreign health workers from Pakistan, the assassination of several U.N. polio vaccine workers, and the suspension of U.N.-supported polio eradication efforts in Pakistan, the deans of several prominent U.S. schools of public health wrote to the Obama Administration stating that "public health programs should not be used as cover for covert operations" and requesting public assurance that cases such as Afridi's would not be repeated.[34] In 2014, the Administration confirmed that "the Director of the Central Intelligence Agency (CIA) directed in August 2013 that the Agency make no operational use of vaccination programs, which includes vaccination workers. Similarly, the Agency will not seek to obtain or exploit DNA or other genetic material acquired through such programs. This CIA policy applies worldwide and to U.S. and non-U.S. persons alike."[35]

---

[31] "Vaccine denial" is defined as refusal to vaccinate, or rejection of recommended vaccinations, usually by the parent or guardian of an eligible child.

[32] Christopher Blanchard, Specialist in Middle Eastern Affairs, contributed to this text box.

[33] Saeed Shah, "U.S. defense chief confirms Pakistan holds doctor with role in bin Laden raid," *McClatchy Newspapers*, January 29, 2012; Shah, "Pakistani who helped CIA gets 33 years," *McClatchy Newspapers*, May 24, 2012; and, Alexander Mullaney and Syeda Amna Hassan, "He Led the CIA to bin Laden—and Unwittingly Fueled a Vaccine Backlash," *National Geographic*, February 27, 2015.

[34] Letter from Pierre M. Buekens, M.D., M.P.H., Ph.D. Dean, Tulane University School of Public Health and Tropical Medicine et al. to President Barack Obama, January 6, 2013.

[35] Letter from Assistant to the President for Homeland Security and Counterterrorism Lisa Monaco, May 16, 2014; and Johns Hopkins School of Public Health, "White House

Geographic Location

Geographical distance from health centers negatively impacts vaccination coverage.[36] Underserved populations within any given country often shoulder a heavier burden of disease, and they may lack access to basic medical care. Notably, vaccine coverage disparities between children in urban and rural areas persist throughout the world, and commonly exacerbate disease spread within a certain geographical area. For example, according to the WHO, in some countries (e.g., Nigeria and Indonesia), coverage of the measles vaccine in rural areas is 33% lower than in urban areas.[37]

Poverty, Socioeconomic Status, and Social Determinants of Health

Vaccination coverage in low-income countries (41%) lags behind coverage in high-income countries (90%).[38] Medical systems in many low-income countries are often underfunded and unable to vaccinate enough children to stop a virus's spread even with donor aid. In addition, researchers have found that inequities in vaccination coverage are associated with individual socioeconomic determinants, such as a family's income level and the educational status of a child's mother.[39] Children born into poverty are almost twice as likely to die before the age of five as those from wealthier families, and researchers suggest that unequal access to vaccines is a key factor.[40] Vaccine coverage for the richest fifth of the population in some countries is up to 58% higher than for the poorest fifth.[41]

Responds to Public Health Deans: the Central Intelligence Agency Makes No Use of Operational Vaccination Programs," press release, May 20, 2014.

[36] C. Edson Utazi, Julia Thorley, Victor A. Alegana, et al., "Mapping vaccination coverage to explore the effects of delivery mechanisms and inform vaccination strategies," *Nature Communications*, vol. 10, no. 1633 (April 19, 2019).

[37] Ibid.

[38] Rebecca Casey, Laure Dumolard, and Carolina Danovaro-Holliday, *Global Routine Vaccination Coverage, 2015*, CDC, November 18, 2016, https://www.cdc.gov/mmwr/volumes/65/wr/mm6545a5.htm.

[39] WHO, Global Vaccine Action Plan 2011-2020, op. cit.

[40] UNICEF, *Sustainable Development Goals: Goal 3 Good Health and Well-Being*, 2017.

[41] Ibid.

Fragile and Conflict Settings

UNICEF reports that 40% of unvaccinated children live in countries affected by armed conflict or other humanitarian challenges.[42] Often, already fragile health care infrastructure is further crippled by armed conflict, which can hinder health workers in carrying out vaccinations and interfere with proper disease treatment and containment.

Humanitarian settings such as refugee and internal displacement camps can also foster conditions (e.g., poor nutrition, overcrowding, and unsanitary conditions) conducive to the rapid spread of infectious diseases.[43] According to UNICEF estimates, as of 2015, half of the 10 countries that had under 50% diphtheria, tetanus, and pertussis vaccine coverage—the Central African Republic, Somalia, South Sudan, Syria, and Ukraine—had experienced conflicts or other humanitarian emergencies.[44] Other conflict-affected countries have seen spikes in VPD cases, such as a 2019 surge in measles cases in the Democratic Republic of Congo (DRC), which has killed more people than the ongoing Ebola outbreak in that country.[45]

U.S. ROLE AND FUNDING

Congress has historically supported global child vaccination programs, both as a component of U.S. foreign assistance and as part of efforts to eradicate infectious diseases that might affect Americans at home or abroad. Through annual appropriations for the Department of Health and Human Services and the Department of State and Foreign Operations (SFOPS), Congress funds global immunization activities through the Centers for Disease Control (CDC), the United States Agency for

[42] UNICEF, *Infographic: Fast Facts on Immunization*, April 2019.

[43] Chimeremma Nnadi, Andrew Etsano, aBelinda Uba, et al., "Approaches to Vaccination Among Populations in Areas of Conflict," *The Journal of Infectious Diseases*, vol. 216 (July 1, 2017).

[44] Eric E. Mast, Stephen L. Cochi, Olen M. Kew, et al., "Fifty Years of Global Immunization at CDC, 166-2015," *Public Health Reports*, vol. 132, no. 1 (January-Febrary 2017), pp. 18-26.

[45] University of Minnesota Center for Infectious Disease Research and Policy, "DRC declares measles outbreak after 1,500 deaths," June 11, 2019.

International Development (USAID), and the Global Alliance for Vaccines and Immunization (GAVI, now called GAVI, the Vaccine Alliance).

The U.S. Agency for International Development (USAID) and the Centers for Disease Control and Prevention (CDC) are the primary U.S. federal agencies involved in international vaccination provision and immunization campaigns. These campaigns support the 2016-2020 Strategic Framework for Global Immunization and the WHO's 2011-2020 Global Vaccine Action Plan, the agencies work with country governments to strengthen immunization programs by bolstering infectious disease surveillance, increasing laboratory capacity, and strengthening public health workforce capacity. The efforts of both agencies align with the 2010 HHS National Vaccine Plan, the Global Health Security Agenda, and the U.N.'s 2030 Sustainable Development Goals.

CDC and USAID also support routine immunizations worldwide through enhanced supply chain management and product procurement assistance. Related efforts are implemented bilaterally and through international partnerships with the WHO, UNICEF, the World Bank, and others. In addition, CDC, along with the Department of Defense, finances the research and development of new vaccines.

Centers for Disease Control and Prevention (CDC)

The CDC has played a central role in controlling vaccine-preventable diseases since it established the CDC Smallpox Eradication Program in January 1966.[46] The Global Immunization Division of the CDC's Center for Global Health is responsible for coordinating CDC's global immunization activities.[47] To support these activities, the CDC provides scientific and public health expertise in infectious disease epidemiology and surveillance by building laboratory capacity and helping to implement evidence-based prevention strategies. CDC also carries out clinical trials and epidemiologic studies.

---

[46] CDC, CDC's 2016-2020 Strategic Framework for Global Immunization, May 2016.
[47] Ibid.

Funding for the CDC's Global Immunization Program is detailed in *Table 2*. The majority of CDC's efforts are focused on polio, with smaller funding allocations for measles and other VPDs. Global vaccination campaigns against polio have lowered the worldwide incidence of polio by 99% compared with that of 1988, and in 2018 only two countries recorded wild polio cases: Afghanistan and Pakistan.[48] Vaccine-derived poliovirus continues to be detected in Nigeria, but as of August 21, 2019, no cases had been confirmed there in three years.[49]

The CDC's programming is based on its 2016-2020 *Strategic Framework for Global Immunization,* which builds on three previous strategic frameworks and outlines five goals:

1. Control, eliminate, or eradicate vaccine-preventable diseases to reduce death and disability globally.
2. Strengthen country ownership, policy and practices, and partnerships.
3. Ensure quality of vaccination delivery to achieve high and equitable coverage.
4. Strengthen surveillance and immunization information to prevent, detect, and respond to vaccine-preventable diseases.
5. Conduct and promote research, innovation, and evaluation.[50]

To implement the strategic framework, the CDC works with USAID, UNICEF, GAVI, and other stakeholders. The strategy is aligned with the HHS National Vaccine Plan 2010, the Global Health Security Agenda, and the WHO Global Vaccine Action Plan 2011-2020.

---

[48] UNICEF, Infographic: Fast Facts on Immunization, April 2019.

[49] In under-immunized populations vaccine-derived polio remains a challenge. An excreted vaccine-virus can continue to circulate for extended periods of time, the longer the virus survives the more genetic changes it undergoes (in rare occurs vaccine-derived poliovirus can mutate into a version that can paralyze an afflicted person). According to the WHO, this occurs when immunization campaigns are poorly conducted, and populations are left susceptible to vaccine- derived or wild poliovirus. WHO experts note the issue is not the vaccine, but low vaccination coverage. WHO, What is vaccine-derived polio? April 2017.

[50] Ibid., and CDC, 2016-2020 Strategic Framework for Global Immunization, May 2016.

In FY2019, Congress appropriated more funding for CDC global immunization programs than the Trump Administration sought and more than was appropriated in prior years (*Table 2*). The Administration's FY2019 and FY2020 budget requests would have reduced funding for global immunization activities and proposed that the CDC "focus its global immunization activities to continue progress towards polio eradication, as well as measles and rubella elimination in countries with the highest disease burden."[51]

Table 2. CDC Center for Global Health Global Immunization Program Funding, FY2015-FY2019 (current U.S. $ millions)

	Year	Polio Eradication	Measles and other VPDs	Total
FY2015	Requested	162	50	211
	Enacted	159	50	209
	% Change Requested to Enacted	-1.85%	0%	-1.08%
FY2016	Requested	169	50	219
	Enacted	169	50	219
	% Change Requested to Enacted	0%	0%	0%
FY2017	Requested	174	50	224
	Enacted	174	50	223
	% Change Requested to Enacted	0%	0%	0%
FY2018	Requested	165	N/A	206
	Enacted	176	50	226
	% Change Requested to Enacted	+6.67%	N/A	+9.71%
FY2019	Requested	165	N/A	206
	Enacted	176	50	226
	% Change Requested to Enacted	+6.67%	N/A	+9.71%
FY2020	Requested	NA	NA	206

Source: CDC Congressional Justifications, 2015-2020; Statements of Conferees, Joint Explanatory Statements accompanying omnibus appropriations measures, 2015-2020, FY2015-2020, appropriations legislation (P.L. 114- 113, 115-31, 115-41, and P.L. 116-6); and CRS correspondence with CDC, July 2019. USAID.

[51] CDC, FY2020 Congressional Justification, March 2019.

To strengthen routine immunization campaigns and community-based disease surveillance, USAID works with foreign countries' ministries of health and provides funding to GAVI. These actions are part of the agency's strategy to prevent child and maternal deaths, which it also supports through capacity building for foreign health systems.[52] For example, in Ethiopia, the agency works with Ethiopia's Ministry of Health to train community volunteers to identify symptoms of vaccine-preventable diseases (e.g., paralysis due to polio) and track "vaccine defaulters" (individuals who do not receive the full schedule of immunizations) to keep them on schedule.

U.S. Funding for Multilateral Initiatives

The United States, through contributions to international organizations and GAVI, provides significant support for multilateral immunization and vaccination programs (*Figure 3*).[53] Such support is intended to complement U.S. bilateral efforts in this arena while enabling the United States to expand its reach and provide opportunities for collaboration and burden sharing.

GAVI, the Vaccine Alliance

GAVI is a multilaterally funded public-private partnership. It was founded in 2000 by the United States, the WHO, the United Nations, the World Bank, and the Bill and Melinda Gates Foundation to expand global access to vaccines and prevent deaths from VPDs. The United States played a central role in the creation of GAVI and continues to be involved in GAVI's governance, strategic planning, and funding. U.S. support of GAVI is intended to accelerate access to vaccines, strengthen vaccine

---

[52] USAID, Acting on the Call: A Focus on the Journey to Self-Reliance for Preventing Child and Maternal deaths, June 2019.

[53] From 2000 to present, the United States has provided approximately 12% of GAVI's total funding. See https://www.gavi.org/investing/funding/donor-contributions-pledges/ for more information.

delivery platforms, and work with country governments to sustain immunization programs.[54]

Which Countries Are Eligible for GAVI Support?[55]

GAVI supports the lowest-income countries. Eligibility for GAVI funds is determined by World Bank data on per capita Gross National Income (GNI). Recipients of GAVI funds must co-finance vaccination campaigns. As GNI grows, governments must finance increasing proportions of vaccine costs. When countries pass GAVI's "eligibility threshold," they phase out of GAVI support and enter a five-year "accelerated transition phase," during which GAVI works with transitioning countries to progressively assume full financial responsibility for their immunization programs. As of 2019, fifteen countries have "graduated" from GAVI support, including Angola, Bhutan, Bolivia, Guyana, Honduras, Indonesia, Kiribati, Mongolia, and Sri Lanka.[56]

U.S. Contributions to GAVI

The United States is GAVI's third largest donor, having provided nearly $2 billion of the $21 billion donated to GAVI since its founding (*Figure 3*).[57]

Congress appropriates U.S. funding for GAVI via USAID's Global Health Programs (GHP) account in annual SFOPS appropriations measures. In turn, the United States holds a seat on GAVI's board, as do the WHO and UNICEF, which also receive U.S. funding (*Figure 4).*

---

[54] GAVI, *Annual Progress Report: 2017*, 2018, https://www.gavi.org/results/gavi-progress-reports/.

[55] GAVI, *Eligibility and transition policy*: June 11, 2015, https://www.gavi.org/about/programme-policies/eligibility- and-transition/.

[56] For a full list of countries that have graduated, see GAVI. *Transitioning out of GAVI support*: 2019, https://www.gavi.org/support/sustainability/transition/.

[57] GAVI, *Investing in GAVI: Cash Receipts 2000-2019*, 2019, https://www.gavi.org/investing/funding/donor- contributions-pledges/cash-receipts/.

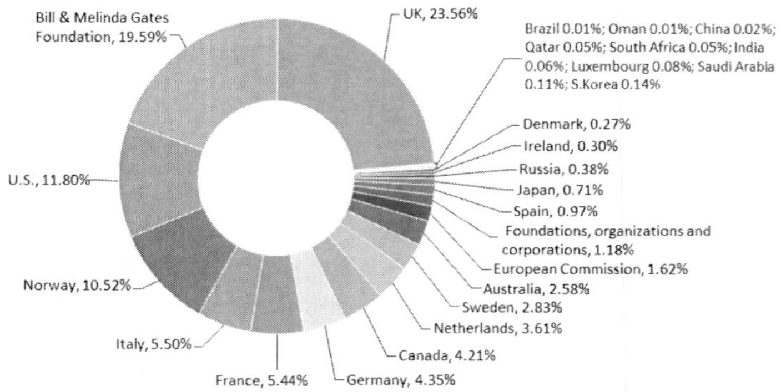

Source: GAVI, Key figures: donor contributions & pledges, Geneva, Switzerland, 2019.

Note: Total amount represents U.S. $21 billion donated to GAVI since 2000.

Figure 3. Donor Contributions to GAVI, 2000-2020.

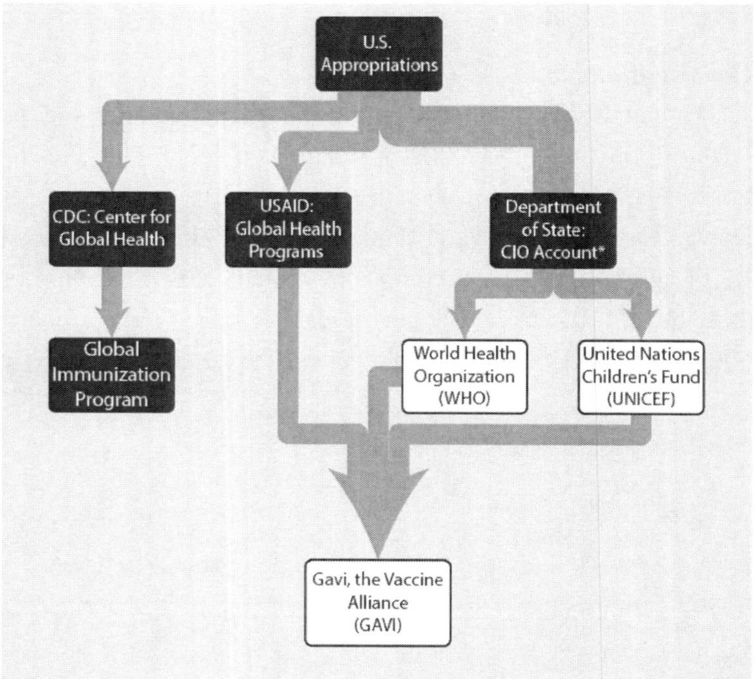

Source: CRS graphic, created by Edward Collins-Chase from information available at https://www.gavi.org/ investing/funding/.

Note: *Department of State Contributions to International Organizations Account.

Figure 4. U.S. Funding for GAVI.

Table 3 details U.S. budget requests and enacted appropriations for GAVI from FY2015 to FY2020.

Table 3. U.S. Funding for GAVI, Global Health Programs Account (FY2015-FY2020) (appropriations, current U.S. $ millions)

Fiscal Year	Administration Request	Enacted
FY2015	200	200
FY2016	235	235
FY2017	275	275
FY2018	290	290
FY2019	250	290
FY2020	250	TBD

Source: GAVI, Investing in GAVI: Cash Receipts 2000-2019, 2019. Department of State and Foreign Operations Congressional Budget Justifications, FY2015-2020, appropriations legislation (P.L. 114-113, 115-31, 115-41, and P.L. 116-6), and CRS correspondence with USAID, July 2019.

Note: TBD = to be determined.

During the Obama Administration, congressional appropriators met the Administration's requests to increase funding for GAVI year on year. In line with the Trump Administration's broad calls for cuts to foreign assistance, the Administration proposed $250 million for GAVI in FY2019 and in FY2020, a $40 million decrease from the FY2018-enacted level. In FY2019, Congress appropriated $290 million for GAVI, the same level as in FY2018.

Outlook and Issues for Congress

Congress has continued to demonstrate interest in supporting child vaccinations for VPDs overseas—for example, by appropriating increasing levels of funding for related programs. However, numerous global outbreaks of VPDs have raised concerns about whether the progress made in preventing and eradicating communicable diseases can be maintained. In light of recent events, and in the context of the FY2020 appropriations process (and beyond), Congress may examine a few additional issues.

One area that could be explored is the effectiveness of global vaccination campaigns as a tool of domestic pandemic preparedness. U.S. government public health officials have argued that the global resurgence of certain vaccine-preventable diseases, particularly measles and mumps, may threaten U.S. public health.[58] Recent outbreaks of vaccine-preventable diseases in the United States have been traced to travelers from Europe and abroad, and the CDC reports that these travelers, coupled with domestic vaccine hesitancy, are the main cause of outbreaks in the United States.[59]

In March 2019, the full Senate Committee on Health, Education, Labor and Pensions (HELP) held a hearing to discuss the reasons behind preventable disease outbreaks, including imported cases of vaccine-preventable diseases linked to international travelers.[60] As these outbreaks continue, Congress may continue to consider its oversight of, and federal government involvement in, issues surrounding vaccines, such as misinformation campaigns and their role in vaccine hesitancy.[61]

Another core area of interest relates to U.S. funding, foreign policy objectives, and foreign aid programs supporting immunization. The U.S. government has long-included vaccination as a core component of foreign policy, and as a foreign aid priority. Recently, the Trump Administration requested cuts to global health funding, including for U.S. agencies involved in global vaccination campaigns.[62] The Administration contends

---

[58] Department of Health and Human Services, "HHS Secretary Azar Statement on National Infant Immunization Week," press release, April 29, 2019. CDC, "CDC Media Statement from Dr. Redfield on National Infant Immunization Week, Safety and Effectiveness of Vaccines," press release, April 29, 2019. Food and Drug Administration, "FDA In Brief: During National Infant Immunization week, FDA reinforces continued confidence in the safety and effectiveness of vaccines, stresses the importance of immunization to prevent diseases," press release, April 29, 2019.

[59] Centers for Disease Control and Prevention, *Measles Cases and Outbreaks*, August 15, 2019.

[60] U.S. Congress, Senate Committee on Health, Education, Labor, and Pensions, *Vaccines Save Lives: What Is Driving Preventable Disease Outbreaks?*, 116th Cong., 2nd sess., March 5, 2019.

[61] James Hohmann, "Growing bipartisan alarm in Congress over measles outbreaks amid falling vaccination rates," *The Washington Post*, March 5, 2019.

[62] See *Table 2* and *Table 3* for detailed figures on Administration requests and congressional appropriations for U.S. foreign assistance for global immunization coverage.

that the funding requests will not affect programs and that "the reduction reflects the Administration's intent to further focus funds on countries, populations, and programs where resources will have the greatest public health impact ... [and] CDC will focus its global immunization activities to continue progress towards polio eradication, as well as measles and rubella elimination in the countries with the highest disease burden."[63] Some experts argue that stagnation in vaccination coverage and the resurgence of some vaccine-preventable diseases are "alarm bells," and have expressed concern about flat support for global vaccine campaigns leading to a continued resurgence of vaccine-preventable diseases.[64] These issues raise questions about burden sharing and the role of other high-income country donors in global immunization funding, as well as factors affecting the efficacy of global campaigns to increase vaccination rates.

---

[63] CDC Congressional Budget Justification p.13, 2018.

[64] Helen Branswell, "Could the world see a resurgence of polio? Experts fear a cautionary tale in measles," *STAT*, August 19, 2019. WHO, *Wild poliovirus type 1—Islamic Republic of Iran*, Disease outbreak news, May 2019. Kimberly Thompson, "Eradication versus control for poliomyelitis: an economic analysis," *The Lancet*, April 2007.

In: Vaccines
Editor: Oliver Huerta
ISBN: 978-1-53619-059-5

Chapter 12

AN OVERVIEW OF STATE AND FEDERAL AUTHORITY TO IMPOSE VACCINATION REQUIREMENTS*

Wen W. Shen

According to the latest available data from the Centers for Disease Control and Protection (CDC), 7 states in the United States are currently in the midst of 10 separate measles outbreaks. With 880 total confirmed cases so far this year, 2019 now has the greatest number of reported cases of measles since 1994 and since measles was declared eliminated in the United States in 2000. These cases, the majority of which involves unvaccinated individuals, follows a number of notable measles outbreaks over the past several years, including an outbreak of 383 cases in 2014 among unvaccinated Amish communities in Ohio and another multi-state outbreak of 147 cases in 2015 linked to an amusement park in California. In addition to measles, for about every 5 years since 2006, outbreaks of other vaccine-preventable diseases, such as mumps, have also been

* This is an edited, reformatted and augmented version of Congressional Research Service Publication No. LSB10300, dated May 22, 2019.

reported in the United States. In light of these outbreaks and their association with unvaccinated individuals, this Sidebar provides an overview of the relevant state and federal authority to require vaccination for U.S. residents.

STATE AND LOCAL AUTHORITY OVER VACCINATION

Under the federalist system of the United States, state governments have the general authority, within constitutional limits, to enact laws "to provide for the public health, safety, and morals" of the states' inhabitants. In contrast to this general police power, as discussed below, Congress's power to legislate is confined to those powers enumerated in the Constitution.

The states' general police power to promote public health and safety encompasses the authority to require mandatory vaccinations. Pursuant to this authority, states and localities have long enacted various compulsory vaccination laws for certain populations and circumstances, including for school children and certain health care workers and in cases of public health emergency. In the early part of the 20th Century, the Supreme Court twice considered constitutional challenges to such mandatory vaccination requirements. Each time, the Court rejected the challenges and recognized such laws to fall squarely within the states' police power. In 1905, the Supreme Court in Jacobson v. Commonwealth of Massachusetts upheld a state law that gave municipal boards of health the authority to require the vaccination of persons over the age of 21 against smallpox, determining that the vaccination program had a "real and substantial relation to the protection of the public health and safety." In doing so, the Court rejected the argument that such a program violated a liberty interest that, under more modern jurisprudence, would likely have been asserted as a substantive due process right. Less than two decades later, in Zucht v. King, parents of a child who was excluded from school due to her unvaccinated status challenged the local ordinance requiring vaccinations for schoolchildren, arguing that the ordinance violated the Equal Protection and Due Process Clauses of the Fourteenth Amendment. Relying on Jacobson, the Supreme Court rejected the constitutional challenges, concluding that "it is within the police power of a State to provide for compulsory vaccination" and that the ordinance did not bestow "arbitrary power, but only that broad discretion required for the protection of the public health."

All 50 states, as well as the District of Columbia, currently have laws requiring specified vaccines for students. This requirement is generally subject to certain exemptions, which vary from state to state. While all student immunization laws grant exemptions to children for medical reasons (e.g., if a child is allergic to vaccines or immunocompromised), most but not all states grant religious exemptions for those whose beliefs counsel against immunization. Sixteen states also provide a broader philosophical exemption for those who object to immunizations because of personal, moral, or other beliefs. While compulsory vaccination requirements have faced legal challenges since Jacobsen and Zucht, courts have consistently rejected these challenges and given considerable deference to the use of the states' police power to require immunizations to protect the public health. A number of relatively recent decisions, for instance, have concluded that a state is not constitutionally required to provide a religious exemption, upholding compulsory vaccination laws that provide only a medical exemption. In states that provide a religious exemption and where parents have filed suit to challenge their unsuccessful invocation of the exemption, courts, applying the relevant state law, have, at times, scrutinized whether their objections to vaccination are based on a sincere religious belief.

FEDERAL AUTHORITY OVER VACCINATION

Although states have traditionally exercised the bulk of authority in this area, Congress, as a result of various enumerated powers in the Constitution, likewise has some authority over public health matters, including regulation of vaccination. This authority derives from, among other sources, the Commerce Clause and the Spending Clause of the U.S. Constitution. The Commerce Clause grants Congress the power "[t]o regulate Commerce with foreign Nations, and among the several States." This authority empowers Congress to regulate "three broad categories of activities": (1) "channels of interstate commerce," like roads and canals; (2) "persons or things in interstate commerce," and (3) activities that substantially affect interstate commerce. The Spending Clause empowers Congress to tax and spend for the general welfare. Under this authority, Congress may offer federal funds to nonfederal entities and prescribe the terms and conditions under which the funds are accepted and used by recipients. This power is generally expansive, but the funding conditions on grants to the states are subject to certain limitations, including that they must be germane to the federal interest in the particular national projects or programs to which the money is directed.

Congress's exercise of these authorities is also subject to certain external constraints. In the context of public health regulations, the key constraints are those grounded in federalism and the protection of individual rights. Pursuant to the principles of federalism, the Supreme Court has interpreted the Tenth Amendment to prevent the federal government from commandeering or requiring state officers to carry out federal directives. In the context of vaccination, this principle prevents Congress from requiring states or localities to pass mandatory vaccination laws, but it does not impede Congress from using its Spending Clause authority to provide incentives (in the form of federal grants) to states to enact laws concerning vaccination. In terms of protection of individual rights, there are few external constraints on Congress's ability to impose mandatory vaccination requirements. Potential due process and equal protection concerns, as noted above, are limited under Jacobsen and Zucht. Moreover, while the First Amendment's Free Exercise Clause seemingly could provide a limit on the federal government's ability to require vaccinations for those who would otherwise refuse on religious grounds, this constitutional concern is mitigated under Employment Division, Department of Human Resources of Oregon v. Smith. In Smith, the Court held that neutral, generally applicable laws (i.e., ones that do not target specific religious groups)— which would include a law mandating vaccination—generally do not violate the Constitution.

Nonetheless, federal statutes can also restrict federal authority with regard to public health regulations. Under the Religious Freedom Restoration Act of 1993 (RFRA), for instance, the federal government is prohibited from substantially burdening a person's sincere exercise of religion, unless the government "demonstrates the application of the burden to the person" represents "the least restrictive means" of advancing a compelling government interest. Thus, to the extent a federal law prescribes certain public health requirements that may impose substantial burdens on a regulated person's exercise of religion, RFRA may require certain religious exemptions to the federal law for the regulated entities. RFRA does not, however, apply to the actions of state governments, as the Court held the law to be unconstitutional as applied to the states because the law exceeded Congress's enforcement authority under the Fourteenth Amendment. As a result, unless a state has chosen to enact a state version of RFRA (as 21 states have), states generally have broad authority under their police power to impose mandatory vaccination requirements without providing a religious exemption.

CONSIDERATIONS FOR CONGRESS

Currently, the federal government has generally limited its role with respect to vaccination to promoting, facilitating, or monitoring the use and/or manufacture of vaccines, such as requiring insurance coverage for recommended vaccinations, providing clinical guidance on vaccinations, and ensuring vaccine safety. Except for certain populations, including immigrants seeking permanent residence in the United States and military personnel, the federal government has not sought to invoke its authority to impose federal vaccination requirements on the populace.

Nonetheless, Congress has "granted broad, flexible powers to federal health authorities who must use their judgment in attempting to protect the public against the spread of communicable disease" under the Public Health Service Act (PHSA). This authority to make and enforce regulations necessary "to prevent the introduction, transmission, or spread of communicable diseases from foreign countries into the States or possessions, or from one State or possession into any other State or possession" could conceivably be used to mandate vaccinations, provided that the authority is not exercised in a way that otherwise violates the Constitution or fails to comply with other statutory requirements, such as the Administrative Procedure Act. Current regulations issued pursuant to this authority, however, are limited to measures that include quarantine and isolation measures to halt the spread of certain communicable diseases.

In addition, Congress's Spending Clause authority empowers it to prescribe certain vaccination requirements that must be implemented by states or localities as a condition of receiving certain federal funds. Currently, Section 317 of the PHSA, among other functions, provides federal immunization grants to numerous states, cities, and territories to implement measures that would improve vaccination rates, including by reducing the out-of-pocket costs for families for vaccines, providing targeted education services, and providing targeted vaccination reminders for patients. The conditions of a Section 317 grant at present do not include vaccination requirements. A bill introduced in the 116th Congress, the Vaccinate All Children Act of 2019, would, however, impose an additional condition requiring a grant applicant to demonstrate that it requires every student enrolled in the state's public elementary and secondary schools to have received the recommended vaccinations. This requirement, which appears germane to one of the federal interests of Section 317 (i.e., to improve vaccination rates), would thus expand the federal government's role in mandating vaccinations through Congress's Spending Clause authority.

In: Vaccines
Editor: Oliver Huerta
ISBN: 978-1-53619-059-5

Chapter 13

MITIGATING THE IMPACT OF PANDEMIC INFLUENZA THROUGH VACCINE INNOVATION*

The Council of Economic Advisers

EXECUTIVE SUMMARY

This chapter estimates the potentially large health and economic losses in the United States associated with influenza pandemics and discusses why the most commonly used vaccine production technologies are unlikely to mitigate these losses. We estimate the value of new vaccine technologies that would make vaccines available more quickly and likely improve their effectiveness in moderating the risks of pandemics. We discuss why private market incentives may be insufficient to develop new vaccine technologies or promote the uptake of existing, faster but more expensive technologies, despite their large expected value to society. And we argue that increased utilization of, and investment in, these new technologies—along with public-private partnerships, to spur

* This is an edited, reformatted and augmented version of The Council of Economic Advisers, dated September 2019.

innovation—may be valuable to decrease the impact of both pandemic and seasonal influenza.

Every year, millions of Americans suffer from seasonal influenza, commonly known as "the flu," which is caused by influenza viruses.1 A new vaccine is formulated annually to decrease infections resulting from the small genetic changes that continually occur in the most prevalent viruses and make them less recognizable to the human immune system. There is, however, a 4 percent annual probability of pandemic influenza resulting from large and unpredictable genetic changes leading to an easily transmissible influenza virus for which much of the population would lack the residual immunity that results from prior virus exposures and vaccinations. The Council of Economic Advisors (CEA) finds that in a pandemic year, depending on the transmission efficiency and virulence of the particular pandemic virus, the economic damage would range from $413 billion to $3.79 trillion. Fatalities in the most serious scenario would exceed half a million people in the United States. Millions more would be sick, with between approximately 670,000 to 4.3 million requiring hospitalization. In a severe pandemic, healthy people might avoid work and normal social interactions in an attempt to avert illness by limiting contact with sick persons. By incapacitating a large fraction of the population, including individuals who work in critical infrastructure and defense sectors, pandemic influenza could threaten U.S. national security.

Large-scale, immediate immunization is the most effective way to control the spread of influenza, but the predominant, currently licensed, vaccine manufacturing technology would not provide sufficient doses rapidly enough to mitigate a pandemic. Current influenza vaccine production focuses on providing vaccines for the seasonal flu and primarily relies on growing viruses in chicken eggs. Egg-based production can take six months or more to deliver substantial amounts of vaccines after a pathogenic, influenza virus is identified—too slowly to stave off the rapid spread of infections if an unexpected and highly contagious pandemic virus emerges.

Egg-based production can also diminish vaccines' efficacy in protecting against influenza infection in both seasonal and pandemic years. Influenza viruses must be adapted to grow in chicken eggs, which can lead to modifications in their surface proteins (antigens) so that the vaccine prepared from them may not match the circulating influenza viruses well. In addition, the length of time needed for egg-based production may impair vaccine efficacy in two ways: the virus selected for vaccine manufacture may no longer be the predominant circulating virus six months later; or, even if the selected virus remains the predominant circulating virus, it may mutate between the time it is identified and the time the vaccine is available six months later, making

[1] In this chapter, we use the terms "influenza" and "flu" interchangeably.

the vaccine less effective. During the severe 2017–18 influenza season, the overall effectiveness of the vaccine against the circulating viruses was 38 percent. The vaccine created for the last pandemic, which occurred in 2009–10, was 62 percent effective in protecting people under age 65 years and 43 percent effective for those age 65 and older—the age group at highest risk of medical complications and death from influenza. And in 2014–15, when there was a mismatch between the virus used for the vaccine and the predominant circulating virus, the vaccine was only 19 percent effective.[2]

Improving the speed of vaccine production and vaccine efficacy are both important goals to mitigate pandemic risks and may also decrease the costs of seasonal influenza. Our analysis shows that innovation to increase the speed of vaccine production is key. Improving vaccine efficacy alone will be of little value in a pandemic if, as is the case with current egg-based production, the vaccine only becomes available after a large number of infections have occurred. Improving efficacy only yields value after greater speed has been achieved.

The CEA finds that technologies that could deliver sufficient doses of vaccine at the outset of an influenza pandemic could produce about a $730 billion benefit for Americans over the course of an average pandemic, primarily due to the prevention of loss of life and health. Combining this increase in production speed with a 30 percent increase over the vaccine effectiveness seen in the last pandemic (2009–10) would generate a larger benefit of about $953 billion— about one half the cost of an average pandemic. The benefits dissipate quickly, however, with each week of delay in the vaccine's availability, as the number of unexposed people to protect diminishes. The cost of a 1-week delay at the baseline vaccine effectiveness from the last pandemic is $41 billion per week, on average, for the first 12 weeks; falls to $20 billion per week for the next 12 weeks; and disappears entirely if the vaccine's availability is delayed by more than 39 weeks, because the outbreak would be over before the vaccine prevented new infections. Adding a 30 percent improvement to the vaccine effectiveness seen in the last pandemic makes the per-week cost of delay $53 billion over the first 12 weeks, on average, falling to $26 billion over the next 12 weeks.

The expected value of having a vaccine available at the outset of a pandemic—that is, the savings discounted by the 4 percent annual probability of having a pandemic—is $29 billion, or $89.63 per American. Adding a 30 percent increase to the baseline pandemic vaccine's effectiveness to the faster production increases the expected value to $38 billion, or $117.07 per American. The expected per capita

[2] We use "efficacy" as a general term to describe how well a vaccine prevents infection and "effectiveness" to describe how well the vaccine performed in historical studies of previous influenza epidemics.

value from increasing the production speed for pandemic vaccines is over four times the current per-dose cost for egg-based vaccines.

Newer technologies, like cell-based or recombinant vaccines, have the potential to cut production times and improve efficacy compared with egg-based vaccines and are currently priced below the expected per capita value of improved production speeds for pandemic vaccines. But these existing technologies have not yet been adopted on a large scale. Besides improving pandemic preparedness, new vaccine technologies may have an additional benefit of potentially improving vaccine efficacy for seasonal influenza. We estimate the economic benefits that these new technologies could generate for each seasonal influenza vaccine recipient, and find that the benefits are particularly compelling for older adults (65+) who are at high risk of influenza complications and death.

We discuss why the private market has not embraced these newer vaccine production technologies and the lack of private incentives to develop and utilize improved vaccine production technologies that could better mitigate pandemic risk. First, there is a key misalignment between the social and private returns from medical research and development (R&D) and capital investment in pandemic vaccines. R&D and investment costs are only recouped by sales when the pandemic risk occurs. Part of the value of vaccines that can mitigate future pandemic risks, however, is their insurance value today that provides protection against possible damage. This insurance value accrues even if the pandemic does not occur in the future, and it implies that the social value of faster production and better vaccines is much larger than its private return to developers. This divergence leads to an underprovision in vaccine innovation because it does not get rewarded for its insurance value. Second, pandemics represent a risk with a small probability of occurring but with large and highly correlated losses across the population. The rarity of influenza pandemics and the fact that the last serious one in this country occurred a hundred years ago may lead consumers and insurers to underestimate the probability and potential impact of a future influenza pandemic. Moreover, the risk cannot be effectively pooled because everyone is at risk concurrently.

Although vaccine innovation is not currently rewarded for its insurance value, public-private partnerships created under a 2006 statute have been key in the development of the newer vaccine production technologies that offer the prospect of improved seasonal influenza vaccines and the accelerated timelines needed for improved pandemic preparedness. Push incentives like public-private partnerships combined with pull incentives—such as the government's preferential purchase of vaccines produced domestically with newer, faster technologies—that may create more efficacious seasonal vaccines, especially for older people, can promote additional cost-effective innovation and lessen the impact of future pandemics.

INTRODUCTION

One hundred years ago (1918–19), an influenza pandemic sickened 500 million people worldwide (about a third of the world's population), killing an estimated 50 million, including 675,000 Americans (Taubenberger and Morens 2006). In that year, the average U.S. life expectancy fell by 12 years (CDC 2018h). Although our ability to combat influenza viruses has greatly improved since then—thanks to the availability of flu vaccines, better public health measures, and antiviral and antibiotic medications—current technology would still be inadequate to combat another severe influenza pandemic.

Influenza is a familiar disease in the United States, with an annual epidemic known as the seasonal flu usually peaking between December and February. Small mutations in seasonal influenza viruses from year to year change the viruses' surface proteins (antigens) that the human immune system recognizes. As a result of these changes, along with natural decreases in peoples' antibody levels over time, the residual population immunity due to prior infection or vaccination is incomplete. Seasonal influenza remains a serious public health problem, causing widespread illness and even death, and exacting substantial economic losses. To lessen the impact, large-scale immunization campaigns are undertaken yearly in the U.S. At the end of February of each year, government health authorities analyze global data sets and identify the influenza viruses that are expected to prevail the following flu season. Private vaccine manufacturers start production with the goal of delivering vaccines against the three or four most likely circulating viruses to healthcare practitioners by early fall.

In contrast, pandemic influenza is more sporadic. Over the past 100 years, there have been only four pandemics, with the most recent instance in 2009, suggesting a 4 percent chance of one occurring in any given year (Uyeki, Fowler, and Fischer 2018). Pandemic viruses have had larger antigenic changes than seasonal influenza viruses. As a result, the population largely lacks residual immunity. Easily transmissible viruses will spread rapidly from person to person, infecting a large fraction of the population in a short period with what can be a more severe form of influenza. Tens of millions of people could become ill, with many requiring hospitalization; and a significant number—especially among the vulnerable elderly population—could die. Aside from the high costs associated with the high rates of illness, missed work, hospitalizations, and deaths, a severe pandemic influenza could disrupt the government's vital defense and security functions by incapacitating large numbers of people with nonfatal and fatal illness and changing the daily behaviors of healthy people who seek to avoid exposure to infection. Because the infection will spread rapidly during the early weeks of a pandemic, when there is a large pool of unexposed people, it is imperative to find ways to mitigate the impact of a pandemic influenza through an early and effective immunization campaign.

Unfortunately, the United States is unprepared to deliver a sufficient number of vaccine doses quickly enough to stop the rapid initial spread of a pandemic virus. Current vaccine production primarily utilizes viral replication in chicken eggs, which can take six months or more to produce substantial doses of vaccine. Egg-based production may also diminish vaccine efficacy in preventing the spread of infection and illness in both pandemic and seasonal influenza. Viruses must be adapted to grow in chicken eggs, so the vaccine prepared from them may not match the original viruses selected for vaccine production. In addition, the lengthy production process can decrease efficacy because of a possible vaccine virus mismatch—the candidate viruses selected for seasonal vaccine manufacture in February may no longer be the predominant circulating viruses in the fall season. Moreover, even if the candidate virus is correctly identified, a circulating virus can change between the time it is first identified and the time the vaccine becomes available six months later.

This chapter estimates the large potential losses to the United States associated with this slow production of vaccines in case of an influenza pandemic. We estimate the value of faster vaccine production technologies and improved vaccine efficacy to mitigate pandemic risks and argue that public-private partnerships along with preferential government purchases of vaccines prepared with newer, faster production technologies may be valuable to overcome the misalignment between private and social returns in the development of adequate risk mitigation for pandemics.

To estimate the value of faster production capability, we used infection propagation scenarios, historical estimates of vaccine effectiveness, and the existing capacity for administering vaccines based on published papers and inputs from the Centers for Disease Control and Prevention (CDC), the Food and Drug Administration (FDA), and the Office of the Biomedical Advanced Research and Development Authority (BARDA). Our main finding is that improving vaccine production speed is the key to mitigating the effects of a pandemic, because under most pandemic scenarios, the predominant egg-based production only delivers vaccines after the peak in influenza infections. Improving the efficacy of vaccines interacts with speed by adding more value the more quickly the vaccines can be produced.

Technologies that could deliver sufficient doses of vaccine at the outset of a pandemic when there are only a small number of infected people could produce about $730 billion in benefits at the level of vaccine effectiveness seen in the last (2009) pandemic in an average pandemic year. Combining this increase in production speed with a 30 percent improvement in the vaccine effectiveness seen in the last pandemic would increase the benefits to about $953 billion. But these savings decline each week that vaccine availability is delayed beyond the onset of the pandemic. The average savings forgone per week of delay during the first 12 weeks with no improvement in efficacy is $41 billion, declining to $20 billion per week during the following 12 weeks. Adding a 30 percent improvement in the effectiveness seen in the last pandemic brings the average savings forgone per week of delay during the first 12 weeks is $53 billion, declining to $26 billion during the following 12 weeks. Savings disappear after week 39, as the pandemic would run its course without vaccine intervention.

The large losses associated with delays in vaccine availability during an influenza pandemic suggest that developing and utilizing faster vaccine production technologies would have great value. Factoring in the 4 percent annual probability of a pandemic occurring in a given year generates an expected savings of $29 billion from faster production that makes vaccines available at the outset of a pandemic and $38 billion from faster production, plus a 30 percent improvement over baseline effectiveness. On a per capita basis, this translates into $89.63 and $117.07 in value, respectively. The current price per dose to adults for standard egg-based vaccines ranges from $17.84 to $19.77, and the price of vaccines made with newer, existing technologies that could increase production speed ranges from $22.79 to $53.37. Hence, utilizing existing, faster vaccine production technologies and developing additional faster production technologies, even if they were a bit more expensive than current vaccines, would make economic sense.

Nevertheless, the development of, and demand for, faster vaccine production technologies have lagged. Newer, existing technologies, like cell-cultured or recombinant vaccines, have the potential to cut production times compared with egg-based vaccines, but they currently only account for 10 to 15 percent and 1 to 2 percent of the market, respectively. In addition to improving pandemic preparedness, new vaccine technologies may have an additional benefit of improving vaccine effectiveness for seasonal flu.

In the face of this slow development, we discuss the lack of appropriate market incentives for developing faster vaccine production technologies to decrease pandemic risk. Part of the value of vaccines that can mitigate future pandemic risks is through their insurance value today. Just as life insurance benefits the vast majority of buyers who survive their policy, being insured against pandemic risk through the development of faster vaccine production and more effective vaccines would still be beneficial in the years when pandemics did not emerge. This insurance value implies that the social return from faster and more effective vaccines is larger than their private return to developers. Because private vaccine innovation currently does not get rewarded for this insurance value, we argue that public-private R&D partnerships and increased government purchase of vaccines produced with faster technologies that may also be more efficacious, will enhance welfare. This combination of what many term push and pull incentives can promote cost-effective innovation and the availability of better vaccines for both seasonal and pandemic influenza.[3]

The rest of the report is organized as follows. The first section describes in more detail the differences between seasonal and pandemic influenza and estimates the losses associated with each, given current vaccine technology. The second section describes the barriers to improving influenza vaccine effectiveness created by the currently prevalent, egg-based vaccine production, and in particular describes why its lengthy production process makes it inadequate for combating pandemic influenza. The next section describes how outcomes can be improved through innovation that speeds up vaccine production and improves vaccine effectiveness over previous years, and by increases in the percentage of people vaccinated. We calculate the potential cost savings in a given pandemic year and the expected savings over time for improved production technologies. The fourth section describes new vaccine technologies that may address the problem of pandemic influenza by shortening production times and produce more effective vaccines than egg-based production for both pandemic and seasonal influenza. We provide our estimates of the value of switching vaccine production to the newer technologies in seasonal influenza years in the subsequent section. The following section discusses the difference in private versus social returns to explain why private markets may fail to provide the innovation needed to improve pandemic influenza preparedness. The final section describes how public-private partnerships have led to the development of the newer, faster vaccine and production techniques and how these partnerships and other government actions can be helpful in promoting innovation and the widespread adoption of new vaccine production technologies.

[3] "'Push incentives' that lower the cost of drug research and development are widely used by governments to support new antibacterial discovery. 'Pull incentives,' which provide a known return on investment and reward successful development, are increasingly viewed as viable mechanisms to engage industry to develop new antibacterial drugs" (CDC 2017b). Also: "Incentives used to engage the participation of commercial parties are generally thought of as either 'push' or 'pull' incentives, with push funding inputs, and pull funding or rewarding outputs" (Institute of Medicine 2010).

ESTIMATING THE COSTS OF SEASONAL AND PANDEMIC INFLUENZA WITH CURRENT VACCINE TECHNOLOGIES

This section describes the differences between seasonal and pandemic influenza. It then estimates the annual cost of each given the current, predominant vaccine production technology.

The Nature of Seasonal and Pandemic Influenza

Influenza, or "the flu," is caused by an infection with a virus that is endemic—that is, one permanently present in some form (but with some variation) in humans and animals. The annual "seasonal flu" typically circulates in the United States from October to May, peaking between December and February (CDC 2018d). Only some of the people who come in contact with the viruses that are circulating that season will contract influenza, and most of those who do will fully recover. However, influenza can cause serious illness, leading to hospitalization and even death, especially among vulnerable populations like senior citizens, young children, pregnant women, and people with certain chronic medical conditions (Grohskopf et al. 2018).

An influenza pandemic is the worldwide spread of a new influenza virus that is different than recent, commonly circulating seasonal influenza viruses. Rates of illness, serious complications, and mortality are higher than for the usual seasonal influenza. In the last 100 years, there have been four major influenza pandemics leading to substantial deaths worldwide: the 1918 pandemic, popularly (but misleadingly) known as the "Spanish Flu," with more than 50 million dead; the 1957 "Asian Influenza," with more than 1 million dead; the 1968 "Hong Kong Influenza," with 1 million dead; and the 2009 "Swine Flu," with 151,700 to 575,400 dead (CDC 2018i).

The difference between the seasonal influenza that we experience every year and a pandemic influenza that we experience infrequently results from the degree of change in the genetic composition of the influenza virus. Every year, mutations in the influenza virus's genetic material, or ribonucleic acid (RNA), change the protein (antigens) on the surface of the virus, which enables the virus to partly evade the immunologic protections people have developed from previous flu vaccinations or virus exposures. Usually, these changes are small, and are described as "antigenic drift." Antigenic drift usually causes enough change in seasonal influenza viruses so that seasonal flu vaccines are updated annually. Large, abrupt changes in the influenza virus's genetic makeup that cause larger changes in the virus's surface proteins are called "antigenic shift." Antigenic shift produces a virus to which most people have limited immune memory, and therefore have little or no immune protection from infection. As a result, the virus has the potential to infect people easily and spread from person to person in an efficient and sustained way. Though only certain groups (e.g., infants, the elderly, and people with underlying medical conditions) are at high risk of serious disease during seasons when the virus has undergone antigenic drift, antigenically shifted viruses put all ages and previously healthy people at risk of serious complications (CDC 2018f). When a virus has undergone an antigenic shift, spreads easily from person to person, and causes serious illness in a broad range of persons, it produces a pandemic (CDC 2017a; NIH 2017).

There are four types of influenza viruses: A, B, C, and D. Only influenza A and B are common causes of disease in humans, and only type A viruses have the potential to cause a pandemic because type B viruses do not undergo antigenic shift (CDC 2017a). Influenza A viruses are divided into subtypes based on the proteins (hemagglutinin, H; and neuraminidase, N) on the surface of the virus. There are 18 known H subtypes and 11 known N subtypes. Each subtype is further divided into clades. Aquatic birds and other animals are hosts to influenza A viruses that do not normally infect people. Random mutations lead to antigenic drift in the viruses' H and N proteins. However, larger genetic changes lead to antigenic shift, for example, when nonhuman viruses exchange genes with one another and with human viruses to gain the ability to infect humans.

The Annual Cost of Seasonal Influenza

In this subsection, we derive the cost estimates from published papers that were based on surveys and medical spending data. These estimates of the cost of medical care, lost productivity, and fatalities for the seasonal flu will allow us to make cost estimates for pandemic flu later in this chapter and to quantify to what extent market incentives could help move vaccine production toward improved production technologies. For the purposes of this estimation, whenever applicable, we adjust the cost estimates from previously published papers for inflation to express them in 2018 dollars. Finally, whenever the age brackets presented in a paper do not fully correspond to the age brackets used in this chapter, we use data for the adjacent/overlapping age brackets and use population-based weights to adjust the numbers for the age brackets presented in this chapter. The distribution of the U.S. population by age is from the Census Bureau's estimates for 2016.

Our main cost estimates come from Molinari and others (2007), who estimated the cost of seasonal influenza to the United States economy and obtained their risk and cost estimates from the meta analysis of papers published in academic journals and other public sources. Their paper estimated the costs for the following age groups: 0–4, 5–17, 18–49, 50–64, and 65 and older. We also use these age groups in this part of our analysis.

The probability of getting the flu in a given year is called the clinical "attack rate," which is a measure of contagiousness and population immunity.[4] Because young children experience more physical contact with other people and have less acquired immunity from past influenza, they face the highest risk of flu infection and illness. The elderly may also have a mild increase in infection risk due to the erosion of their immune response.

A person who becomes ill with the flu can have several possible outcomes. The person may or may not decide to seek medical help, such as

[4] "Attack rate" is also sometimes used to designate the probability of being infected by the influenza virus, and would include those who become sick and show symptoms (clinical attack rate) plus those who remain asymptomatic.

an outpatient visit. A subset of ill people require hospitalization, and some of these people die. As shown in Table 1, these adverse scenarios are unevenly distributed across age groups, with the youngest and the oldest age groups generally being at highest risk. Additionally, each age group has a proportion of "high-risk" individuals who have other medical conditions that make the flu illness more serious and more likely to result in complications, resulting in higher medical costs. The percentage of people at high-risk generally rises with age.

Table 1. Seasonal influenza: Associated risks

	Age group					
Measure	0–4	5–17	18–49	50–64	65+	Population-weighted average
Proportion of U.S. population (%)	6.2	16.6	42.4	19.6	15.2	100.0
Attack rate (%)	20.3	10.2	6.6	6.6	9.0	8.4
Proportion (high-risk) (%)	5.2	10.6	14.9	33.0	51.2	22.7
Probability (outpatient visit)						
Low-risk individuals (%)	45.5	31.8	31.3	31.3	62.0	36.9
High-risk individuals (%)	91.0	63.5	62.5	62.5	82.0	67.4
Probability of hospitalizations (%)	1.4	0.1	0.4	1.9	4.2	1.3
Probability of death (%)	0.004	0.001	0.01	0.1	1.2	0.2

Sources: Molinari et al. (2007); CEA calculations.

When estimating the costs incurred due to illness, we again use data from Molinari and others (2007) and inflate the costs to 2018 dollars. For the value of lost productivity, we multiply the number of workdays missed by the value of a productive day ($151.88 per day).[5] Medical costs include the cost of medicine and the cost of a doctor's visit or hospital stay. They are summed for each person, and cases are grouped by the highest level of care used (e.g., each hospital case includes inpatient, outpatient, and pharmaceutical costs for that person). Table 2 presents cost estimates associated with various flu illness outcomes across all age groups. It

[5] This is an update to 2018 of the value used by Molinari et al. (2007). Lost productivity attributed to children and the elderly captured lost days of work of their caretakers, who are typically parents and family members.

presents the fact that both people who recover from the flu (the first three categories) and people who go on to die (the fourth category) incur medical costs and productivity costs from missing work while ill.

In addition, we must account for the value of the lives lost. For influenza fatalities, we assign a monetary value based on calculations of the value of a statistical life (VSL) for different age groups derived by Aldy and Viscusi (2008).[6] Using the probabilities given in Table 1 and the direct costs of various outcomes given in Table 2, and adding in the cost of fatalities using age- based VSL valuations, we calculate the cost of seasonal influenza. Given the 2017 U.S. population of 325.7 million, the probability distributions presented in Table 1 suggest that a typical seasonal flu would cause illness in 27 million; of these, 368,000 will need to be hospitalized but will survive and 59,000 will die. The vast majority of the fatalities, about 89 percent, will be among the population over 65 years of age. We estimate the total cost of seasonal influenza to be $361 billion per year, in 2018 dollars, due largely to the value of lives lost.[7] Of this total cost, $30 billion is incurred as the immediate cash cost, which equals the sum of medical expenditures and lost productivity due to work missed while sick.[8]

---

[6] The CEA (2017) applied a similar approach to valuing fatalities adjusted for age brackets in evaluating the opioid epidemic. The VSL summarizes willingness to pay for small changes in the risks of premature death (OMB 2003). This measure is widely used by government agencies to evaluate policies. We use the VSL to place a monetary value on the extra risks of death due to the influenza virus. Throughout this chapter we refer to the monetary value of the fatality risks as a component of the "costs" of influenza and to the monetary value of reductions in fatality risks as "cost savings" or "benefits."

[7] Molinari et al. (2007) estimated this cost to be significantly lower, largely because they used lower VSL assumptions and their estimate was 2003 dollars.

[8] There is also the possibility of lost productivity during epidemics resulting from healthy people avoiding work out of fear they will be infected by coworkers. Molinari did not include this cost. This sort of absenteeism may be especially common among healthcare providers (Qureshi et al. 2005) and would be most pronounced in a severe pandemic. Because reliable estimates of how big this effect is during seasonal and pandemic influenza epidemics are not available, we do not add this effect to the estimates we derived from Molinari.

Table 2. Costs associated with various flu illness outcomes, 2018 Dollars

	Age group					Population- weighted average
Outcome	0–4	5–17	18–49	50–64	65+	
Case not medically attended						
Medical cost (all risk)*	5.08	5.08	5.08	5.08	5.08	5.08
Lost productivity (all risk)	151.88	75.94	75.94	75.94	151.88	92.20
Outpatient visit						
Low-risk medical costs	282.62	160.77	211.54	253.85	409.54	245.95
Low-risk lost productivity	151.88	151.88	151.88	303.77	455.65	227.93
High-risk medical costs	971.39	1,098.31	1,226.92	1,240.46	805.54	1,128.22
High-risk lost productivity	911.31	607.54	303.77	607.54	1,063.19	566.98
Hospitalization						
Low-risk medical costs	18,412.33	25,408.34	32,174.19	37,745.28	19,378.64	29,342.16
Low-risk lost productivity	1,215.07	1,366.96	1,822.61	1,974.50	1,974.50	1,762.30
High-risk medical costs	138,085.70	70,938.24	80,760.40	69,907.62	28,346.19	72,548.85
High-risk lost productivity	4,708.41	3,493.34	3,189.57	3,645.22	2,733.92	3,353.56
Fatalities						
Low-risk medical costs	48,768.98	48,768.98	129,184.15	200,665.62	70,989.01	115,991.85
Low-risk lost productivity**	1,215.07	1,366.96	1,822.61	1,974.50	1,974.50	1,762.30
High-risk medical costs	453,461.15	453,461.15	128,429.38	201,117.47	55,864.84	205,686.86
High-risk lost productivity**	4,708.41	3,493.34	3,189.57	3,645.22	2,733.92	3,353.56
VSL (millions)***	5.76	5.76	12.34	7.75	5.29	8.87

Sources: Molinari et al. (2007); Aldy and Viscusi (2008); CEA calculations.

Note: Cost estimates shown are per person per influenza incident, assuming the individual is symptomatic.

*Costs for those who did not seek medical attention assumes average over-the-counter medication costs per case.

**Molinari did not calculate the lost productivity (work days missed) while ill of the eventual fatalities. We used the lost productivity costs incurred by the hospitalization group as a lower-bound value. ***Value of Statistical Life (VSL).

Cost Estimates of Pandemic Influenza

If pandemic influenza were to hit the United States, the assumptions from Table 1 would need to be revised because pandemic influenza would result in a higher attack rate and a greater risk of adverse outcomes compared with seasonal influenza. Relying on Biggerstaff and others (2015) and Meltzer and others (2015), who estimated hypothetical pandemic influenza scenarios informed by past pandemic flu outcomes, we consider four pandemic flu scenarios: those having a high or low attack rate (which we refer to as high/low contagiousness scenarios) and those having a high or low risk of medical complications, including death (high/low severity rate).

For the high and low contagiousness scenarios, we assume population-weighted average attack rates of 30 percent and 20 percent (Biggerstaff et al. 2015). Rates vary by age group (Meltzer et al. 2015). Though overall attack rates are increased compared with seasonal influenza, the attack rate for pandemic flu is lower among older people relative to other age groups because the elderly may have already experienced a similar flu strain in the past and have residual immunity. In the high-contagiousness scenario, the rates range from a high of 39 percent in the 11–20 age group down to a low of 20 percent among people over 60. In the low- contagiousness scenario, rates range from a high of 29 percent in age 11–20 group down to a low of 12 percent for people over 60. In the high-contagiousness scenario, each infected person infects another 1.65 previously unexposed people, and in the low-contagiousness scenario, each infected person infects another 1.3 previously unexposed people, on average.

Figure 1 plots the so-called pandemic curve, which is the evolution of new infections over weeks that follow, for both scenarios. Following Biggerstaff and others (2015), we assume that in week 0, at the start of the flu pandemic in the United States, the first 100 people are infected.

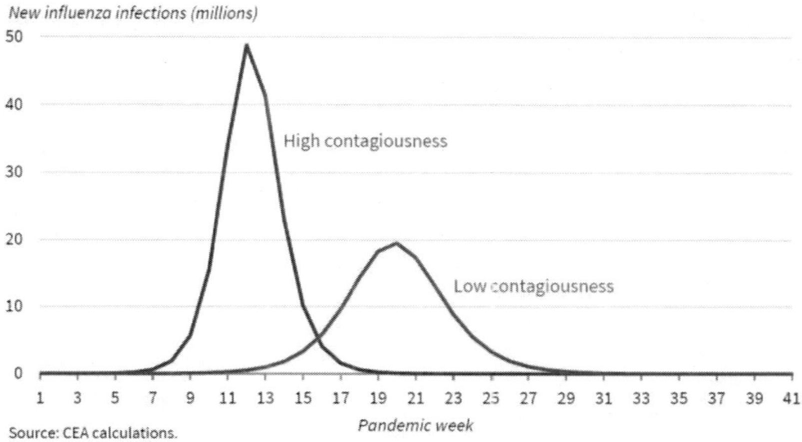

Figure 1. New Infections per Pandemic Week without Vaccination.

In the figure, both plots have a bell shape. At the outset, infected people come into contact with a large number of previously unexposed people who lack immunity to the virus, some of whom become infected. As the pandemic progresses, a higher fraction of the population would have been exposed and developed immunity, and there are fewer new people to become infected. For this reason, the number of new infections initially increases, peaks, and then declines with time.

In the high-contagiousness scenario, the number of newly infected people peaks in week 12 and then gradually declines to zero by week 27. The total number of infected people equals 187,959,100 in the United States. In the low-contagiousness scenario, the number of new infections peaks later, in week 20, and gradually declines to zero by week 42. The total number of infected people is also lower than for the high-contagiousness scenario and equals 127,346,700.

Following Biggerstaff and others (2015), we break the higher risks of adverse outcomes (hospitalizations and fatalities) in pandemic influenza into low- and high-severity scenarios. Biggerstaff and colleagues calculated the risk of hospitalization and death by age group based on historic pandemics.[9]

Table 3. Probability of hospitalizations and fatalities conditional on pandemic influenza infection

Severity		**Age group**			**Population-weighted**
		0–19	20–59	60+	average
Low	Probability of hospitalization (%)	0.08	0.23	3.48	0.88
	Probability of death (%)	0.01	0.02	0.28	0.07
High	Probability of hospitalization (%)	0.30	0.90	14.00	3.53
	Probability of death (%)	0.04	0.11	1.75	0.44

Sources: Biggerstaff et al. (2015); CEA calculations.

Note: Biggerstaff's probabilities of adverse events conditional on becoming symptomatic are halved since the infected population is approximately twice the symptomatic population.

Table 4. Cost outcomes for the four pandemic flu scenarios

Scenario	**Low contagiousness**	**High contagiousness**
Low severity		
Number of hospitalizations	669,889	1,071,650
Number of fatalities	53,674	85,868
Total costs (billions of dollars)	412.61	649.68
Total immediate cash cost (billions of dollars)	54.76	85.14
High severity		
Number of hospitalizations	2,690,569	4,304,752
Number of fatalities	336,321	538,094
Total costs (billions of dollars)	2,399.61	3,786.14
Total immediate cash cost (billions of dollars)	158.58	250.33
Average total costs (billions of dollars)	1,812.01	
Average immediate cash cost (billions of dollars)	137.20	
Average total costs per capita (dollars)	5,563.43	
Average immediate cash cost per capita (dollars)	421.26	

Sources: Molinari et al. (2007); CEA calculations.

[9] Biggerstaff et al. (2012) estimate the probability that a person with a flu-like illness would seek medical care using data from a large-scale telephone survey conducted by the Centers for Disease Control and Prevention (CDC) during the 2009 pandemic influenza season.

These age groups were different than the groups utilized by Molinari and others (2015) for the seasonal flu. In addition, Biggerstaff and colleagues assumed that half of all infections would be asymptomatic and therefore, only applied the risk of adverse outcomes to the half of infected people who were sick (symptomatic) with the flu. The probabilities for low- and high-severity scenarios are presented in Table 3.

Utilizing age-weighted averages of the costs of adverse events derived from Molinari and others (2007) (Table 2, supra), we estimate the total costs (fatality costs utilizing VSL, plus immediate cash costs) for the four pandemic scenarios that we have described and an average of the four. These costs, as well as the number of illnesses and fatalities, for each of the four scenarios are presented in Table 4.

Nearly 54,000 to over half a million people could die in the United States. Hospitalizations, which disrupt peoples' ability to participate in the workforce, would range from 669,889 to 4,304,752. Total pandemic costs would be between $413 billion in the low-contagiousness/low-severity scenario and $3.79 trillion in the high-contagiousness/high-severity scenario, with an average total cost of $1.81 trillion. These cost numbers are substantially higher than the $361 billion total cost of seasonal flu that we estimated above. The bulk of these costs is due to the VSL values attributed to fatalities. The immediate cash costs of the pandemic (ignoring VSL) range from almost $55 billion for the low- contagiousness/low-severity scenario to $250 billion for the high-contagiousness/high- severity scenario. It is possible that absenteeism by healthy people who, fearing infection, avoid contact with sick fellow workers, could be substantial in a pandemic with high attack rates and illness severity, resulting in higher immediate costs. The costs imposed by disease avoidance behaviors rise with the prevalence of infectious diseases (Philipson 2000). We do not calculate these costs because there are few reliable estimates of how big this effect might be.[10]

[10] See note 8 supra.

Current Barriers to Vaccination Programs' Effectiveness

Vaccination programs can mitigate the costs of influenza pandemics. But the impact of vaccines is limited by four factors: the speed with which vaccines can be manufactured for emergent viruses; the effectiveness of the vaccine in preventing infection; the number of doses that can be manufactured, distributed, and administered in a given period; and the percentage of the population that is vaccinated. Current methods of influenza vaccine manufacturing constrain the first three of these four factors and limit the effectiveness of vaccination programs as a response to pandemics. The low percentage of people vaccinated is another obvious problem.

Limitations of the Vaccine Manufacturing Timeline

The main method of producing flu vaccines currently in use relies on production in chicken eggs and takes six months or more to produce adequate doses of vaccine. Every year, influenza centers in more than 100 countries conduct influenza surveillance. They select and send representative viruses to five Collaborating Centers for Reference and Research on Influenza around the world that are sponsored by the World Health Organization (WHO). After reviewing the results of the surveillance, laboratory, and clinical studies, WHO recommends which viruses to include in the vaccine for the upcoming seasonal virus season. This occurs in February for the Northern Hemisphere. In the United States, the FDA makes the final decision about which viruses to use in the vaccine (CDC 2018l).

These candidate vaccine viruses (CVVs) are altered (adapted) so that they can be grown efficiently in chicken eggs, isolated, and then provided to private vaccine manufacturers. The manufacturers replicate the CVVs in large numbers of eggs, harvest and inactivate the viruses, and then purify the viral surface proteins (antigens) for the vaccine. The FDA tests and approves vaccines before release and shipment (CDC 2018e).

Essentially, the same 6-month, egg-based process is used to make vaccines in the case of pandemics (WHO 2009). The pandemic curves in Figure 1 suggest that the vaccine would arrive too late to avert a meaningful number of infections and deaths. The experience with the 2009 A(H1N1)pdm09 pandemic is illustrative. The first human infections by the virus were noted in April 2009. Within a week, the CDC began to identify candidate viruses for vaccine manufacture. Increased disease surveillance, stockpiling of antiviral medications, and procurement of respiratory protective equipment were undertaken. In June 2009, WHO officially declared a global pandemic, and cases were reported in all 50 States and Puerto Rico. Despite efforts by the FDA and CDC to speed approval, a new monovalent vaccine for the H1N1 pandemic virus was not approved until September 15. The national vaccination program did not start until October 2009, the same month that influenza activity peaked. During the first six weeks of the program, vaccine supplies were limited, and use was targeted to high-risk populations. Widespread vaccination for anyone who wanted it only became available in December, months after the pandemic peaked (CDC 2010).

Low Vaccine Effectiveness

There is considerable variation from year to year in how much the flu vaccine reduces the risk of contracting the seasonal flu and flu-related illnesses. Figure 2 shows that over the past 14 years, influenza vaccine effectiveness has ranged between 10 and 60 percent. Much of the variability depends on which viruses predominate in a given year. For reasons that are discussed below, egg-based production is least effective against $A(H_3N_2)$ viruses. Hence, during this past 2017–18 season, which was an $A(H_3N_2)$-dominated season, the egg-based vaccine was 38 percent effective overall but just 22 percent effective against the circulating A(H3N2) (Rolfes et al. 2019). The vaccine did even worse among persons

65 or older, with, respectively, 18 percent and 17 percent effectiveness against any influenza strain and A(H_3N_2) viruses (Flannery et al. 2018).

Although the rarity of pandemics makes it hard to determine vaccine effectiveness during pandemics, the monovalent A(H1N1) vaccine prepared during the most recent pandemic in 2009 was 62 percent effective for people less than age 65 and 43 percent effective for people age 65 and older (Borse et al. 2013).

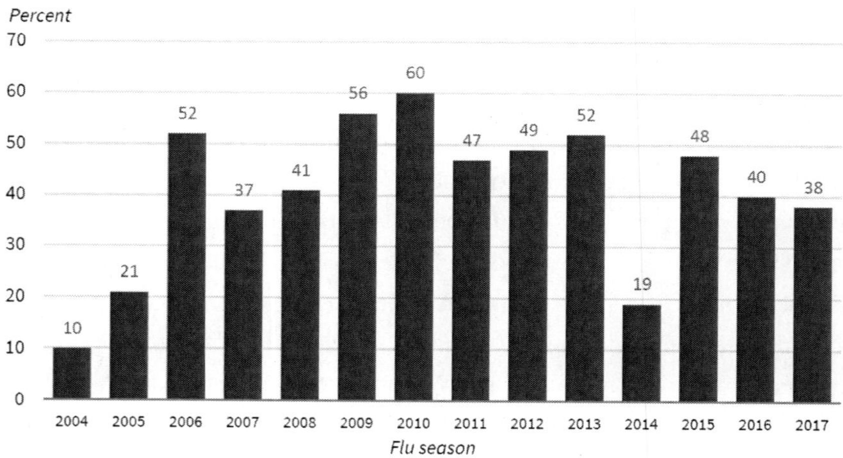

Source: CDC 2019.

Note: Each flu season is from October of the year indicated to May of the following year.

Figure 2. Seasonal Influenza Vaccine Effectiveness.

Efficacy Problems Stemming from Egg-Based Vaccine Production

Egg-based production creates two types of problems with creating effective vaccines that match the circulating virus. First, human viruses must be adapted to grow efficiently in chicken eggs. This process may alter the CVVs' antigens so that they differ from the circulating viruses' antigens, thereby reducing the vaccine's effect. This occurs in all influenza virus types but is most evident in A(H3N2) viruses—the virus type that predominated during 22 of the last 40 flu seasons (CDC 2018n). Mutations in the genes that code for H3 are especially likely to be induced by adaptation to grow in chicken eggs, resulting in decreased vaccine effectiveness (Skowronski et al. 2014). In addition, the A(H3N2) virus grows poorly in eggs, making it difficult to obtain candidate vaccine viruses. Despite WHO's and governmental efforts to select optimal candidate vaccine viruses, "the evolution of A(H3N2) subtype viruses in recent years has resulted in viruses that limit the availability of optimal egg-based vaccine strains" (Barr et al. 2018).

Second, the length of time needed for egg-based production could reduce vaccine efficacy. There can be antigenic drift in the circulating virus between the time it is isolated and prepared for vaccine manufacture in February and the flu season the next fall. The A(H3N2) viruses are more likely to change in ways that have an impact on vaccine effectiveness than are A(H1N1) or B viruses (CDC 2018n). Another problem with long lead times is that the wrong virus could be selected for vaccine production. A pathogenic virus may not appear until later in the season, making it difficult to prepare a candidate vaccine virus in time for vaccine production. In 2014–15, mismatched H3 viruses were first detected in March, a month after the February candidate virus selection. But it did not become clear that they would be the predominant H3 virus until later in the season, and it was not clear that H3 viruses would be the predominant virus for the 2014–15 flu season until it started (CIDRAP 2014). The result was a major mismatch between the seasonal vaccine and the predominant circulating virus—and the vaccine was only 19 percent effective (see Figure 2 above).

Although a mismatch between the vaccine and the so-called wild virus circulating during a flu season reduces efficacy, current vaccines still provide some protection against flu illness (CDC 2018m) and decrease the severity of the illness (CDC 2018n), due to immunologic similarity between the viruses. In addition, seasonal vaccines are designed to protect against the three (trivalent vaccine) or four (quadrivalent vaccine) viruses that are predicted to be most prevalent during the upcoming flu season. The trivalent vaccine includes two type A viruses, an A(H1N1) and an A(H3N2), and one type B virus. The quadrivalent vaccine adds a second type B. When there is a less-than-ideal match against one virus, the vaccine may protect well against the other viruses.

Mismatches and lengthy vaccine production times can become severe issues during a pandemic, when the seasonal flu vaccine that is routinely prepared will be ineffective against the newly emerged, and substantially different, pandemic virus. The 2009 A(H1N1)pdm09 pandemic virus was first detected in April—months after the seasonal vaccine viruses, including a different, seasonal A(H1N1) virus, had been selected. The bulk of the monovalent vaccine against the pandemic virus was unavailable for the first few months of the pandemic— after the peak of infections (Weir and Gruber 2016).

Low Vaccination Rates

Low vaccination rates limit a vaccine's ability to protect the public, no matter how effective the vaccine is. In the 2009 pandemic, the percentage of people vaccinated with the monovalent vaccine varied by age group from 16 to 43 percent but was only 27 percent overall (Borse et al. 2013). Over the past eight seasonal flu seasons, the percentage vaccinated for children (6 months to 17 years) averaged 58 percent, and for adults (18 and above) averaged 41 percent (CDC 2018b, 2018c). Overall, the average population-wide vaccination rate for the seasonal flu was only 45 percent, but was higher for the most vulnerable groups, young children and older adults. Average vaccination rates for each age group over the past 8 influenza seasons (2010–11 to 2017–18) are reported in Table 5. A recent survey found two categories of major reasons that people cite for not getting the seasonal flu vaccine: concerns about vaccine safety (36 percent worried about vaccine side effects and 31 percent believed the vaccine could give them the flu); and doubts about the need for and effectiveness of vaccines (31 percent say vaccines do not work well, 30 percent say they never get the flu, and 27 percent do not believe you can get very sick from the flu) (NORC 2018). These misconceptions about vaccine safety—vaccines do not cause the flu and vaccine side effects are rare, usually mild (unless there is a serious allergic reaction), and generally limited to one or two days (CDC 2018g)—and the potential seriousness of influenza infection persist despite major public education campaigns.

Table 5. Average Vaccination Rates over the Past Eight Seasonal Influenza Years

	Age group						
	0.5–4	5–12	13–17	18–49	50–64	65+	Population-weighted average
Vaccination rate (%)	68.7	58.9	43.3	31.2	44.1	64.7	44.7

Sources: CDC 2018b, 2018c.

Note: Simple average is shown for vaccination rates by age group.

Improving Pandemic Outcomes by Improving the Speed of Production, Vaccine Efficacy, and the Number of People Vaccinated

We now revisit the pandemic flu scenarios described earlier in this chapter and analyze what would happen if the speed of vaccine production increased, effectiveness improved over prior years, and the percentage of the population vaccinated increased.[11] We start with the 2009 pandemic as a baseline. Vaccine production took about 24 weeks. The age group from 6 months to 9 years old received 2 vaccine doses, 4 weeks apart. Vaccine effectiveness was 0 percent after the first dose and 62 percent after the second. Every other age group received a single dose. Effectiveness was 62 percent, except for people 65 or older, for whom it declined to 43 percent. Overall, only 27 percent of the population was vaccinated (Borse et al. 2013). As noted above, this is substantially below the 45 percent average vaccination rate for the seasonal flu. Like Biggerstaff and others (2015), we assume in our calculations that during a pandemic, "demand for

[11] Pandemics often have multiple waves. For simplicity, we look only at the impact on the first wave. Improved vaccine availability should have maximum impact on the first wave because once it is being produced, it would be available for any subsequent waves.

vaccine would be such that 80 percent of the U.S. population" would be vaccinated.[12] Though 80 percent is a high figure compared with historical norms, we believe it is reasonable in the setting of a severe pandemic with high infection and illness rates. The large number of people who cite doubts that they will get the seasonal flu or that it will cause serious illness as a reason to avoid the seasonal flu vaccine (NORC 2018) would be more inclined to be vaccinated in a pandemic with high attack rates and high rates of complication. Moreover, multiple studies have demonstrated that there is high prevalence-elasticity of demand for vaccines for infectious diseases, meaning that as the prevalence of influenza rises in a pandemic, the demand for vaccine will also rise (Philipson 2000). We also allow for a 2- week delay in protection against the virus after administration of the vaccine to account for the time it takes people to mount an immunologic reaction to the vaccine. Finally, we adopt the assumption by Biggerstaff and others (2015) that 30 million vaccine doses can be administered per week.[13]

There is a well-developed, worldwide system of surveillance to uncover threatening viruses. This allows vaccine manufacture to begin before the outbreak of a pandemic, during what is officially called "the recognition interval . . . when increasing numbers of human cases or clusters of novel influenza A infection are identified anywhere in the world, and the virus characteristics indicate an increased potential for ongoing human-to-human transmission" (CDC 2014). During the 2009 pandemic, the process started within a week of the first two infections reported in the U.S.—8 weeks before the pandemic was officially declared.

[12] The objectives of vaccination coverage proposed in the United States—80 percent in healthy persons and 90 percent in high-risk persons—are sufficient to establish herd immunity, while those proposed in Europe—only 75 percent in elderly and high-risk persons—are not sufficient. Current levels of annual vaccination coverage in the U.S. and Europe are not sufficient to establish herd immunity (Plans-Rubió 2012).

[13] Biggerstaff et al. (2015) studied two different scenarios: that the vaccination program could administer either 10 million doses per week, the maximum doses administered per week during seasonal flu programs; or 30 million doses per week, "an untested assumption." We utilize the higher figure on the assumption that in the event of a pandemic, resources to produce and administer vaccines will be mobilized far in excess of what is utilized for the seasonal flu. Moreover, new developments like an oral flu vaccine now in development, which are discussed below, could significantly increase the number vaccinated by making the administration easier and by appealing to patients who resist taking shots.

We use this timeline as our early virus discovery scenario. There is, however, a possibility, for natural or nefarious reasons, that a pandemic virus would not be apparent until later, when a larger number of infections are noted. Therefore, we also consider an alternate scenario—late virus discovery—where vaccine production would not begin until the onset of a pandemic, which is defined in our model as the first 100 confirmed infections (Biggerstaff et al. 2015).[14]

In the early virus discovery scenario, innovations that increase the speed of vaccine production from the current egg-based baseline of 24 weeks down to 8 weeks would move vaccine availability from pandemic week 16 to the outset of the pandemic (pandemic week 0). Faster production in the late virus discovery scenario would move vaccine availability from pandemic week 24 to pandemic week 8.

We also consider the impact of innovation that results in a 30 percent improvement over the baseline 2009 vaccine effectiveness while keeping production speed constant or improving it.[15] A total of 30 percent is a reasonable lower bound improvement because, as we discuss below, early studies of existing recombinant vaccine production have demonstrated this improvement. In addition, it approximates the high-efficacy vaccine (80 percent) that Biggerstaff and others (2015) posit would be available in a future pandemic.[16]

Figure 3 plots the number of new infections per week with no vaccine; a vaccine using baseline egg-based production technology; vaccines using innovations that improve production speed; and vaccines where improved

---

[14] This is officially called "the initiation interval, . . . when human cases of a pandemic influenza virus infection are confirmed anywhere in the world with demonstrated efficient and sustained human-to-human transmission." The 2005 WHO global pandemic plan describes six phases or intervals for defining a pandemic—the investigation, recognition, initiation, acceleration, deceleration, and preparation for subsequent pandemic wave intervals (CDC 2014).

[15] Because baseline effectiveness was zero percent for children receiving a first dose, we assume an increase of 40 percentage points in efficacy for the first dose (as assumed by Biggerstaff et al. 2015) and move from 62 to 81 percent (a 30 percent increase) for the second dose.

[16] Biggerstaff et al. (2015) studied two vaccine efficacy scenarios, the first of which had lower efficacy (62 percent) based on the vaccine effectiveness of standard, unadjuvanted, vaccine in the 2009 pandemic. Our 30 percent increase in over that effectiveness approximates his alternate high vaccine efficacy value of 80 percent, which assumed the use of high-antigen concentrations or the addition of adjuvant to vaccine that are likely to be used in a pandemic setting.

production speed is combined with improved vaccine effectiveness, in four different scenarios under the alternative contagiousness possibilities of a 20 percent attack rate and a 30 percent attack rate and the alternative scenarios for early and late virus discovery.[17] The area between the curves represents the number of infections averted by the current egg-based vaccine and by vaccines improved by innovations. The aggregate number of infections for the four different scenarios with early and late virus discovery and low and high contagiousness are presented in Table 6.

It is apparent that improving the speed of vaccine production is more important for decreasing the number of infections than improving vaccine efficacy. The long production time of the current egg-based vaccine limits its impact on pandemics because the vaccine only becomes available after infections peak in every scenario except the early discovery, low-contagiousness scenario where it becomes available shortly before the infections peak. Figure 3 and Table 6 demonstrate that improving effectiveness at current production speeds only makes a difference in the most favorable, early discovery, low-contagiousness scenario. At current production speeds moving from no vaccine (essentially zero percent effectiveness) to our baseline effectiveness of 62 percent for people below 65 and 43 percent for those 65 and older only averts a substantial number of infections—18.97 million—in the most favorable, early discovery, low-contagiousness scenario and makes little difference in the other three scenarios. This is illustrated in Figure 3, where the yellow curves for the current vaccine are not easily visualized because they are virtually superimposable on the green, no vaccine curves. The yellow vaccine curve is only visible in the bottom left panel of Figure 3, the early discovery, low-contagiousness scenario. The numbers in Table 6 confirm this and also demonstrate that a 30 percent increase over the baseline effectiveness alone, with no change in production speed, makes little or no difference in the same three scenarios and only averts a substantial number of

---

[17] A separate line for improving vaccine effectiveness at current production speeds was omitted for the sake of visual clarity. It did not differ significantly from the yellow curve representing baseline production speed and effectiveness.

infections—about 8 million— in the early discovery, low-contagiousness scenario.

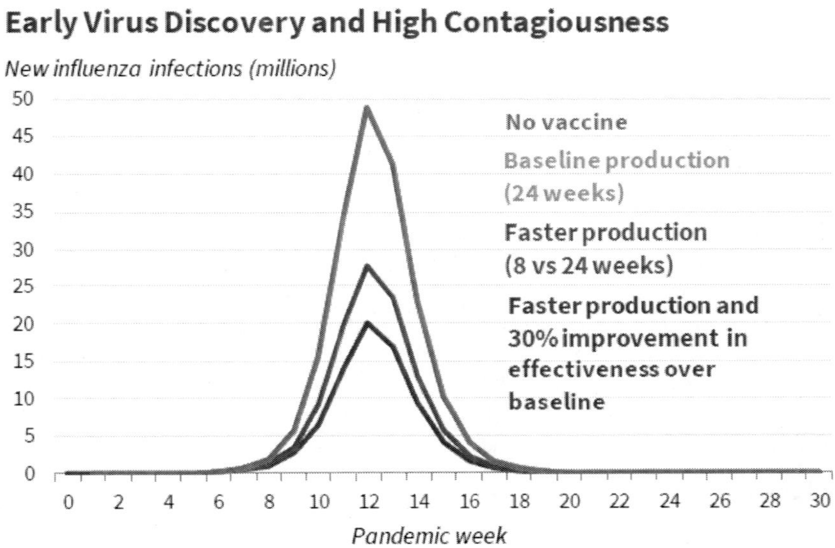

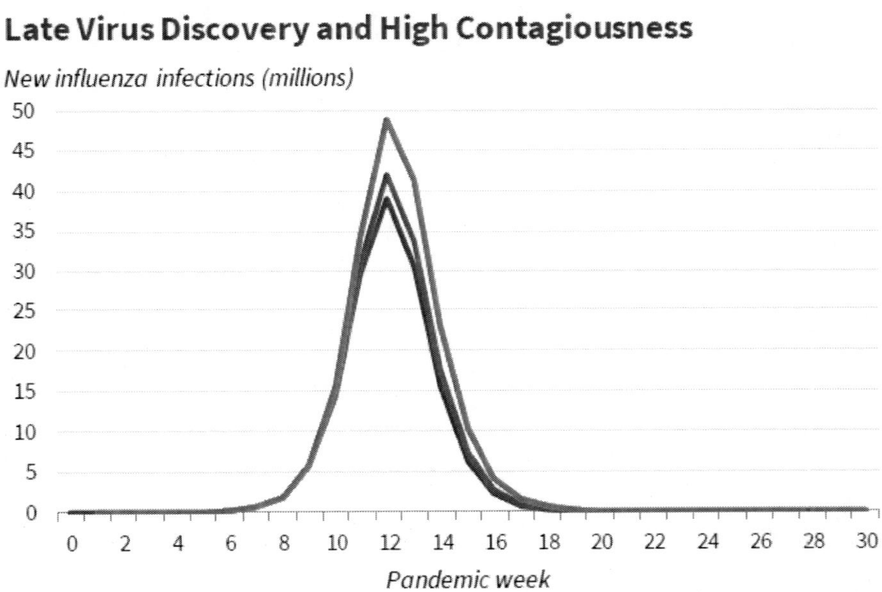

Figure 3. (Continued)

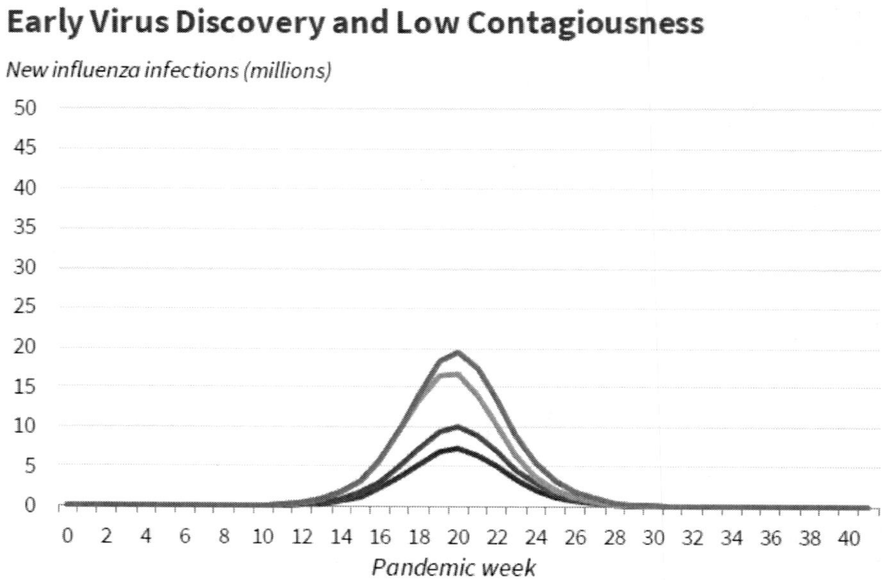

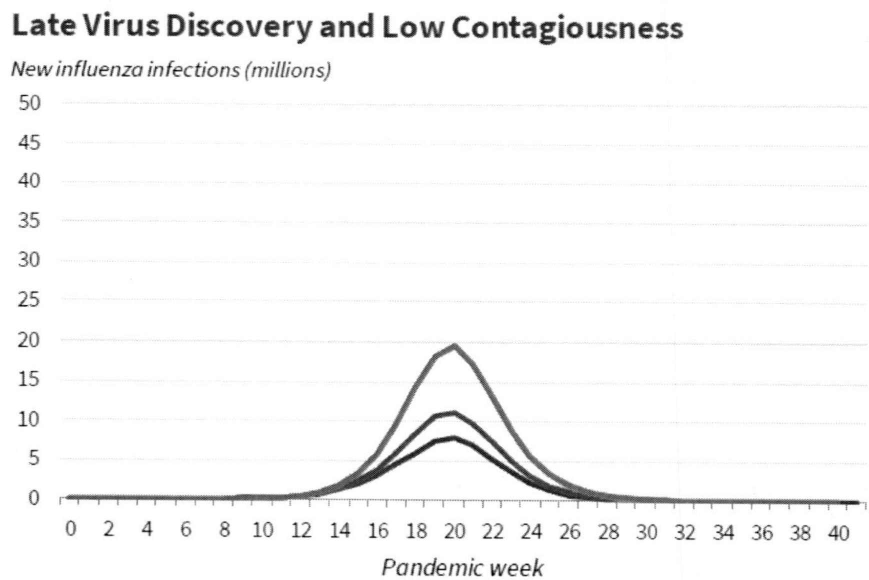

Source: CEA calculations.

Figure 3. New Infections per Pandemic Week with and without Vaccination under Different Scenarios.

Table 6. Infections in four pandemic scenarios with adjustments for faster production and improved effectiveness (thousands of infections)

Virus discovery	Low contagiousness	High contagiousness
Early virus discovery (vaccine available pandemic week 15 baseline)		
No vaccine	127,347	187,959
Baseline production	108,377	187,885
Improvement over baseline effectiveness	100,641	187,856
Faster production	66,792	107,657
Faster production and improved effectiveness	48,302	77,810
Late virus discovery (vaccine available pandemic week 24 baseline)		
No vaccine	127,347	187,959
Baseline production	126,873	187,959
Improvement over baseline effectiveness	126,792	187,959
Faster production	74,511	158,820
Faster production and improved effectiveness	54,912	146,908

Source: CEA calculations.

Note: Faster production indicates decreasing production time from 24 weeks to 8 weeks. We assume an improved effectiveness by 30 percent.

Improving the speed of production from the baseline 24 weeks to 8 weeks with no improvement over baseline effectiveness averts substantial numbers of infections in all four scenarios. Once faster production is in place, improving vaccine effectiveness substantially reduces the number of infections in all four scenarios, as evidenced by the blue curves in Figure 3 and the numbers in Table 6.

Next, we calculate the benefits (cost savings) that could be achieved by week of vaccine availability starting at pandemic week 0. We assume that each of the four pandemic flu scenarios (high/low contagiousness and high/low severity) occurs with an equal probability, to generate an average number of infections, complications, and resulting costs. Figure 4 plots the benefits monetized in dollars per year, conditional on a pandemic occurring, as a function of the week in which the first 30 million vaccine doses become available. Starting with the benefits if a vaccine was available at the outset of the pandemic (week 0), we demonstrate the benefits forgone (cost) by each week of delay in vaccine availability. We plot benefits with the baseline 2009 pandemic vaccine effectiveness described above and with a 30 percent improvement over baseline effectiveness.

Figure 4 shows that with no improvement over the 2009 baseline pandemic vaccine effectiveness, making vaccines available at the outset of the pandemic could generate $730 billion in benefits. A 30 percent improvement over baseline effectiveness raises the benefits to $953 billion—or about one half of the total cost of an average pandemic shown in Table 4. But these cost savings decline quickly as a function of the delay in vaccine availability relative to the start of the pandemic. They decline to $0 after week 39 because the vaccine would be too late to prevent new infections.[18] The benefits forgone per each week of delay during the first 12 weeks with baseline effectiveness is $41 billion, declining to $20 billion during the following 12 weeks. When a 30 percent effectiveness improvement is added in, the benefits forgone per each week of delay during the first 12 weeks is $53 billion, declining to $26 billion during the following 12 weeks.

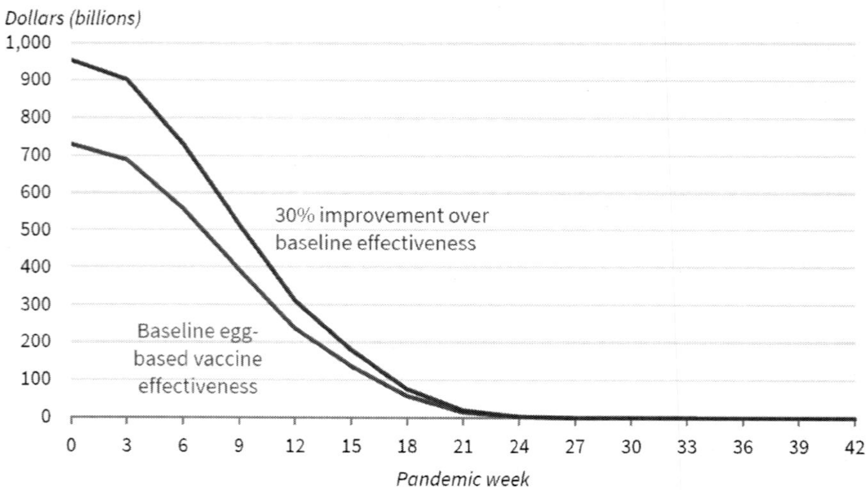

Source: CEA calculations.

Figure 4. Annual Benefits by Week of Vaccine Availability in a Pandemic.

[18] Because the last infections would occur in pandemic week 41, vaccines would not have any impact after pandemic week 39 due to the two weeks needed after vaccination to elicit immunity.

To determine the value of an improvement in the speed of pandemic vaccine production, we calculate the expected cost savings resulting from making a vaccine available at the outset of a pandemic. Given the 4 percent annual probability of a pandemic occurring in a given year, we multiply the savings at pandemic week 0, illustrated in Figure 4 above, by the likelihood of a pandemic. This generates an expected cost savings of $29 billion from faster production that makes vaccines available at the outset of a pandemic and $38 billion from faster production, plus a 30 percent increase over baseline effectiveness (Table 7). On a per capita basis, this translates into $89.63 and $117.07 in value per American, respectively. We also calculate $112.04 and $146.34, respectively, in value per vaccinated person, assuming, as we did above, that 80 percent of the population would be vaccinated during a pandemic. These values are well above the current price per dose for standard egg-based vaccines, which range from $17.84 to $19.77 (CMS 2018), and suggest that society should be willing to pay a premium over four times more than current vaccine prices for improved influenza vaccines. As is discussed below, newer, potentially faster and more effective vaccine production technologies already exist that cost less than the expected values of improved pandemic vaccines. But these technologies have not yet been widely utilized.

Table 7. Expected benefits from improved vaccines in a pandemic

Measure of benefit	**Improved speed, 30% effectiveness improvement**	**Improved speed, baseline vaccine effectiveness**
Total cost savings (billions of dollars)	953.27	729.81
per capita (dollars)	2,926.82	2,240.75
per vaccinated person (dollars)	3,658.53	2,800.94
Total expected savings (billions of dollars)	38.13	29.19
per capita (dollars)	117.07	89.63
per vaccinated person (dollars)	146.34	112.04

Source: CEA calculations.

Newer Technologies to Produce More Effective Vaccines More Quickly

Currently, about 85 percent of influenza vaccines are produced with egg-based manufacturing, which has been in use for more than 70 years. Two newer methods to produce vaccines are available: cell-cultured vaccines, which account for 10 to 15 percent of the market; and recombinant vaccines, which account for 1 to 2 percent. These new production methods may offer better antigen matching because they avoid egg adaptation issues, and faster production allows later selection of CVVs closer to the flu season, thereby minimizing the problem of genetic drift in circulating viruses or viruses arising unexpectedly after the CVVs are selected (Barr et al. 2018). Although vaccines produced with these new methods are more expensive than egg-based vaccines, costs should come down with process optimization and economies of scale.

In 2012, the FDA approved a cell-cultured, influenza vaccine, Flucelvax, in which egg-isolated CVVs were grown in cultured mammalian cells instead of chicken eggs. Four years later, the FDA approved an update to Flucelvax using cell-grown CVVs in cell-cultured vaccine production. Hence, the entire process, from virus isolation to virus growth and vaccine preparation, now occurs in mammalian cells. This eliminates the egg adaptations needed to grow influenza viruses in chicken eggs and may produce more effective vaccines that contain virus antigens closer to the wild types that are circulating (CDC 2018a). This new vaccine, which contained a virus derived from a purely mammalian cell culture, was used for the first time this past 2017–18 season. A CDC/FDA study of Medicare beneficiaries who are older than 65 shows that the cell-based vaccine was 10.4 percent more effective than the most commonly used quadrivalent egg-based vaccine during the 2017–18 flu season in which an A(H3N2) virus predominated (Lu 2018). But another study, by Kaiser Permanente Northern California of its members age 4–64 during the same 2017–18 season, found no significant difference in the effectiveness of cell-culture vaccine compared with standard egg-based vaccine (Klein et al. 2018).

Cell-culture manufacture is also potentially faster and more flexible than egg-based manufacturing. Manufacturing can start later than the current February egg-based date to account for viruses that are identified later on and antigenic drift in the original CVVs. In addition, cell-based production provides the potential for a faster start-up in the event of a pandemic. Unlike eggs, cells for Flucelvax production can be frozen to ensure that a supply of cells is available for vaccine production if there is an unexpected need like a pandemic virus (Klein et al. 2018; FDA 2013).

The second new method of producing influenza vaccines using recombinant technology was approved in 2013. It does not require the growth of influenza virus in mammalian cells or eggs. Instead, the vaccine, Flublok, is produced by taking the genes that code for the hemagglutinin (H) proteins from wild-type viruses, inserting them into viruses that infect insects' cells, and utilizing the insect cells to rapidly produce the influenza vaccine H protein (antigen), which is then harvested from the insect cells and purified. Like the cell-based technology, the recombinant method does not use eggs at all, and thus its effectiveness will not be limited by the selection of viruses that adapt for growth in eggs. Dunkle and others (2017) estimated that the recombinant vaccine was substantially more effective than the quadrivalent egg-based vaccine during the 2014–15 season—an A(H3N2) predominant year—among adults who were 50 years of age or older, reducing the probability of illness by 30 percent. They cautioned that the recombinant vaccine contains higher antigen concentrations per dose (45 micrograms/dose) than standard dose egg-based vaccines (15 micrograms/dose) and that "it is uncertain whether a higher antigen content or genetic fidelity to the recommended strain was responsible for the better relative vaccine efficacy" in the trial (Dunkle 2017, p. 2435). This question is particularly important considering the finding in the FDA/CDC study of cell-cultured vaccines discussed above that just as cell-cultured vaccine is more effective (10.4 percent), high dose, egg-based trivalent vaccine was also 8.4 percent more effective than the standard egg-based vaccine, and there was no significant difference between the cell-cultured and the high dose, egg-based vaccines' effectiveness (Lu 2018). Regardless, it does highlight another advantage of both non-egg-based vaccine production techniques, especially recombinant vaccines, that they are more efficient at producing viral antigens than is the egg-based process. Dunkle and others (2017) advised repeating trials of recombinant vaccine in other flu seasons to see if the results will be replicated when there are different predominant circulating viruses.

Perhaps the biggest advantage of the recombinant vaccine manufacturing is speed, because it can produce vaccines within six to eight weeks once a pathogenic virus is identified and isolated, matching the speed gain in our simulation above, as opposed to six months with the egg-based process (Dunkle et al. 2017). This will be useful in creating vaccines for unexpected, pandemic viruses. It should also be faster than cell-cultured vaccines, given that it does not need to await the development of cell-based CVVs (Weir and Gruber 2016). Its major limitation is that its 9-month shelf life is shorter than those of other flu vaccines (CDC 2018k).

Medicare currently pays $22.79 and $53.37, respectively, for cell-cultured and recombinant vaccines (CMS 2018). These are both well below the expected values of improved pandemic vaccines calculated above. It seems clear that investment to expand manufacturing capacity for recombinant vaccine is warranted. The same will be true for cell-cultured vaccine manufacture if it proves to be appreciably faster than egg-based production.

Another production process, self-amplifying mRNA (SAM) vaccine manufacturing, which is patented but does not yet have an FDA-approved product, could shorten the vaccine manufacturing timeline even further. The SAM vaccine has been shown to be effective in mice (Hekele et al. 2013). Per interviews with government experts on influenza vaccines, both recombinant and SAM vaccines hold great promise for substantially shortening the vaccine manufacturing timeline and may provide the flexibility to engineer what would be a significant advance in the fight against influenza—a "universal" influenza vaccine.

Seasonal vaccines target a part of the influenza H surface antigen—the head—that varies from year to year. But there is another part of the antigen that is consistent across influenza strains and does not change—the stem. Although more research will be required, recent advances suggest that a successful vaccine against this part is possible. The potential benefits are clear. Unlike current vaccines that are strain-specific, a universal vaccine would not need to be reformulated on an annual basis and could be available to provide rapid protection in an emerging influenza pandemic. If it provides a durable immune response, seasonal vaccines would not need to be administered each year. This is an area of active research by both the NIH's National Institute of Allergy and Infectious Diseases and private companies (NIH 2018).

The Value of Switching to New Vaccine Technologies for Seasonal Influenza

Switching to existing cell-cultured or recombinant vaccines and investing in production capacity may also be justified by savings that could be achieved in seasonal influenza years.

Avoiding the Loss of Efficacy due to Egg Adaptations

Assuming that the results from the most optimistic early studies hold up, a cell-cultured vaccine could improve vaccine effectiveness by about 10.4 percent, and a recombinant vaccine could improve effectiveness by 30 percent over egg-based vaccine in years when A(H3N2) is the predominant virus by avoiding egg adaptations. We assume no change in effectiveness in non- A(H3N2) years, but, because effectiveness could improve for years when other viruses also predominate, our estimate should be considered a lower bound. To estimate the probability of a future prevalence of the A(H3N2) virus, we can consider the past outcomes. A(H3N2) viruses predominated during 12 out of the past 20 flu seasons and 22 out of the last

40 flu seasons.[19] Taking the longer-term view, the probability of the A(H3N2) virus dominating in any of the future years is 55 percent.[20] We then estimate the cost savings from the new-technology vaccines based on the 10.4 and 30 percent reductions in the number of illnesses that would occur in an A(H3N2) season among people who are vaccinated (as estimated from Table 5).

Table 8 presents expected savings in each age group for the entire U.S. population and per vaccine given our improved vaccine effectiveness assumptions from avoiding egg-adaptation in A(H3N2) seasonal flu years. The table shows that the cost savings are the highest for the oldest age group due to the high rate of adverse outcomes from influenza. The expected savings from a switch to new-technology vaccines is about $3.1 billion per year for cell-based vaccines and $8.9 billion for recombinant vaccines.

Table 8. Expected benefit due to improved effectiveness from avoiding egg adaptations in seasonal influenza years

	Age group					**Total savings (millions of dollars)**
Measure of benefit	0–4	5–17	18–49	50–64	65+	
Cell-based vaccines Savings (millions of dollars)	38.2	13.9	63.8	319.2	2652.1	3087.1
Savings per vaccinated person (dollars)	2.77	0.48	1.48	11.34	82.58	15.69
Recombinant vaccines Savings (millions of dollars)	110.2	40.0	184.0	920.8	7650.2	8905.2
Savings per vaccinated person (dollars)	7.99	1.40	4.27	32.72	238.22	45.25

Source: CEA calculations.
Note: Data are from seasonal influenza.

On a per-vaccinated-person basis, the value of the new seasonal vaccines, pricing in the improvement over historical vaccine effectiveness,

[19] We thank the CDC for providing this information to us.
[20] 22/40 = 55 percent.

could be $15.69 higher per dose for cell-based vaccines and $45.25 per recombinant dose. The value of these new vaccines is greatest for the 65+ age group—$82.58 per cell-based dose, and $238.22 per recombinant dose. Medicare currently pays up to $53.37 per dose of recombinant quadrivalent vaccine (Flublok), $22.79 per dose for cell-cultured quadrivalent vaccine (Flucelvax) and between $17.84 and $19.77 for standard-dose, egg-based vaccines (CMS 2018).[21] Medicare pays $53.37 for the high-dose, egg-based vaccine (Fluzone), the same as recombinant vaccine but substantially more than cell-based vaccine. Both high-dose egg and cell-based vaccines showed significantly improved effectiveness over standard egg-based vaccines this past season, but the improvement was not statistically different between them (Lu 2018).

The Value of Faster Vaccine Production for Seasonal Flu

The calculations above only account for improvement in efficacy due to the absence of antigen mismatch that results from egg adaptation. Cell-cultured and recombinant vaccines have so far been prepared with the same candidate viruses (minus the adaptation changes) selected for egg-based production in February of each year by the FDA's Vaccines and Related Biological Products Advisory Committee (VRBPAC). But recombinant and possibly cell-culture manufacturers do not need the six months required for egg-based production. Modifying the official calendar so that additional recommendations for the influenza-strain come closer to the actual flu season could enable vaccine manufacturers with short lead times to make more effective vaccines by avoiding antigenic drift that occurs between February and the flu season or inaccurate initial candidate virus selection.

The framework for later candidate virus selection is already in place. Worldwide surveillance is continuous throughout the year, and the results

---

[21] Medicare payment allowances for seasonal influenza vaccines are 95 percent of the average wholesale price, except where the vaccine is furnished to a hospital outpatient, when it is based on a reasonable cost (CMS 2018).

are published in the CDC's *Weekly Influenza Surveillance Report*. A placeholder in the VRBPAC's calendar for a May–June update already exists, although it seems to have been implemented only once, for the H1N1 Swine Flu pandemic strain in 2009 (Weir 2017).

Updates after the initial February CVV selection would allow manufacturers with short lead times to differentiate their products in the market while enhancing surge capacity to deal with pandemics. A strain selection update does not mean that the FDA should decertify the previously certified CVVs. Rather, it would enhance vaccine consumers' (doctors, hospitals, drugstores, and clinics) choices. Consumers can already choose between authorized egg-based trivalent, quadrivalent, high-dose and adjuvanted vaccines, as well as cell-cultured and recombinant vaccines, all based on the February viruses. A late-entry vaccine would present one more authorized choice. If their speed and flexibility allowed them to produce superior vaccines—something that would need to be validated over time by reporting vaccine effectiveness—the financial rewards for the rapid-production techniques would support the building of additional surge capacity to confront a pandemic.

Only limited data are available on the frequency of substantial drift between February and the start of the flu season and on the degree of mismatch between the vaccine viruses and the viruses circulating during flu season. Using CDC data that are available about the past 13 seasonal flu years, however, we conduct the following thought experiment to illustrate the possible market advantage from starting vaccine production later in the season and therefore being better able to match the vaccine to the prevailing strain. In the past 13 seasonal flu years,[22] there were three years with a substantial mismatch between the predominant circulating virus and the virus in the vaccine.[23] Using this 23 percent probability, we can determine what savings would be expected from improving the vaccine

[22] One of the past 14 years, 2009, was a pandemic year, in which the CDC reported that there was not a significant amount of the seasonal vaccine virus circulating during flu season—the predominant circulating virus was the pandemic A(H1N1) virus (CDC 2010). Although this represents a complete mismatch, we dropped 2009 because it was not a typical seasonal flu year, leaving 13 seasonal flu seasons in the past 14 years.

[23] In two years when there were no direct data on the degree of mismatch but vaccine efficacy was high, we assumed there was little mismatch.

effectiveness observed in mismatch years (10, 19, and 21 percent) up to the effectiveness that would be seen in a year with a good match. The average effectiveness observed in the 10 match years over the past 13 flu seasons was 47 percent. This is consistent with CDC estimates that seasonal vaccine effectiveness ranges between 40 and 60 percent in years when the circulating virus is well matched to the vaccine (CDC 2018n).

The total savings and savings per vaccinated person expected from faster vaccine production, enabling vaccine production to be closer to the actual season and better vaccine matches to the circulating viruses, are presented in Table 9.

Table 9. Expected Benefits from Improved Vaccine Effectiveness in Years with the Wrong Strain Forecast

	Age group					Total
Measure of benefit	0–4	5–17	18–49	50–64	65+	
Expected savings (millions of dollars)	184.5	67.0	308.1	1,541.9	12,811.0	14,912.5
Expected savings per vaccinated person (dollars)	13.37	2.34	7.15	54.80	398.91	75.77

Source: Molinari et al. (2007); CEA calculations.

Note: The total expected savings per vaccinated person is the population-weighted average.

According to this calculation, the decreased mismatches result in an expected $75.77 savings per vaccinated person. The most impressive benefits are for the 65+ age group—$398.91 per elderly vaccinated person.

If this suggested adjustment to the FDA's calendar led to a documented improvement in seasonal vaccine efficacy, faster production technologies would likely increase their market share, which would have the additional benefit of contributing, at little cost, to the Nation's ability to rapidly respond to a pandemic. There are many similarities between a surprise emergence of a seasonal influenza virus and the emergence of pandemic virus (although pandemics, by definition, have higher mortality and/or higher transmission rates). Both cause a surge in morbidity and mortality that can be mitigated by shorter vaccine production timelines.

It is likely that vaccine efficacy improvements from less antigen mismatch due to egg adaptation and antigenic drift during prolonged production periods will both result from innovative vaccine technologies. We cannot say they would be perfectly additive, because the egg adaptations and antigenic drift will vary from year to year depending on the predominant viruses and are likely independent of each other.

Why the Private Market Might Not Sell Pandemic Insurance

We have shown that new technologies that speed vaccine production and avoid the need for egg adaption could have substantial benefit in the event of an influenza pandemic and may, if preliminary studies can be replicated, have value for seasonal flu. However, adoption of existing new manufacturing techniques and the development of other innovative technologies has been slow. Here, we discuss the lack of a market for innovative technologies to better mitigate pandemic risk.

Mitigating the losses from pandemic flu is dependent on medical innovation that speeds up vaccine production or increases vaccine effectiveness. The problem with such innovation is that medical R&D into vaccines that better mitigates the risk of a pandemic is only recouped by sales when the pandemic risk occurs. However, part of the value of vaccines that mitigate future pandemic risks is their *insurance value* today. This value accrues even if the pandemic does not occur in the future. To illustrate, most life insurance buyers do not die in a given year but still get value from holding the policy as it mitigates risk in case of death. Similarly, faster vaccine technologies and more effective vaccines would be valuable even when the pandemic did not occur because they mitigate the risks of illness and losing one's life to a possible pandemic. The new vaccine technology would provide insurance against pandemic risk both in terms of monetary losses and losses in one's health.

This insurance value of vaccine technologies implies that the social value of faster vaccine production is larger than its private return to developers, which is based on sales when the pandemic occurs once every 25 years or so.[24] This divergence leads to an underprovision in vaccine innovation because it does not get rewarded for its insurance value. As a result, manufacturers have little incentive to move from the current dependence on egg-based production, which is unable to ramp up production quickly enough, or to target the vaccines closely enough, to mitigate a pandemic. This divergence might become less important if and when the value of newer, existing technologies (cell-based, recombinant) or as-yet-undeveloped vaccine technologies can be conclusively demonstrated for seasonal flu vaccines.

A second barrier to a private market solution is that pandemics represent a risk with large and highly correlated losses across the population, against which it is inherently difficult to get the market to provide private insurance. Insurance works by pooling risk between a few affected people and a large number of people who are not affected by the risk insured against. Unlike the usual insurance scenario, where one person's risk of a car accident has little or no influence on the risk of an accident of other insured motorists with whom she pools the risk, a pandemic (similar to a hurricane) is an instance where a large number of people are simultaneously affected. The risk cannot be pooled because everyone is at risk concurrently. Whenever risks are correlated, private insurance has less value. To illustrate, consider a risk such as a pandemic that either does not affect anyone or affects nearly everyone. If the insurance company is to stay solvent and pay out claims when the pandemic occurs, its premiums must be close to the actual loss on a per capita level. This makes the premiums so expensive that the insurance is not valuable; why pay a dollar to receive a dollar if the risk occurs? The basic issue is that insurers must meet self-imposed and regulatory solvency requirements for the policies that they issue so that they have sufficient

[24] We realize that positive externalities of vaccination (vaccination protects me plus those around me from contracting disease) could also be counted in social value; but for the purposes of this chapter, we do not separately estimate these effects.

capital to compensate for a given level of losses. Kousky and Cooke (2012) demonstrate that the requisite premiums to cover disastrous events can become so high that consumers are not willing to pay large homeowners' premiums. The central issue is that there is little or no pooling of risk when risks are highly correlated. Because pandemic vaccine demand would be hard to insure, it would limit the demand for the superior vaccine technology developed.

A third barrier may be that insurance decisions are often based on past experiences and emotions (Kunreuther, Pauly, and McMorrow 2013). Though people frequently overestimate the likelihood of uncommon events, they sometimes underestimate the likelihood of tail events—rare, high-impact events—based on the "availability heuristic," which leads people to estimate the probability of an event by how easy it is to recall episodes of the event (Barberis 2013). In the case of pandemic flu, there have only been four episodes over the past 100 years, and only one of them, the 1918 flu, resulted in widespread illness and death in the United States. In addition, people may conflate the high expected costs of pandemic flu with the far- more-common, lower-cost, seasonal flu. It is not surprising that people might underappreciate the economic and health risks posed by pandemic flu and not invest in ways to reduce these risks.

Finally, insurers may also undervalue the economic and health risks of pandemics. "Pandemic exposure can present significant tail risk to insurers. The life and health insurance industries will be most severely impacted. However, the property/casualty (P/C) industry could see substantial losses from secondary impacts" (NAIC 2018). Nevertheless, there is inadequate private demand for developing and investing in vaccine technologies to deal with the pandemic flu threat. Insurers undervalue the risk to economic stability and growth and do not value the positive impact investment and research into pandemic flu prevention could have in other medical areas (Sands, Mundaca-Shah, and Dzau 2016).

Given the underprovision of pandemic risk mitigation by the private sector, the public sector has a role in stimulating the development of, and demand for, newer vaccine technologies that are better able to provide pandemic preparedness. Public-private partnerships that stimulate such innovation may enhance welfare.

THE ROLE OF THE PUBLIC-PRIVATE PARTNERSHIPS IN MOVING TOWARD FASTER, MORE FLEXIBLE, AND MORE EFFECTIVE NEW VACCINE PRODUCTION TECHNOLOGIES

All influenza vaccines in the United States are privately manufactured by a handful of firms. Most resources are invested in egg-based production, which has been the predominant method of vaccine production for 70 years. Moving to different production methods requires large capital expenditures in a market with low profit margins earned by vaccine producers.

Public measures have been key in advancing vaccine innovation. The Pandemic and All- Hazards Preparedness Act, enacted in 2006, established the Biomedical Advanced Research and Development Authority (BARDA) within the Office of the Assistant Secretary for Preparedness and Response at the U.S. Department of Health and Human Services to facilitate research and development of countermeasures for chemical, biological, radiological, and nuclear threats, including the development of vaccines for the risks posed by pandemic influenza (HHS 2018).[25] The statute supported public-private partnerships to achieve pandemic preparedness. Public-private partnerships were key in the development of cell-cultured and recombinant protein-based vaccines. Seasonal and pandemic flu preparedness are closely linked, given that vaccine production for seasonal flu viruses is the foundation for vaccines production for pandemic flu.

About half of flu vaccines administered in the United States are to people covered by government health insurance. Hence, the government has a strong interest in purchasing the most cost-effective seasonal flu vaccines. Public-private partnerships can continue to push cell-cultured

---

[25] Public Law 109-417, 109th Congress: Pandemic and All-Hazards Preparedness Act, Washington.

and recombinant protein vaccine technologies or other, as-yet-unknown innovations, to offer greater flexibility and perhaps improved effectiveness than egg-based vaccines while supporting accelerated timelines for vaccine composition updates to cope with changes in seasonal flu viruses and to respond to the inevitable, future pandemic viruses. One promising approach being developed by a private company, supported by a contract with BARDA, is a recombinant, oral flu vaccine. Preliminary results suggest that it is at least as effective as standard vaccines (Hackett 2018). An oral vaccine would be easier to administer because it does not require specialized personnel and could increase vaccination rates among people who resist getting injections—the NORC (2018) survey reported that among people not planning on getting a flu vaccine, 13 percent cited fear of needles and shots as a major reason and 15 percent as a minor reason. This creates the possibility that more than the 30 million doses a week that we used in our model above could be administered and higher vaccination rates achieved, resulting in improved health benefits and decreased economic costs.

Another promising area of public-private collaboration is the development of a universal influenza vaccine, which was described above when discussing new vaccine technologies. The National Institute of Allergy and Infectious Diseases has stated that developing a universal vaccine "will require a global collaborative effort among government agencies, industry, philanthropic organizations, and academia that incorporates interdisciplinary approaches and new technological tools" (NIH 2018).

If the improvements of cell-culture and recombinant technologies over the effectiveness of egg-based vaccine production can be replicated over several influenza seasons with documented cost savings, or other innovative technologies come to the fore, government purchases will likely switch to the more cost-effective products. This increased demand should pull private, domestic production toward better vaccine manufacturing technologies, decreasing the impact of both seasonal and pandemic influenza.

CONCLUSION

Pandemic influenza is a low-probability but high-cost problem that should not be ignored. The current influenza vaccine manufacturing infrastructure in the U.S. is dependent on egg-based production that is too slow to produce adequate doses of vaccines for unexpected pandemic outbreaks and may impair vaccine efficacy. This could lead to tremendous, avoidable costs. This chapter has outlined the importance of innovation in reducing these costs. Improving the speed of vaccine production is key. Once shorter production timelines are achieved, improving vaccine efficacy can also have an important impact. Faster vaccine production that would make sufficient doses of vaccine available at the outset of a pandemic could generate $730 billion in benefits. If combined with improvements in vaccine effectiveness, the benefits would rise to $953 billion. The expected value of improving pandemic vaccine production speed is many times the cost of existing influenza vaccines, suggesting that investment in and adoption of faster, more effective production technologies is worthwhile. New, non-egg-based vaccine production methods able to deliver sufficient doses of vaccine faster in the case of a pandemic, saving millions of lives and billions of dollars, already exist and could be improved upon with additional innovation. These new vaccine technologies may also result in improvements to the past effectiveness of seasonal flu vaccines, ultimately lowering the costs of the annual flu season. The Federal government has played a role through public-private partnerships in the development of these new vaccine technologies. The government should continue to partner with the private sector to develop and adopt new vaccine technologies that mitigate the risks of pandemic influenza and improve outcomes for the seasonal flu. When the value of these new technologies is confirmed, government can move to purchase the most cost-effective vaccines available.

References

Aldy, J., and W. Viscusi. 2008. "Adjusting the Value of a Statistical Life for Age and Cohort Effects." *Review of Economics and Statistics* 90, no. 3: 573–81.

Barberis, N. 2013. "The Psychology of Tail Events: Progress and Challenges." *American Economic Review: Papers & Proceedings* 103, no. 3: 611–16.

Barr, I., R. Donis, J. Katz, J. McCauley, T. Odagiri, et al. 2018. "Cell Culture-Derived Influenza Vaccines in the Severe 2017–2018 Epidemic Season: A Step towards Improved Influenza Vaccine Effectiveness." *Nature Partner Journal Vaccines* 3, no. 44.

Biggerstaff, M., M. Jhung, L. Kamimoto, L. Balluz, and L. Finelli. 2012. "Self-Reported Influenza-Like Illness and Receipt of Influenza Antivirual Drugs During the 2009 Pandemic, United States, 2009–2010." *American Journal of Public Health* 102, no. 10: e21–e26.

Biggerstaff, M., C. Reed, D. Swerdlow, M. Gambhir, S. Graitcer, et al. 2015. "Estimating the Potential Effects of a Vaccine Program Against an Emerging Influenza Pandemic, United States." *Clinical Infectious Diseases* 60, no. 1: s20–s29.

Borse, R., S. Shrestha, A. Fiore, C. Atkins, J. Singleton, et al. 2013. "Effects of Vaccine Program Against Pandemic Influenza A (H1N1) Virus, United States, 2009–2010." *Emerging Infectious Diseases* 19, no. 3: 439.

CEA (Council of Economic Advisers). 2017. "The Underestimated Cost of the Opioid Crisis." https://www.whitehouse.gov/sites/whitehouse.gov/files/images/The%20Underestimated%20Cost%20of%20the%20Opioid%20Crisis.pdf.

CDC (Centers for Disease Control and Prevention). 2010. "The 2009 H1N1 Pandemic: Summary Highlights, April 2009–April 2010." https://www.cdc.gov/h1n1flu/cdcresponse.htm.

———. 2014. "Updated Preparedness and Response Framework for Influenza Pandemics." https://www.cdc.gov/mmwr/preview/mmwrhtml/rr6306a1.htm.

———. 2017a. "How the Flu Virus Can Change: 'Drift' and 'Shift.'" https://www.cdc.gov/flu/about/viruses/change.htm.

———. 2017b. "Transatlantic Taskforce on Antimicrobial Resistance (TATFAR): Drug Development Incentives." https://www.cdc.gov/drug resistance/tatfar/news/drugdevelopment.html.

———. 2018a. "Cell-Based Flu Vaccines." https://www.cdc.gov/flu/protect/vaccine/cell-based.htm.

———. 2018b. "Estimates of Flu Vaccination Coverage among Adults—United States, 2017–18 Flu Season." https://www.cdc.gov/flu/fluvax view/coverage-1718estimates.htm.

———. 2018c. "Estimates of Flu Vaccination Coverage among Children—United States, 2017– 18 Flu Season." https://www.cdc.gov/flu/fluvaxview/coverage-1718estimates-children.htm.

———. 2018d. "The Flu Season." https://www.cdc.gov/flu/about/season/flu-season.htm

———. 2018e. "How Influenza (Flu) Vaccines Are Made." https://www.cdc.gov/flu/protect/vaccine/how-fluvaccine-made.htm.

———. 2018f. "How Is Pandemic Flu Different from Seasonal Flu?" https://www.cdc.gov/flu/pandemic-resources/basics/about.html.

———. 2018g. "Misconceptions About Seasonal Flu and Flu Vaccines." https://www.cdc.gov/flu/about/qa/misconceptions.htm.

———. 2018h. "The 1918 Flu Pandemic: Why It Matters 100 Years Later." https://blogs.cdc.gov/publichealthmatters/2018/05/1918-flu/.

———. 2018i. "Pandemic Influenza – Past Pandemics." https://www.cdc.gov/flu/pandemic-resources/basics/past-pandemics.html.

———. 2018j. "Preliminary Estimates of 2017–18 Seasonal Influenza Vaccine Effectiveness against Laboratory-Confirmed Influenza from the US Flu VE and HAIVEN Networks." https://www.cdc.gov/vaccines/acip/meetings/downloads/slides-2018-06/flu-02-Flannery-508.pdf.

———. 2018k. "Recombinant Influenza (Flu) Vaccine." https://www.cdc.gov/flu/protect/vaccine/qa_flublok-vaccine.htm.

———. 2018l. "Selecting Viruses for the Seasonal Influenza Vaccine." https://www.cdc.gov/flu/about/season/vaccine-selection.htm.

———. 2018m. "Summary of the 2016-2017 Influenza Season." https://www.cdc.gov/flu/about/season/flu-season-2016-2017.htm.

———. 2018n. "Vaccine Effectiveness: How Well Does the Flu Vaccine Work?" https://www.cdc.gov/flu/about/qa/vaccineeffect.htm.

———. 2019. "Seasonal Influenza Vaccine Effectiveness, 2004–2018." https://www.cdc.gov/flu/professionals/vaccination/effectiveness-studies.htm.

CIDRAP (Center for Infectious Disease Research and Policy). 2014. "CDC's Flu Warning Raises Questions About Vaccine Match." *CIDRAP News*, December 5. http://www.cidrap.umn.edu/news-perspective/2014/12/cdcs-flu-warning-raises- questions-about-vaccine-match.

CMS (Centers for Medicare and Medicaid Services). 2018. "Seasonal Influenza Vaccines Pricing: Payment Allowances and Effective Dates for the 2018–2019 Flu Season. September 5." https://www.cms.gov/Medicare/Medicare-Fee-for-Service-Part-B-Drugs/McrPartBDrugAvg SalesPrice/VaccinesPricing.html.

Dunkle, L., R. Izikson, P. Patriarca, K. Goldenthal, D. Muse, et al. 2017. "Efficacy of Recombinant Influenza Vaccine in Adults 50 Years of Age or Older." *New England Journal of Medicine* 376, no. 25: 2427–36.

Flannery, B., J. Chung, E. Belongia, H. McLean, M. Gaglani, et al. 2018. "Interim Estimates of 2017–18 Seasonal Influenza Vaccine Effectiveness—United States." *American Journal of Transplantation* 18, no. 4: 1020–25.

FDA (Food and Drug Administration). 2013. "The Evolution, and Revolution, of Flu Vaccines." https://www.fda.gov/ForConsumers/ConsumerUpdates/ucm336267.htm.

Grohskopf, L., L. Sokolow, K. Broder, E. Walter, A. Fry, et al. 2018. "Prevention and Control of Seasonal Influenza with Vaccines: Recommendations of the Advisory Committee on Immunization

Practices—United States, 2018–19 Influenza Season." *Morbidity and Mortality Weekly Report* 67, no. 3: 1–20.

Hackett, D. 2018. "Oral Tablet H1 Influenza Vaccine vs Fluzone." https://www.precisionvaccinations.com/vaxart-vxa-a11-oral-flu-vaccine-met-phase- 2-clinical-study-end-points.

Hekele, A., S. Bertholet, J. Archer, D. Gibson, G. Palladino, et al. 2013. "Rapidly Produced SAM® Vaccine against H7N9 Influenza Is Immunogenic in Mice." *Emerging Microbes and Infections* 2, no. 8: e52.

HHS (Department of Health and Human Services). 2018. "Pandemic Influenza." https://www.medicalcountermeasures.gov/barda/pandemic-influenza.aspx.

Institute of Medicine. 2010. "The Public Health Emergency Medical Countermeasures Enterprise: Innovative Strategies to Enhance Products from Discovery through Approval: Workshop Summary." https://www.ncbi.nlm.nih.gov/books/NBK50757/.

Klein, N., B. Fireman, K. Goddard, O. Zerbo, J. Asher, et al. 2018. "Vaccine Effectiveness of Flucelvax Relative to Inactivated Influenza Vaccine during the 2017–18 Influenza Season in Northern California." *Open Forum Infectious Diseases* 5, no. 1: S764.

Kousky, C., and R. Cooke. 2012. "Explaining the Failure to Insure Catastrophic Risks." *Geneva Papers on Risk and Insurance-Issues and Practice* 37, no. 2: 206–27.

Kunreuther, H., M. Pauly, and S. McMorrow. 2013. *Insurance and Behavioral Economics: Improving Decisions in the Most Misunderstood Industry*. New York: Cambridge University Press.

Lu, Y. 2018. "Relative Effectiveness of Cell-Cultured versus Egg-Based Influenza Vaccines, 2017–18." https://www.cdc.gov/vaccines/acip/meetings/downloads/slides-2018- 06/flu-03-Lu-508.pdf.

Meltzer, M., M. Gambhir, C. Atkins, and D. Swerdlow. 2015. "Standardizing Scenarios to Assess the Need to Respond to an Influenza Pandemic." *Clinical Infectious Diseases* 60: S1–S8.

Molinari, N., I. Ortega-Sanchez, M. Messonnier, W. Thompson, P. Wortley, et al. 2007. "The Annual Impact of Seasonal Influenza in the

U.S.: Measuring Disease Burden and Costs." *Vaccine* 25, no. 27: 5086–96.

NAIC (National Association of Insurance Commissioners). 2018. "Pandemics." https://www.naic.org/cipr_topics/topic_pandemics.htm.

NIH (National Institutes of Health). 2017. "Influenza Vaccines." https://www.niaid.nih.gov/diseases-conditions/influenza-vaccines.

———. 2018. "Universal Influenza Vaccine Research." https://www.niaid.nih.gov/diseases- conditions/universal-influenza-vaccine-research.

NORC (National Opinion Research Center–University of Chicago). 2018. "41 Percent of Americans Do Not Intend to Get a Flu Shot This Season." http://www.norc.org/NewsEventsPublications/PressReleases/Pages/41-percent-of- americans-do-not-intend-to-get-a-flu-shot.aspx.

OMB (Office of Management and Budget). 2003. "Circular A-4." https://www.whitehouse.gov/sites/whitehouse.gov/files/omb/circulars/A4/a-4.pdf.

Qureshi, K., R. Gershon, M. Sherman, T. Straub, E. Gebbie, M. McCollum, M. Erwin, and S. Morse. 2005. "Health Care Workers' Ability and Willingness to Report to Duty during Catastrophic Disasters." *Journal of Urban Health: Bulletin of the New York Academy of Medicine* 82, no. 3: 378–88.

Plans-Rubió, P. 2012. The Vaccination Coverage Required to Establish Herd Immunity against Influenza Viruses. *Preventive Medicine* 55, no. 1: 72–77. https://www.ncbi.nlm.nih.gov/pubmed/22414740.

Philipson, T. 2000. "Economic Epidemiology and Infectious Diseases." In *Handbook of Health Economics*, vol. 1, edited by A. Culyer and J. Newhouse. Amsterdam: Elsevier.

Rolfes, M., B. Flannery, J. Chung, A. O'Halloran, S. Garg, et al. 2019. "Effects of Influenza Vaccination in the United States during the 2017–2018 Influenza Season." *Clinical Infectious Diseases*.

Sands, P., C. Mundaca-Shah, and V. Dzau. 2016. "The Neglected Dimension of Global Security—A Framework for Countering Infectious-Disease Crises." *New England Journal of Medicine* 374, no. 13: 1281–87.

Skowronski, D., N. Janjua, G. De Serres, S. Sabaiduc, A. Eshaghi, et al. 2014. "Low 2012–13 Influenza Vaccine Effectiveness Associated with Mutation in the Egg-Adapted H3N2 Vaccine Strain Not Antigenic Drift in Circulating Viruses." *PloS One* 9, no. 3: e92153.

Taubenberger, J., and D. Morens. 2006. "1918 Influenza: The Mother of All Pandemics." *Emerging Infectious Diseases* 12, no. 1: 15–22.

Uyeki, T., R. Fowler, and W. Fischer. 2018 "Gaps in the Clinical Management of Influenza: A Century since the 1918 Pandemic." *Journal of the American Medical Association* 320, no. 8: 755–56.

WHO (World Health Organization). 2009. "Pandemic Influenza Vaccine Manufacturing Process and Timeline." https://www.who.int/csr/disease/swineflu/notes/h1n1_vaccine_20090806/en.

Weir, J. 2017. *Influenza Virus Vaccine Strain Selection: 2018 Southern Hemisphere.* https://www.fda.gov/downloads/AdvisoryCommittees/CommitteesMeetingMaterials/BloodVaccinesandOtherBiologics/VaccinesandRelatedBiologicalProductsAdvisoryCommittee/UCM586391.pdf.

Weir, J., and M. Gruber. 2016 "An Overview of the Regulation of Influenza Vaccines in the United States." *Influenza and Other Respiratory Viruses* 10, no. 5: 354–60.

About the Council of Economic Advisers

The Council of Economic Advisers, an agency within the Executive Office of the President, is charged with offering the President objective economic advice on the formulation of both domestic and international economic policy. The Council bases its recommendations and analysis on economic research and empirical evidence, using the best data available to support the President in setting our nation's economic policy.

www.whitehouse.gov/cea
September 2019

In: Vaccines
Editor: Oliver Huerta
ISBN: 978-1-53619-059-5

Chapter 14

Influenza (Flu) Vaccine (Inactivated or Recombinant): What You Need to Know*

U.S. Department of Health and Human Services, Centers for Disease Control and Prevention

Why Get Vaccinated?

Influenza Vaccine Can Prevent Influenza (Flu)

Flu is a contagious disease that spreads around the United States every year, usually between October and May. Anyone can get the flu, but it is more dangerous for some people. Infants and young children, people 65 years of age and older, pregnant women, and people with certain health conditions or a weakened immune system are at greatest risk of flu complications.

* This is an edited, reformatted and augmented version of Vaccine Information Statement, Publication No. 42 U.S.C. § 300aa-26, dated August, 2019.

Pneumonia, bronchitis, sinus infections and ear infections are examples of flu-related complications. If you have a medical condition, such as heart disease, cancer or diabetes, flu can make it worse.

Flu can cause fever and chills, sore throat, muscle aches, fatigue, cough, headache, and runny or stuffy nose. Some people may have vomiting and diarrhea, though this is more common in children than adults.

Each year *thousands of people in the United States die from flu*, and many more are hospitalized. Flu vaccine prevents millions of illnesses and flu-related visits to the doctor each year.

Influenza Vaccine

CDC recommends everyone 6 months of age and older get vaccinated every flu season. *Children 6 months through 8 years of age* may need 2 doses during a single flu season. *Everyone else* needs only 1 dose each flu season.

It takes about 2 weeks for protection to develop after vaccination.

There are many flu viruses, and they are always changing. Each year a new flu vaccine is made to protect against three or four viruses that are likely to cause disease in the upcoming flu season. Even when the vaccine doesn't exactly match these viruses, it may still provide some protection.

Influenza vaccine *does not cause flu.*

Influenza vaccine may be given at the same time as other vaccines.

Talk with Your Health Care Provider

Tell your vaccine provider if the person getting the vaccine:

- Has had an allergic reaction after a previous dose of influenza vaccine, or has any severe, life- threatening allergies.
- Has ever had Guillain-Barré Syndrome (also called GBS).

In some cases, your health care provider may decide to postpone influenza vaccination to a future visit.

People with minor illnesses, such as a cold, may be vaccinated. People who are moderately or severely ill should usually wait until they recover before getting influenza vaccine.

Your health care provider can give you more information.

RISKS OF A VACCINE REACTION

- Soreness, redness, and swelling where shot is given, fever, muscle aches, and headache can happen after influenza vaccine.
- There may be a very small increased risk of Guillain-Barré Syndrome (GBS) after inactivated influenza vaccine (the flu shot).

Young children who get the flu shot along with pneumococcal vaccine (PCV13), and/or DTaP vaccine at the same time might be slightly more likely to have a seizure caused by fever. Tell your health care provider if a child who is getting flu vaccine has ever had a seizure.

People sometimes faint after medical procedures, including vaccination. Tell your provider if you feel dizzy or have vision changes or ringing in the ears.

As with any medicine, there is a very remote chance of a vaccine causing a severe allergic reaction, other serious injury, or death.

WHAT IF THERE IS A SERIOUS PROBLEM?

An allergic reaction could occur after the vaccinated person leaves the clinic. If you see signs of a severe allergic reaction (hives, swelling of the face and throat, difficulty breathing, a fast heartbeat, dizziness, or weakness), call *9-1-1* and get the person to the nearest hospital.

For other signs that concern you, call your health care provider.

Adverse reactions should be reported to the Vaccine Adverse Event Reporting System (VAERS). Your health care provider will usually file this chapter, or you can do it yourself. Visit the VAERS website at *www.vaers.hhs.gov* or call *1-800-822-7967. VAERS is only for reporting reactions, and VAERS staff do not give medical advice.*

THE NATIONAL VACCINE INJURY COMPENSATION PROGRAM

The National Vaccine Injury Compensation Program (VICP) is a federal program that was created to compensate people who may have been injured by certain vaccines. Visit the VICP website at www.hrsa.gov/vaccinecompensation or call 1-800-338-2382 to learn about the program and about filing a claim. There is a time limit to file a claim for compensation.

HOW CAN I LEARN MORE?

- Ask your healthcare provider.
- Call your local or state health department.
- Contact the Centers for Disease Control and Prevention (CDC):
    - Call 1-800-232-4636 (1-800-CDC-INFO) or
    - Visit CDC's www.cdc.gov/flu

In: Vaccines
Editor: Oliver Huerta

ISBN: 978-1-53619-059-5

Chapter 15

FOOT AND MOUTH DISEASE AND VACCINE USE*

United States Department of Agriculture

Foot-and-mouth disease (FMD) is a severe and highly contagious viral disease. The FMD virus affects cows, pigs, sheep, goats, deer, and other animals with divided, or split, hooves. Animals with FMD typically develop a fever and blisters on the tongue and lips, in and around the mouth, on the mammary glands, and around the hooves. Other signs of illness include depression, anorexia, excessive salivation, lameness, and reluctance to move or stand. Most affected adult animals will not die from FMD, but the disease leaves them weakened, resulting in reduced meat/milk production. Younger animals may not survive.

As part of its overall mission to protect American agriculture, the United States Department of Agriculture's (USDA) Animal and Plant Health Inspection Service works to ensure the continued health of the nation's livestock and poultry healthy. USDA works to keep foreign

* This is an edited, reformatted and augmented version of Factsheet of the United States Department of Agriculture, Animal and Plant Health Inspection Service, dated May 2018.

animal diseases out of the country and to deal with outbreaks of serious animal diseases. If a foreign animal disease like FMD occurs in the U.S., USDA would be the lead Federal agency responding to the outbreak, working closely with state animal health agencies and other agencies.

FMD is a worldwide concern as it can spread quickly and cause significant economic losses. A single detection of FMD could close international export markets for meat, dairy and other products, causing billions of dollars in lost trade for the United States. If FMD is found in the United States, USDA with its partners would need to act quickly to eradicate the disease and keep it from spreading throughout the country.

FMD Vaccination

One of the most powerful tools for combatting an FMD outbreak is vaccination. FMD vaccination is a safe and standard practice used in many parts of the world where the disease is commonly detected and controls the spread of infection by reducing the amount of virus being shed by animals and by controlling clinical signs of illness.

Vaccinated animals may still become infected, but would not be able to spread the disease to other animals. Vaccinated animals will not develop signs of clinical disease and can move normally through production channels. It is safe to consume the meat and milk of FMD exposed or vaccinated animals.

In the event of an FMD outbreak, USDA would evaluate the size, scope and species involved, as well as the availability of the proper vaccine, before deciding if vaccination is appropriate. Vaccination could be used to help slow the spread of an FMD outbreak or to protect specific animals, depending on the situation.

If an outbreak takes place, USDA and State authorities will determine how and where FMD vaccine is to be deployed working under the joint incident command structure. USDA will control the vaccine supply. Animals will be vaccinated under the direction of USDA accredited veterinarians, who will ensure that vaccinated animals are properly identified.

If we used vaccine to control an FMD outbreak, we would use high potency vaccines manufactured by USDA-approved companies. Vaccine is given to cattle, swine, sheep, and goats by intramuscular injection, typically in the neck area. However, USDA is assessing whether needle-free vaccine guns may be used, which would be faster, use less vaccine, and provide higher carcass quality.

In addition to vaccination, enhanced biosecurity and surveillance testing, strategic depopulation, movement controls and quarantines, and other virus-spread control methods can also help end outbreaks. USDA's priority is to as quickly as possible eradicate the disease and restore the livestock industry to full production and exports.

LIMITS OF FMD VACCINATION

Vaccination is not a "magic bullet" practice that solves all FMD problems. While it is useful in certain circumstances, there are limits. There are seven known types and more than 60 subtypes of the FMD virus. Immunity to one type does not protect an animal against other types or subtypes. This means that to be effective, vaccines must be closely matched to the virus strain circulating in livestock. In assessing the potential effectiveness of vaccine, USDA would need to determine which strain of the virus is causing an outbreak before determining which vaccine would control it.

Time is also a concern. FMD vaccine provides immunity for up to six months. Cattle, sheep, and goats require a single vaccine dose for full immunity, while swine require two doses two weeks apart. Animals would need to be re-vaccinated every six months for as long as vaccination is being used as a control measure.

FMD vaccination could impact export markets as well. Many countries will not accept live animals or untreated products from a country or region where FMD is present.

Vaccine use is often considered an indication that there is a risk of FMD in the livestock population, and therefore trade in various commodities may be limited when vaccine is used, or even when vaccinated animals remain present in a country or region.

USDA does not use vaccine proactively to prevent FMD. It is impossible to know which strain of the virus we might face, and extremely expensive to revaccinate the millions of cattle, pigs, sheep and goats throughout the country every six months. This could also severely limit our trade opportunities, which our producers depend upon for their livelihoods.

USING FMD VACCINE

The United States, Canada and Mexico established the North American Foot and Mouth Disease Vaccine Bank years ago so the countries would have a ready stock of FMD vaccine in case of an outbreak. The bank contains a variety of FMD vaccines concentrates, which can rapidly be processed into finished vaccine by manufacturers when the vaccine is needed. If one of the countries has an outbreak and needs to use FMD vaccine, the bank provides vaccine, assuming there is an appropriately matched vaccine in the inventory. The vaccines in the bank are all high potency inactivated vaccines, which means they do not contain live virus and are shown to be effective in cattle, swine, sheep and goats.

However, the current quantities in the bank are only sufficient to address small outbreaks. If countries use all the doses from the bank, they would need to rely on vaccine manufacturers to provide a continuous supply to conduct a vaccination campaign. It takes at least 14 weeks for newly manufactured vaccine to be available.

If an appropriately matched vaccine is not available in the bank, it may take longer to have any vaccine available. An appropriate vaccine would need to be developed and tested before it could be manufactured and used. This could take many months.

The vaccines are all DIVA_ (differentiate infected from vaccinated animal) capable, meaning that certain testing can distinguish between naturally-infected and vaccinated animals. DIVA capability would allow us to move live animals and their products within the U.S. during an outbreak, and support recovery of trade after the outbreak has been contained.

It is possible that in a prolonged outbreak, retail sale of FMD vaccine would be mandated in affected areas to ensure containment of the disease. In this situation, the livestock producer would buy the vaccine from a federally accredited veterinarian rather than receiving it from USDA.

FMD Vaccine and the Food Supply

In countries where FMD is common, meat and animal commodities from vaccinated animals are consumed every day without public health concerns. During a widespread FMD outbreak where vaccination is used, animal and public health officials may determine that meat and milk from vaccinated and recovered animals can be sent into the food supply.

Post-Vaccination

Because countries may limit trade as long as FMD-vaccinated animals remain in the country, eventually the vaccinated animals may need to be removed from the national herd before trade can be fully restored. This may be done through normal attrition or through targeted depopulation, depending on the circumstances and how we used vaccination.

For More Information

To learn more about FMD and emergency response and find helpful resources on these topics, go to:

- www.aphis.usda.gov/animalhealth/animal-disease-information/fmd
- www.aphis.usda.gov/fadprep

USDA is an equal opportunity provider and employer.

In: Vaccines
Editor: Oliver Huerta
ISBN: 978-1-53619-059-5

Chapter 16

OPIOID VACCINES*

United States Government Accountability Office

WHY THIS MATTERS

The ongoing opioid epidemic in the United States impacts lives on both a personal and national level. More than 10 million people abused opioids in 2017, with more than 47,000 opioid-related deaths — a nearly six-fold increase since 1999. Opioid vaccines could offer advantages over current treatment options.

THE TECHNOLOGY

What Is It?

Opioid vaccines are medical therapies designed to block opioids, such as heroin and fentanyl, from entering the brain or spinal cord, thus

* This is an edited, reformatted and augmented version of the United States Government Accountability Office Publication, No. GAO-19-706SP, dated September 2019.

preventing addiction and other negative effects. While none are approved for use yet, they could be useful for at-risk individuals, patients in drug recovery programs, or first responders who might accidentally come into contact with deadly opioids that can be absorbed through the skin. This approach offers advantages over some current treatment methods, including requiring minimal medical supervision and no potential for abuse.

How Does It Work?

When opioid molecules bind to receptors in the central nervous system (the brain and spinal cord), they can cause psychotropic effects (e.g., hallucination, euphoria), addiction, and overdose. Opioid molecules have specific chemical structures. Opioid vaccines are designed to trigger an immune response to these structures when injected into a patient. Similar to vaccines for infectious diseases, such as polio or measles, when a patient is treated with an opioid vaccine, their immune system learns to identify the targeted opioid as a dangerous foreign substance so it can respond if that opioid enters the bloodstream in the future.

After the body has learned to target an opioid molecule, it naturally forms antibodies that can bind to it. These opioid- specific antibodies stick to opioid molecules in the bloodstream, forming a unit that is too large to enter the central nervous system.

Without entering the central nervous system, the molecule is not able to produce the negative effects associated with opioids. The antibody-bound opioid will eventually be excreted via urine without harming the exposed individual.

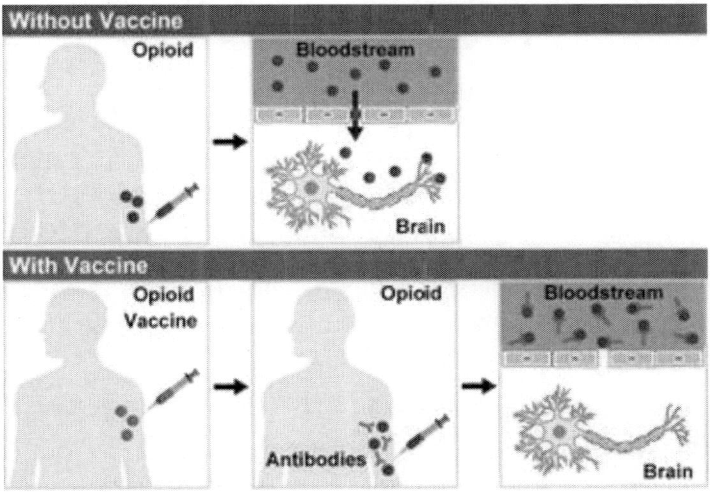

Source: GAO. | GAO-19-706SP.

Figure 1. When an opioid enters the bloodstream (top), it crosses into the brain, where it can act on the target receptor to cause psychotropic effects, addiction, and overdose. Opioid vaccines (bottom) trigger the body to create antibodies that bind to opioid molecules and prevent them from entering the central nervous system, thus preventing negative effects.

How Mature Is It?

As of 2019, the Food and Drug Administration (FDA) has not approved any opioid vaccines for use. While opioid vaccine studies were initially proposed as early as the 1970s, clinical trials have thus far been unsuccessful.

Currently, at least three early-stage clinical trials of potential opioid vaccines are underway, including one that the Walter Reed Army Institute of Research is conducting on a heroin vaccine.

Recently the National Institutes of Health and the National Institute of Allergy and Infectious Diseases released a broad agency announcement to fund the development of opioid vaccines against heroin and fentanyl. This funding is set to begin in August 2020. Other academic researchers continue to publish studies focusing on development and preclinical testing of opioid vaccines.

OPPORTUNITIES

- Treat at-risk patients. Unlike some current treatment options, opioid vaccines do not carry the risk of abuse. This could allow for more effective treatment of patients at high risk of abusing another medication, such as methadone.
- Medical advantages. The vaccines have a long duration (months to years) of action and require limited medical supervision.
- Compatible with other therapies. Vaccines currently in development are targeted to illicit use of opioids such as heroin and fentanyl, and therefore do not interfere with most drug treatment or pain management therapies.
- Protection against accidental exposure. Vaccines could be administered prophylactically to individuals at risk of accidental exposure to opioids, such as law enforcement, military, and first responders.

CHALLENGES

- Lack of broad-based effect. Current opioid vaccines are designed against the specific chemical structure of each opioid; therefore, multiple vaccines would be needed to provide broad-spectrum immunity. In addition, opioids such as fentanyl can be easily altered into a series of similar molecules called analogs, further complicating vaccine development.
- Less effective in immune-compromised patients. Patients with opioid use disorders often have other infections and altered immune responses that may limit the effectiveness of vaccines.
- Mechanism not well understood. The current biological mechanism of opioid vaccines is not as well understood as that of vaccines for infectious diseases.

- Patient consent. Consent issues could arise for people who might receive an opioid vaccine. For example, some might question a parent's right to compel their child to take a vaccine against a non-infectious agent, or an addicted person's ability to understand potential long-term effects of an opioid vaccine.
- Interference with medical care. If vaccines were developed against legal opioids that are used for pain management, vaccinated individuals would have a reduced risk of addiction but would also be unable to use those medications as effective treatments.
- Insurance and payment. Recent refusals to provide insurance to individuals who carry naloxone, used to counter opioid overdose, highlight the insurance issues surrounding opioid-related treatments. Would insurance cover an opioid vaccine? What might be the baseline costs?

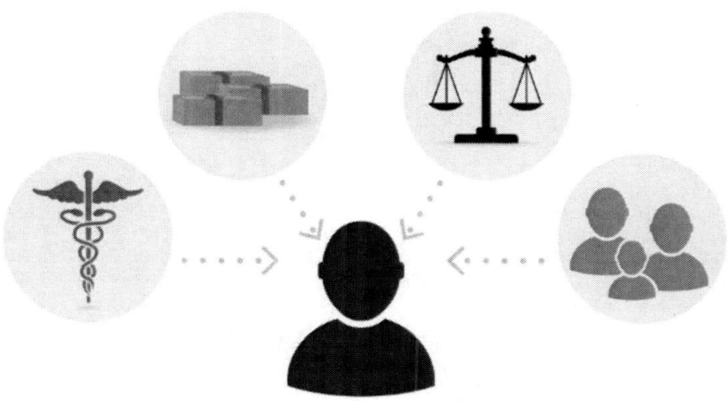

Source: GAO. | GAO-19-706SP.

Figure 2. Opioid vaccines will likely have a wide range of social and economic effects that could impact the individual.

POLICY CONTEXT AND QUESTIONS

PGS use in forensic analyses is increasing, but PGS results reportedly can be used with only limited confidence under certain circumstances. Some key questions for consideration include:

- In what situations is PGS useful, and when should it be avoided or used with caution?
- What are the gaps in empirical evidence that need to be filled to increase confidence in PGS results for use in criminal or civil trials, and what is the cost and feasibility of addressing these gaps?
- How are federal agencies evaluating and using PGS, and what should the federal role be?
- What additional validation work is needed to expand use of PGS?

REFERENCES

Banks, Matthew L., Margaret E. Olson, and Kim D. Janda. "Immunopharmacotherapies for Treating Opioid Use Disorder." *Trends in Pharmacological Sciences* 39, no. 11 (2018): 908-11. doi:10.1016/j.tips.2018.08.001.

Janda, Kim D., and Jennifer B. Treweek. "Vaccines Targeting Drugs of Abuse: Is the Glass Half-empty or Half-full?" *Nature Reviews Immunology* 12, no. 1 (2011): 67-72. doi:10.1038/nri3130.

Liang, X., Liu, R., Chen, C., Ji, F., & Li, T. (2016). Opioid System Modulates the Immune Function: A Review. *Translational perioperative and pain medicine*, 1(1), 5–13.

"NOT-AI-19-052: Broad Agency Announcement (BAA): Development of Vaccines for the Treatment of Opioid Use Disorder BAA-DAIT-75N93019R00009." *National Institutes of Health*. August 01, 2019.

Pravetoni, Marco, and Sandra D. Comer. "Development of Vaccines to Treat Opioid Use Disorders and Reduce Incidence of Overdose." *Neuropharmacology*, 2019, 107662. doi:10.1016/j.neuropharm.2019.06.001.

INDEX

A

B

C

D

E

F

G

H

I

L

M

N

O

P

R

S

T

U

V

W